Health Services

POLICY AND SYSTEMS FOR THERAPISTS

2nd Edition

Robert W. Sandstrom PhD, PT
Department of Physical Therapy

Helene Lohman OTD, OTR/L
Department of Occupational Therapy

James D. Bramble PhD
Department of Pharmacy Sciences
Center for Health Services Research
School of Pharmacy and Health Professions
Creighton University
Omaha, Nebraska

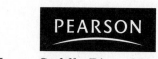

PEARSON

Upper Saddle River, New Jersey

Library of Congress Cataloging-in-Publication Data

Sandstrom, Robert W., 1957-
   Health services : policy and systems for therapists / Robert
Sandstrom, Helene Lohman, James Bramble. — 2nd ed.
         p.; cm.
   Includes bibliographical references and index.
   ISBN-13: 978-0-13-514652-1
   ISBN-10: 0-13-514652-6
   1. Medical policy—United States.   2. Public health—United States.   3. Physical therapy—Practice.
4. Occupational therapy–Practice.   I. Lohman, Helene.   II. Bramble, James D.   III. Title.
   [DNLM: 1. Health Services Accessibility—organization & administration—United States.
2. Health Policy—United States.   3. Occupational Therapy—organization & administration—United States.
4. Physical Therapy (Specialty)—organization & administration—United States. W 76 S221h 2009]
   RA395.A3S366 2009
   362.1068—dc22
                                                                                        2008021783

Publisher: Julie Levin Alexander
Executive Editor: Mark Cohen
Development Editor: Melissa Kerian
Assistant Editor: Nicole Ragonese
Marketing Manager: Katrin Beacom
Marketing Assistant: Lauren Castellano
Marketing Specialist: Michael Sirinides
Production Manager: Wanda Rockwell
Media Project Manager: Stephen Hartner
Creative Director: Jayne Conte
Cover Design: Bruce Kenselaar
Cover Image: Getty Images, Inc.
Composition/Full-Service Project Management: Nitin Agarwal, Aptara®, Inc.

Credits and acknowledgments borrowed from other sources and reproduced, with permission, in this textbook appear on appropriate pages within text.

Pearson Education LTD.
Pearson Education Singapore, Pte. Ltd
Pearson Education, Canada, Ltd
Pearson Education–Japan

Pearson Education Australia PTY, Limited
Pearson Education North Asia Ltd
Pearson Educación de Mexico, S.A. de C.V.
Pearson Education Malaysia, Pte. Ltd

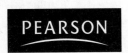

www.pearsonhighered.com

10 9 8 7 6 5 4 3
ISBN-13: 978-0-13-514652-1
ISBN-10:   0-13-514652-6

Brief of Contents

Contents

Preface

The central purpose of this book remains unchanged from the first edition, published in 2003. We have striven to produce a comprehensive introduction to the policies and systems by which and in which occupational therapists, physical therapists, and therapist assistants find their work and provide their care. In doing so, we have made several changes in response to the users and reviewers of the book. We are very grateful to those persons who have given of their time and expertise to help us improve this edition. The changes are as follows:

- The book's structure has been shortened from 15 to 12 chapters. The chapters on health care personnel and the mental health system have been eliminated, and content from those chapters that we thought to be important has been included in the two chapters on the health care system. The two chapters on access and cost have been condensed into one chapter.
- All chapters have had updates and revisions to their content and emphasis that reflect changes in policy and the health care system since the publication of the first edition. We have emphasized application to therapy practice. A notable change from the first edition is the inclusion of content on therapy services in special education environments.
- Facts and details have been updated throughout the book. We have increased the use of tables and figures in order to present content in a clear manner.
- A case example with focus questions has been added at the beginning of each chapter to apply concepts to the clinical environment. Cases are also presented within other chapters.
- Active learning exercises, most of which are web based, have been created and are interspersed throughout the book.
- An appendix has been created which contains tables that outline the historical and legislative time lines of the policies addressing social disablement that are presented in Chapter 4.
- Key terms for each chapter are defined in the glossary.

Special thanks go to Melissa Kerian, Mark Cohen, Brian Baker, Nitin Agarwal and the people of Pearson Education for their advice, assistance and support of this project. We hope that students, faculty, and clinicians will find the book of value as they do their daily work.

R. W. S.
H. L.
J. D. B.
Omaha, Nebraska
June 30, 2008

Reviewers

Second Edition

Patty Cahoj, PT, MS, DPT, GCS
Assistant Professor, Physical Therapy
Missouri State University
Springfield, Missouri

Gail Fisher, MPA, OTR/L
Clinical Associate Professor, Occupational Therapy
University of Illinois at Chicago
Chicago, Illinois

Margo Gross, OTR/L, LMT, LMFT
Assistant Professor, Graduate Program in Occupational Therapy
Sacred Heart University
Fairfield, Connecticut

Becky Keith, PT, MSHS
Coordinator, Physical Therapist Assistant Program
Arkansas State University
State University, Arkansas

Lori Khan, PT, MS, DPT
Assistant Professor and Program Director,
Physical Therapist Assistant Program
Washburn University
Topeka, Kansas

Jeffrey Loveland, OTD, MS, OTR/L
Associate Professor and Director, Occupational Therapy
James Madison University
Harrisonburg, Virginia

Bill McGehee, PT, MHS, ACCE
Assistant Professor and Academic Coordinator of Clinical Education,
Physical Therapy and Health Science
Bradley University
Peoria, Illinois

M. Beth Merryman, PhD, OTR/L
Associate Professor, Occupational Therapy
Towson University
Towson, Maryland

Tim Nanof, MSW
Legislative Representative
American Occupational Therapy Association
Bethesda, Maryland

Barbara Sanders, PT, PhD, SCS
Chair, Physical Therapy
Texas State University
San Marcos, Texas

Laurie A. Walsh, PT, JD
Associate Professor, Physical Therapy
Daemen College
Amherst, New York

Elizabeth Wark PT, DPT, MBA
Assistant Professor, Physical Therapy
Medical College of Georgia
Augusta, Georgia

Jennifer E. Wilson, PT, MBA
Assistant Professor, Physical Therapy
Nazareth College
Rochester, New York

First Edition

Elizabeth M. Kanny, PhD, OTR/L
Associate Professor and Head
Division of Occupational Therapy
University of Washington
Seattle, Washington

Kathleen Lewis, MAPT, JD
Associate Professor
Department of Physical Therapy
Wichita State University
Wichita, Kansas

1

Disablement, Policy, and Systems

CHAPTER OBJECTIVES

At the conclusion of this chapter, the reader will be able to:

1. Explain the interaction between policy, systems, and everyday practice in occupational therapy and physical therapy.
2. Define power and describe how policy is used to create and distribute power in a society.
3. Compare and contrast the uses of private policy and public policy as a method to effect social change.
4. Discuss the experience of disablement using the medical disablement, social disability, and universalism models.
5. Differentiate medical care and human services systems as components of the health care system for persons with disabilities.
6. Explain the development of the health care system in the 20th century and the effect of this development on the physical therapy and occupational therapy professions.

KEY WORDS: Biomedical Model, Disablement, Dualism, Health Services, Marginalization, Social Disability, Universalism

Case Example

Susan is a 22-year-old single woman who works full time in a low wage job as a hotel house-keeper. Her employer does not offer health insurance to employees. Susan does not qualify for any public insurance program. Susan is among the 47 million Americans without health insurance. She does not have a regular health care provider.

Susan lives with her grandmother, Sarah, who is age 70. Sarah worked for many years at a local factory and has been retired for the last five years. She receives a small pension and a Social Security payment each month. Sarah has health insurance through the Medicare program. Her low monthly income qualifies her to receive assistance from the Medicaid program for her Medicare deductibles. This benefit is important, since last year Sarah had surgery and was hospitalized. Sarah did not pay any out-of-pocket costs for her surgery.

Susan's mother, Ann, was injured in a motor vehicle accident three years ago and is unable to find work in her community. Since then, she has lost her job and has spent most of her life savings on medical expenses and monthly bills. She is waiting for a decision on her application for permanent disability status from Social Security. This would permit her to qualify for health insurance through Medicare and a disability benefit. She would like to work, but she has had difficulty finding vocational training options in her small community to help her learn new skills.

Case Example Focus Questions:

1. Compare and contrast the experiences of Susan, Sarah, and Ann. Who is better off and why?
2. Describe the social responses to their circumstances. Why do you think that the responses are different?

INTRODUCTION

Policies and systems are established to improve the lives of people and the overall community. This book is about an important and complex set of policies and systems in the United States: **health services**. Health services include the organizational, financing, and operational delivery of medical care and certain human services to persons who experience disease, illness, injury, and **disablement**. We are most interested in the health services that affect disablement because this book is intended for physical therapists and occupational therapists. Specifically, we are going to explore the policies that support and direct therapy care, as well as the systems that organize these services. It is our intent that as you become better informed about health services, you will become a better advocate for your patients and profession in order to improve existing policies and systems.

This chapter will introduce broad concepts regarding the development and implementation of health services affecting both occupational therapy and physical therapy. While our two professions are different, we are often similarly affected by policy. The next two chapters will introduce and explore the three foundational principles of health care policy: access, cost, (Chapter 2) and quality (Chapter 3). Chapter 4 discussed public policies designed to address social disablement (i.e., marginalization and discrimination against persons experiencing disability). In Chapter 12, we present information about advocacy, or how you can understand and potentially change the policies that we are going to discuss in this book. As you will learn, these policies have profound effects on the financing and organization of health care, including therapy services. First, we begin in this chapter by discussing the social structures that generate the policy and systems affecting therapists and persons with disabling conditions. Second, we will discuss different theoretical models of disablement and how they can explain different policies and systems.

We begin this chapter by introducing and discussing the issue of power as it affects health services. Specifically, we will discuss how power is distributed in American society through two policy-creating mechanisms: government (the public sector) and private enterprise. Next, we will study different viewpoints about what it means to experience disablement. One's perspective on disablement affects the type of policy that is created and how its effectiveness is evaluated. Third, we will integrate the concepts of a medical care system and a human services system into our discussion. All of these systems affect the organization of health services for persons who are experiencing temporary or permanent disablement. We will conclude the chapter with a historical review of the development of the U.S. health care system in the 20th century.

POLICY AND POWER

In the 20th century, many policies and systems were established to improve the health and well-being of the population. Not all of these health services were provided equally or comprehensively. Some of the health services offered were very effective. For example, the Medicare program virtually guaranteed access to medical care for people over age 65 and for people with permanent disablement. Other health services policies were ineffective; for instance, an insurance system that permits a large number of working Americans to be without health insurance is essentially a failure (see Chapter 2). Other policies have not yet been developed, such as a financing system for long-term care of the growing population of elderly Americans. Our policy-making system is unique in the world.

The lack of uniformity in health services in the United States can be traced to our system of policy **dualism** (see Table 1–1 ■). Both the government and private enterprise are involved in the financing, organization, and delivery of health services, including occupational and physical therapy. In addition, the government has a large regulatory role (e.g., licensure of providers). The sources of these two forms of health services policy-making are the core documents of our republic and the dominant economic system, free-market capitalism. Physical and occupational therapy services are shaped by each source of power.

As noted in Table 1–1, health services originate from two sources of *power* in the United States: public and private. The allocation of resources and the organizational ability of government and the free-enterprise system create the foundation for health services in the United States. As we will discuss in later chapters, government uses its taxing and regulatory authority to create access to medical and rehabilitation

Table 1–1.   Dualism and American Health Services Policy

	Government	*Free Enterprise*
Source of power	Constitution	Capitalistic markets
Role	Financing	Financing
	Regulation	Organization and delivery
	Organization and delivery	

services and, in some cases, to provide them to persons in need. Health services are also large economic enterprises (see Chapter 2). Both not-for-profit and for-profit enterprises have privately invested in the delivery and financing of health care, including therapy services. The generation of profit from this investment creates economic power that influences the health services system. The tension and interplay between private policy and public policy affecting health services are dynamic and political.

While policy is often affected by government decisions and economic investment, effective and fair health services policy must consider those who are powerless. The lives of many persons who experience disablement are characterized by poverty, unemployment, lack of adequate housing and transportation, impaired access to medical care services, and barriers to equal social and economic opportunity in the broader society. Policies reflect the distribution of power in the decision-making process and the values and ethics of the broader society. Just policy considers the life and circumstances of the powerless and creates opportunities for empowerment and advancement for all persons in the society (Banja and DeJong 2000; Purtilo 1995).

In sum, *policies* are expressions of power that allocate and organize resources to address identified needs in a society. As we will discuss later, *systems* are established that respond to policy decisions. Just policies affirm the human rights of those who are powerless and provide a pathway for advancement. In the next section, we will discuss in more detail the sources of power that drive health services: government, private enterprise, and moral/ethical principles.

SOURCES OF POWER

Government

In the United States, the power of the government is established in the Constitution and other core documents. The United States was founded in a revolt against the authority of central government, based on the idea of promoting individual liberty. In general, the American democratic republic is a system of limited and distributed government. The American system distributes power among three branches: executive, legislative, and judicial. Government authority is further divided between the national government and the states. Laws enacted by legislative bodies require executive approval and are reviewable by the courts. All of these decisions are reported, analyzed, and commented upon by a free press to the governed citizenry. American citizens have a right to address their government, and public policymakers are held responsible for their decisions by election on a regular basis. As a result, government power is expected to be used cautiously, for understood reasons, and only when necessary.

When it does act, government power is coercive (Weiner and Vining 1992). Government has the power to unilaterally ascertain, restrict, permit, or direct resources of private individuals and organizations. Through the establishment and enforcement of laws and regulations, government can force behavioral change on individuals and organizations that may not agree with the policy or that would not implement the same policy on their own. We also need to recognize the important role of government in establishing the "playing field" for private enterprise. Laws are government policies that establish private property and regulate markets which help to create the conditions that allow competition and the efficient, effective allocation of economic resources, including health services. When and under what circumstances can government use this power?

We can summarize two reasons for government action: failure of the private market to work as expected and a consensus among the governed populace for government action (Weiner and Vining 1992). In certain circumstances, private markets are perceived to be ineffective in meeting individual or community needs. For example, government provides the resources and ensures that roads and bridges are available to meet the transportation needs of society. It is accepted that it would be ineffective for each individual or community to privately organize and maintain a system of roads and bridges that permit people to work, shop, trade, or use recreational resources. It is a government responsibility to perform this service. Government action is also expected to address concerns raised by the will of the people. For example, the Americans with Disabilities Act of 1990 (see Chapter 5) was enacted to improve the civil rights of all Americans with disabilities and reflected the social consciousness that this was the "right thing to do." It would be very difficult, if not impossible, for civil rights to be achieved in all communities unless government power were used.

Political Process

The will of the people is exercised through the political process at all levels of government. Chapter 12 will introduce you to the principles and application of advocacy related to the political process. It is useful now, however, to discuss the political process as it relates to the distribution of power. It is within the political process that priorities are determined and actions taken or not taken by government to address societal concerns. Even if government power is not used, it does not mean that priorities are not being established. It means that these priorities will be established in the private sector.

Political power derives from electoral activity, position, and the power of persuasion. Elections determine the representatives who will make decisions regarding policy. Elections reflect a perspective on the proper role of government in solving solving societal issues (e.g., health care problems). In Table 1–2 ■, two contrasting political perspectives on the role of government are presented. A libertarian perspective views the primacy of the individual and freedom from government intervention as important. Health care is viewed as an earned reward for work, and persons who have difficulty receiving health care are best served by private charity. In contrast, egalitarian philosophy emphasizes the society (its rules, attitudes, and barriers) as the source of societal problems. Government action is encouraged from this perspective to improve overall freedom. Health care is looked upon as a

Table 1–2. Political Perspectives on the Role of Government in Personal Health Care

	Libertarian	*Egalitarian*
Source of Responsibility	Individual	Society
Health Care	Earned Reward	Prerequisite for Work
Treatment of Poor	Private Charity	Government Programs

Source: Long M. J. "Social Values and the Medical Care System." In *The Medical Care System: A Conceptual Model.* Ann Arbor: Health Administration Press, 1994, pp. 23–40.

prerequisite for work and government programs as the solution to improve the health care system. While not presented in this table, a utilitarian perspective on health care that emphasizes the greatest good for the greatest number of people was discussed by Long (1994). This viewpoint is the foundation for many public health initiatives (see Chapter 11) that improve health by ensuring clean water or proper vaccinations against communicable disease. Elections determine a dominant perspective, although in our political debates it is common to hear views that blend both perspectives. Policymakers have decision-making power by virtue of their position, whether elected or appointed by an elected official. Persuasion is commonly demonstrated by the influence of interest groups as expressed through lobbying on legislative matters. This system is carried over to regulators who develop regulations concerning medical care policy.

Private Enterprise

Private enterprise creates power by the investment of capital and the organizational ability of individuals and institutions that create systems each day to exchange economic resources in a marketplace. The American system of capitalism provides opportunities for individual success and allows unsuccessful enterprises to fail. In this economic system, private enterprises accept the risk of failure, create strategy, innovate, and implement services that meet the needs of consumers. People who successfully do this have a proprietary advantage, a form of economic power. This proprietary advantage creates business activity, initiates competition, allocates economic resources efficiently, and creates wealth.

Active Learning Exercise

Reflect upon your personal political philosophy. Would you describe yourself as a libertarian, an egalitarian, or someone with a position somewhere in between? Think about the issue of providing mandatory national health insurance for all Americans. To what extent does the social issue affirm or change your perspective?

Decisions that meet the demands of the marketplace in an efficient manner result in rewards to the owner of the resources, that is, a profit. Profits are used to pay creditors, create new investment, and provide for the personal well-being of the owners (Helfert 1997). Profits create economic power. Investment and the incentive to invest provide the economic resources to build hospitals and clinics, hire therapists, educate the next generation of providers, and deliver critical medical care services to the ill or injured.

The generation of economic resources also finances the government. Individuals and businesses pay taxes that support governmental action. While government and private sources of power are different, we must recognize that they are symbiotic and, at times, complementary. This relationship fuels the reality of interest-group politics; the necessary advocacy of specialized, private groups for governmental action; and political action committees, groups that privately finance the candidates for government office who support their perspectives. The American Physical Therapy Association (APTA) and the American Occupational Therapy Association (AOTA) have long recognized this reality at all levels of government and expend considerable time and resources to involve members in the political process.

ETHICS AND VALUES

As we have already indicated, many people experience disenfranchisement from the mainstream of society. Socioeconomic disadvantage, discrimination, and isolation from opportunities affect the lives of people who are "different" from the majority in the community. Persons with disabilities have historically experienced these circumstances (Banja 1997). Policies that affect everyone, including the powerless, should be fair and equitable. Laws and private policies reflect the basic values and ethics of the society and must be considered along with economic power and government authority in any debate on health services. Long (1994) describes four values that form the ethical base for health policy in the United States: freedom, equality, rewards, and treatment of the poor. Table 1–3 ■ outlines the four principles and provides an example of a contemporary health services policy issue that is an application of the principles developed by Long.

Table 1–3. Ethical Considerations of Health Services Policy

Ethical Principle	Contemporary Issue
1. Freedom	Medicare therapy cap
2. Equality	46 million uninsured Americans
3. Rewards	Universal or employment-based health insurance
4. Treatment of the poor	Medicaid program changes

Adapted from M. Long, *The Medical Care System: A Conceptual Model* (1994).

Freedom is a social construct that describes our relationship to one another and our ability to make and act upon individual decisions. Related to the ethical principle of autonomy, the ability to make choices about health care and the right to have access to services are examples of policy matters related to the principle of freedom. Should people have the freedom to choose their health care provider without limitations from a managed care plan? Should Medicare beneficiaries have the same therapy benefit, irrespective of the type of provider (e.g., private outpatient clinic or hospital)?

Related to the ethical principle of beneficence, the principle of equality defines the sharing and disbursement of rewards and responsibilities in society. Who is entitled to receive health care services? How will health care services be distributed to people? The large number of Americans without health care insurance illustrates that we do not have a system that guarantees equal access to health care (see Chapter 2).

The principle of rewards addresses this question: Is health care a basic right, or is it payment for contributions to the greater social good? Our core government documents do not define health care as a basic right of citizenship. Over the last half-century, certain groups have advocated several proposals (most recently in 1994) to create a basic right to health care. Despite these efforts, a universal, national health insurance plan for all Americans has not been enacted.

Finally, according to Long (1994), health care policy must address the issue of the powerless and the poor. Treatment of the poor is an issue of social justice. A civil and just society will have policies and systems that provide for the care and treatment of all people, not only the economically advantaged or socially elite. Government intervention in health care has often been predicated on meeting the needs of historically disadvantaged groups (see Chapters 8 and 9).

In sum, health services are affected by competing and complementary sources of power in society: government, private enterprise, and moral/ethical values. This is a dynamic and changing situation that is created by multiple stakeholders making independent decisions each day. This system reflects the American decision to distribute power widely on important issues like health care. Unlike other industrialized nations, the United States has not decided to centralize its health care system. Health care in the United States is, however, political, and the decisions made by private enterprises and government affect the experience of disablement for millions of Americans. Let us now turn our attention to the experience of disablement and discuss how changing perspectives on this issue have affected the development of health services for persons with disabilities.

EXPERIENCE OF DISABLEMENT

The special interest of this book is how policy and systems affect people with disabilities and the people who care for them. Physical therapy and occupational therapy exist as professions to serve a societal need for people experiencing disablement. The incidence and prevalence of temporary and permanent disablement creates a human and social need for assistance, new opportunities for independence, and community.

The experience of disablement creates foundational paradigms for the understanding of what needs to be done and the organization of rehabilitation health services. Disablement is experienced as a biomedical problem, an economic challenge, and a sociopolitical issue. Disablement is a major social problem. It is estimated that disablement affects 49 million Americans at an annual cost of $300 billion to the American economy (Brandt and Pope 1997). The size and prevalence of disablement means that solutions require the involvement of major social institutions.

Disablement is common to the human experience and has existed since antiquity. It is only in the last 150 years, however, as Western society has industrialized, that formal attempts have been made to define disablement and to develop a major organized social response beyond the family unit. In the United States, a fundamental principle for defining and determining this social response is the individual's ability or inability to work (Alson 1997; Kennedy and Minkler 1998). The inability of a person to work jeopardizes the ability of the person and his or her family unit to be self-sustaining. As a result, a broader social response is needed to provide the individual and family unit with support. At odds with this idea is the societal expectation that everyone capable of self-support and work will do so. Society can ill afford a policy that provides generous benefits to individuals and family units that are capable of working for self-support.

Ability to work as an establishing principle for defining disablement creates three new questions for policymakers: Who can work or not work? What types of services are needed by people who cannot work? What can society afford to provide to those who are unable to support themselves and their family units? The first two questions have been addressed to medical care providers. The third question is a matter of continuing contention within and between private and public policymakers.

Answers to these questions are affected by the prevailing definition of the disablement experience. The basic characteristics of three major perspectives of disablement are summarized in Table 1–4 ■. Historically, the biomedical model has been the dominant model of thinking about disablement in the United States. The social disability model has arisen in complement to and, in some cases, opposition to the biomedical model. Universalism challenges the notion that disablement is a special or separate policy issue. All three models affect the organization and delivery of therapy services to persons with disability in the United States.

Table 1–4. Disablement Models

	Medical Rehabilitation	*Social Disability*	*Universalism*
Source of disablement	Person	Social attitudes and policies	Both
Experience of disablement	Structure and function of body	Discrimination and isolation	All persons have potential
Response	Medical care	Human services	Integrated system

Biomedical Model

In order to determine eligibility for benefits, policymakers have turned to health care providers to determine the type and extent of disablement. Since the late 19th century, medical doctors have been granted power to determine and certify who is disabled and who, within the guidelines of the policy, may receive benefits. This policy decision resulted in the "medicalization" of disablement (Craddock 1996a; Williams 1991). As the scientific rationale for medical practice grew exponentially in the 20th century, disablement became increasingly viewed as a biomedical problem.

The focus of the **biomedical model** is to explain the patient's experience by understanding the source of the problem in terms of basic science and cellular pathology. This perspective emphasizes the role of the physician. The expansion of science and the acceptance of the biomedical model fostered a sophisticated and expensive medical care system with an emphasis on the identification and cure of pathology. Disablement was understood as a problem of medical pathology.

The biomedical model has limits, however, in its ability to explain disablement. Disablement is not "curable." Disablement often begins at the point where medical practice has limited effectiveness to eliminate disease or reverse injury. The manifestations of the pathology are not acute. Instead, they are usually chronic. A definition of disablement and the ultimate determination of success in treating disablement go beyond the terms used in treating acute illness, that is, morbidity and mortality. By the mid-1960s and thereafter, with the emergence of the Nagi model (Nagi 1965), new biomedical models emerged to explain the experience of disablement.

These models of "medical disablement" broaden our understanding of the manifestations of disease and injury. Impairments, functional limitations, and disability define the organ/tissue, whole person, and societal role effects of chronic illness and disablement (Brandt and Pope 1997). The philosophy of medical disablement supports policies that develop systems to address these concerns. Physical therapy and occupational therapy services that improve function and address pain, weakness, contracture, and similar problems can be defined as "medically necessary" and, therefore, are reimbursed through medical care insurance. This policy supports the provision of necessary services for those who are recovering from recent or recurring illness or injury.

The definition of "medical necessity" also limits independent therapist action and direct access to therapy services by the public. Many insurance plans, including public plans, require physician certification of therapy services in order for persons with disablement to access therapy care. The medicalization of therapy services has also organized complex systems that employ therapists within the medical care system, typically dominated by physicians. We will explore this system in detail in Chapters 9 and 10. In sum, the medicalization of disablement has made it possible for many people to receive therapy services funded through medical care insurance. The dominance of the medical model, however, has also limited direct access to rehabilitation therapy care for persons with medically stable, disabling conditions. While providing many employment opportunities, the medical rehabilitation model also constrains the distribution of therapists to the medical care system.

Although the medical disablement model broadens the understanding of disablement to include more than pathology, the focus of the disablement experience remains on the individual. This conceptualization reinforces the importance of the patient–provider relationship to the exclusion of broader societal influences on the experience of disablement. As a result, some theorists reject the biomedical model as an inadequate explanation of disablement. Since medicine has limits to its effectiveness in treating chronic and disabling conditions, they argue, improvements in lifestyle and the barriers that affect people with disabling conditions must be addressed by different mechanisms.

Social Disability Model

Social disability thinking has developed as "a dynamic social phenomenon that has as much to do with cultural norms and socioeconomic status as it is due to the individual's physiologic condition" (Kennedy and Minkler 1998). Social disability theory can be traced to the responses of people with chronic disease and illness to the limits of the biomedical model in explaining their experience and to the American civil rights movement of the 1960s (Craddock 1996b). The social disability movement has instigated the development and study of disability as a culture and caused the rethinking of the policy response to disablement.

From the perspective of social disability theory, medical disablement models are ineffective in explaining the situation of people who are physiologically stable but have ongoing disablement, social, and human services needs. Social disability theorists argue that the focus of medical disablement models on the person as the source of disability reinforces three negative stereotypes (Kennedy and Minkler 1998; Williams 1991). First, there is an excessive reliance on the health care provider as a source of solutions for disablement. Second, the biomedical model emphasizes a continual need for the person with a disabling condition to assume a "sick role" in order to receive services. Finally, the understanding of the disablement experience from a pathophysiologic perspective ignores other powerful social influences. From the social disability perspective, the source of disablement is not the pathophysiologic condition of the person, but the sociopolitical environment.

Rather than originating as a pathologic event, disablement is created as the result of a social process of **marginalization** of persons with disabilities by the larger society and its policies. Marginalization of persons with disabilities results in stigmatization by others (Williams 1991; Zola 1989). The inability to work weakens the economic power of people with disabilities, and, as a result, their political voice weakens. Those who are not disabled begin to view the expensive and special services required for full social participation by people with disabilities as a drain on other pressing social needs. Persons with disabilities are then forced to compete for limited social resources, but experience barriers in their attempts to do so. In sum, one social disability theorist writes that disability "becomes a problem when it causes a person to consume rather than produce economic surplus" (Kennedy and Minkler 1998). From this perspective, disablement is not found in the person with physical or mental impairments. Disablement is created by a pattern of social and economic discrimination by the majority of the population against one group through a mechanism of isolation and exclusion.

The effect of the social disability model on policy has led to the enactment of numerous civil rights laws over the last 25 years that address discrimination against persons with disabilities. Policies have also been enacted to support a human services system that empowers persons with disabilities to live more full and productive lives in the community. For example, the Rehabilitation Act of 1973 created Centers for Independent Living and state vocational rehabilitation programs that provide services to address the issues of community integration and socioeconomic discrimination. We will cover many of these programs and laws in Chapter 4.

It is important to note that the medical rehabilitation system and the human services system are distinct systems. Although both serve persons with disability, there is little formal integration and varying levels of coordination of policies and services between them. As we have discussed, their philosophical foundations, policy histories, and organizations are quite different. The problem of division, experienced in both theory and practice, is addressed by the concept of **universalism**.

Universalism

The historical development of disablement policy in the United States has created two separate systems. The medical rehabilitation system is organized using the biomedical model focusing on the person as the source of disablement and directing interventions, including therapy services, at improving the quality of life from this perspective. The human services system is based on a social disablement model that identifies the policies and attitudes of the society as the source of disablement. Services that empower the person with disability through expanded civil rights, access to employment, improved housing, and transportation are provided by organizations supported by policies that address social disablement.

Both of these models and systems emphasize the experience of separation and difference for persons with disability. Universalism attempts to explain disablement not as a condition that affects a few individuals who require specialized medical or human services, but rather as a situation to be recognized by the entire population at risk for disablement (Zola 1989). All of us live in a temporary state of nondisablement. The universalism philosophy advocates that most people will be affected by disability at some point during the aging process. As a result, policies should be developed to integrate all persons and to educate the population about living with a disability. Universalism addresses the fundamental problem of the marginalization of those with disabling conditions, whether on biomedical, social, economic, or political terms.

Universalism attempts to bridge the gap between the biomedical and social disability models. Integrated and coordinated policy that addresses the biologic, social, economic, and political reality of disablement is needed to truly address the experience of disablement. Ideally, an integration of medical and human services would be of the greatest benefit for persons who are experiencing disablement (Leutz, Greenlick, and Capitman 1994; Leutz 1999). There are few current examples of this form of pragmatic policy and systems development for persons with disabling conditions in the United States.

Internationally, there has been progress in conceptualizing the experience of disablement from a perspective that integrates both medical and social disablement models (Hurst 2003; Vrkljan 2005). The implementation of the International Classification of Functioning, Disability and Health (ICF) is an important development for therapists to understand and utilize when assessing patient status, effectiveness of treatment, and population health. The ICF was introduced in 2001 as a revision of the 1980 World Health Organization International Classification of Impairments, Disability and Handicap (ICIDH). The ICF describes "how people live with their health condition" (WHO 2007). The ICF assesses body structure and function, activities, and participation and contextual factors—i.e., the environment and personal factors (Jette 2006). Body structure and function, activities, and participation are similar to the previously described conditions of impairments, disabilities, and handicap in the ICIDH (similar also to the medical model we discussed earlier). Environmental conditions include social variables (e.g., attitudes and services, systems, and policies) as they affect persons with disabilities. The ICF has been influential in several of these domains and shows progress as a useful measure of both medical and social disablement.

THERAPISTS AND THE HEALTH CARE SYSTEM

The practices of occupational therapy and physical therapy have been shaped and transformed both by various models of conceptualizing disability, as well as by the sociopolitical process that defines the priorities of the society and the health care resources needed to address these priorities (see Table 1–5 ■). Today, it is difficult to comprehend the state of health care delivery at the beginning of the 20th century. At that time, health care was a small, unregulated, and privately funded enterprise. The number of health care providers was relatively few, and the nation lacked uniform educational standards. Competing philosophies of treatment (e.g., allopaths vs. homeopaths) applied care in a largely unregulated and unscientific environment. Limited technologies were available to diagnose or treat disease. Acute illnesses (e.g., infectious disease) were the predominant problems. Most care was provided in private homes or, for the poor, in substandard hospitals designed to quarantine illness. A small public health structure existed only in a few urban areas. Disablement was not a major health care issue and the social response was limited primarily to families.

The first half of the 20th century witnessed the development of a private health care system dominated by allopathic medicine. Other providers (e.g., homeopaths, naturopaths, and chiropractors) were marginalized. This development was supported by the growth of a bioscientific understanding of disease, the

Table 1–5. Development of U.S. Health Care in the 20th Century

	1900	1950	2000
Philosophy of Care	Competing Philosophies/ Little Science	Dominance of Allopaths/Rise of Bioscientific Model	Increasing Interdependence/Increased emphasis on understanding the sociology and economics of health care
Funding	Private Pay	Private Pay/Small Insurance Industry	Large Insurance Programs/Small Private Pay
Primary Location of Care	Home	Hospital	Outpatient Settings
Role of Government	None	State Regulation	Federal Insurance Programs
Concept of Disablement	No Social Response	Medical Problem	Medical and Social Response
Status of OT and PT	Nonexistent	Rationalized within organizations; Dominated by medicine	Growth of private practice; Work in acute and postacute care environments
Primary Societal Health Policy Objective	Standardize and Improve Quality	Improve Access to Care	Restrain Growth in Cost

standardization of educational qualifications of providers, the emergence of new technologies, and the establishment of environments (i.e., the hospital and strong political activity) to support these technologies, especially at the statehouse level. Private health insurance emerged in mid-century as a way to provide a benefit to workers. Private pay, however, dominated the financing of health care. Both physical therapy and occupational therapy were established in the health care system during this period, but came to be dominated by medicine and rationalized within hospital organizations.

The second half of the 20th century saw significant changes, especially in the financing of health care. The enactment of Medicare/Medicaid in 1965 and the development of managed care in the late 1980s into the 1990s marked the entrance of both government and corporations into the operations of health care delivery. Both of these programs greatly increased the amount of money available to fund health care; but as concerns about the high cost of health care rose, the power of these entities increased in determining how and where this money was spent. This led to an expansion in the size and scope of the health care system, followed by a reorganization and reintegration of health care services. Health care was no longer provided in hospitals, but in a number of settings in the outpatient and "postacute" environments. Chronic diseases, many associated with the modern lifestyle, emerged as dominant problems. Occupational therapy and physical therapy grew with the health care system and emerging problems. A private practice emerged in both professions during the latter half of the century. To varying degrees, therapists achieved freedom from the dominant position of allopathic medicine, although medicine retains an influential position in relation to both professions. Health care has become increasingly a federal political issue, despite the fact that the country has rejected several attempts at national health insurance or a national health care system.

As can be noted from this review, both occupational therapy and physical therapy have grown and adapted as occupations with the changes in the health care system. The future of both professions, especially their autonomy, will be affected by these social forces and the continuing and emerging needs of society (Domholdt 2007; Sandstrom 2007). In this book, we are going to introduce the structure of the policies and systems in and with which therapists do their work. Coupled with an appreciation for the historical context of this work, the book should give the reader several perspectives on the future opportunities and challenges facing these professions.

CONCLUSION

In this chapter, we have introduced the principles that affect the creation of policy and systems to deliver rehabilitation services to people with disabilities, as well as the practice of occupational therapy and physical therapy. Policy is about distributing power to maintain the status quo or to effect needed social change. The power to develop health services policy has three sources: government, private enterprise, and ethics/values. Policy development and implementation is a political process. Much of the remainder of this book will discuss the effects of policy decisions made in both private and public forums.

Health services policy that addresses disablement has developed in response to the dominant perspective that has defined the disabling experience. The medical model focuses on the person as the source of disablement. Important in determining eligibility for medical and social benefits, this model has reinforced the development of an acute and postacute health care system and a financing system for the rehabilitation health care system to address these needs. The social disability model finds the source of disablement in the community and society. This model has fostered the development of a community-based system of services for persons with disability that is explored in Chapter 4.

Access, cost, and quality are three foundational principles that drive all health policy, including policies that affect occupational therapy and physical therapy. An ideal system would maximize access to high-quality health care at a reasonable cost. In the upcoming chapters, we will review the successes and challenges for U.S. health services policymakers as they attempt to achieve these objectives.

CHAPTER REVIEW QUESTIONS

1. Define the relationship between power and policy.
2. What are the sources of power in the policy-making process?
3. Who is involved in policy formation, and how is policy formed?
4. Identify the uses and limitations of private policy and public policy in meeting social need and effecting social change.
5. How does "ability to work" affect policy toward persons with disabilities?
6. Compare and contrast the characteristics of the biomedical and social disablement models.
7. Define the source of disablement according to the social disability model.
8. What is universalism?
9. How have perspectives on the experience of disablement affected the development of system responses to disablement?

CHAPTER DISCUSSION QUESTIONS

1. Some people advocate for government action to improve health care. Others believe that private market solutions are the choice for increasing access to quality and affordable health care for more Americans. What are the pros and cons of each of these philosophies on health services policy?
2. Compare and contrast the positions of the social disability and medical disability models of disablement. Which of these models do you believe is most effective in meeting the needs of persons with disability? Why?
3. Physical therapy practices primarily within the model of medical disablement. Occupational therapy also practices within the context of social disability. How does the orientation of each profession affect the type of services provided?

REFERENCES

Alston, R. J. 1997. Disability and health care reform: Principles, practices and politics. *J Rehabil* 63(3): 15–19.

Banja, J. D. 1997. Values, function and managed care: An ethical analysis. *J Head Trauma Rehabil* 12 (1): 60–70.

Banja, J. D., and G. DeJong. 2000. The rehabilitation marketplace: Economics, values, and proposals for reform. *Arch Phys Med Rehabil* 81: 233–39.

Brandt, E. N., and A. M. Pope, eds. 1997. *Enabling America: Assessing the role of rehabilitation science and engineering.* Washington DC: National Academy Press.

Craddock, J. 1996a. Responses of the occupational therapy profession to the perspective of the disability movement. Part 1. *Br J Occup Ther* 59(1): 17–21.

———. 1996b. Responses of the occupational therapy profession to the perspective of the disability movement. Part 2. *Br J Occup Ther* 59(2): 73–78.

Domholdt, B. 2007. The meanings of autonomy for physical therapy. Invited commentary. *Phys Ther* 87(1): 106–108.

Helfert, E. 1997. *Techniques of financial analysis: A modern approach.* 9th ed. Chicago: Irwin Press.

Hurst, R. 2003. The International Disability Rights Movement and the ICF. *Disabil Rehab* 25(11–12): 572–76.

Jette, A. 2006. Toward a common language towards function, disability and health. *Phys Ther* 86(5): 726–734.

Kennedy, J., and M. Minkler. 1998. Disability theory and public policy: Implications for critical gerontology. *Int J Health Law* 28(4): 757–76.

Leutz, W. 1999. Five laws for integrating medical and social services: Lessons from the United States and the United Kingdom. *Milbank Q* 77(1): 77–110.

————, M. R. Greenlick, and J. Capitman. 1994. Integrating acute and long term care. *Health Affairs* 13(4): 59–74.

Long, M. J. 1994. *The medical care system: A conceptual model.* Ann Arbor: AUPHA Press.

Nagi, S. Z. 1965. Some conceptual issues in disability and rehabilitation. In *Sociology and Rehabilitation,* 110–113, ed. M. B. Sussman. Washington DC: American Sociological Association.

Purtilo, R. 1995. Revisiting the basics of professional life. *PT Magazine* 3: 81–82.

Sandstrom, R. 2007. The meanings of autonomy for physical therapy. *Phys Ther* 87(1): 98–105.

Vrkljan, B. 2005. Dispelling the disability stereotype: Embracing a universalistic perspective on disablement. *Can J Occup Ther* 72(1): 57–59.

Weiner, D. L., and A. R. Vining. 1992. *Policy analysis: Concepts and practices.* Englewood Cliffs, NJ: Prentice Hall.

Zola, I. 1989. Toward the necessary universalizing of a disability policy. *Milbank Q* 67 (suppl 2, pt. 2): 401–28.

2
Access and Cost of Health Care

CHAPTER OBJECTIVES

At the conclusion of this chapter, the reader will be able to:

1. Distinguish the different components that define access to health care services.
2. Describe the role of health care insurance with regard to accessing health care services.
3. Explain the relationship of health care insurance, access to health care services, and a person's health status.
4. Explain the concept of direct access to health care services.
5. Identify and discuss the major components of health care revenue in the United States.
6. Discuss the major components of health care expenditures in the United States.
7. Explain the economic, demographic, and systems reasons for the growth in health care costs.
8. Discuss the effects of different payment mechanisms on health care costs.
9. Compare and contrast the methods of financing for health care in the United States and several other countries.

KEY WORDS: Access, Direct Access, Enabling Factors, Need Factors, Uninsured, Capitation, Case Rate, Fee-for-Service, Financing, Global Budgeting, Gross Domestic Product, Markets

Case Example

Steve worked for many years in a factory before losing his job in a series of layoffs. Without a job to help provide insurance coverage, Steve was now one of the millions of uninsured. During the time that he had health insurance, Steve regularly visited his primary care physician. Now, without any health care coverage and feeling relatively healthy, Steve decided to postpone his regular visits due to the extra out-of-pocket costs and use this money for other expenditures.

Steve eventually found part-time employment, but it did not provide health care benefits. Steve's limited financial resources could not support either the high cost of health care insurance premiums or the potential out-of-pocket cost associated with a physician. Thus, he continued not to seek health care services or obtain health care insurance in lieu of other financial needs. When he did not feel well, he treated himself with over-the-counter medications and rest.

During this time, Steve began experiencing pain in his back and stomach, but believed he must have done something to injure himself at work. The pain persisted, and over-the-counter medication and rest did not have any lasting effect. He started losing weight; however, since the pain in his stomach was worse after meals, he decided he just was not eating enough. Over time, friends noticed that Steve's skin and the whites of his eyes were yellowing—a sign of jaundice. Still worrying about having no insurance, Steve continued to postpone care. Eventually the pain was so bad that he reluctantly decided he must see his physician, even though he was unsure how he would pay for the visit. After examinations and a number of tests, Steve was diagnosed with pancreatic cancer.

Case Example Focus Question/Discussion:

1. Describe Steve's access to health care services and how his care was affected by his access.
2. Discuss what activities, policies, or programs might have influenced Steve's ability to receive timely care.

INTRODUCTION

The three-legged stool of health care policy in the United States is access, cost, and quality. These three major constructs are commonly used in describing and evaluating the health care system (Barton 1999). A set of relatively simple questions can illustrate the importance that each of these constructs has in our discussion of health care services. For example, when an individual is in need of medical attention, is the needed care for complete recovery both available and accessible in a timely manner? Does the person receive the necessary referrals for medical care from the appropriate provider? Is the health care provided appropriately? Are the desired outcomes achieved? How much will the health care cost? How will the provider be paid, and who will pay for the health care received? The focus of this chapter is on issues surrounding the access and cost of health care, while quality is addressed in Chapter 3.

The conversation about access to the health care system often is centered on the presence or absence of health insurance. While a lack of health insurance is the largest barrier to access, it is not the only barrier that individuals face as they enter the health care system. The high cost of health care services is the root of many of the barriers associated with health care delivery. This chapter addresses some of the complexities surrounding both the access to, and the cost of, health care services.

ACCESS TO HEALTH CARE SERVICES

Unlike the situation in much of the industrialized world, access to health care in the United States is not a guaranteed right (Fuchs 1993). Thus, a person's ability to access needed health care services is a perennial issue for health care providers and policymakers. There are many different dimensions worthy of consideration in conceptualizing access to health care services. For example, Penchansky and Thomas's (1981) conceptualization of access that examines the fit between the characteristics of the health care system and the expectations of patients is presented in Table 2–1 ■. Penchansky and Thomas examine this fit along five dimensions: availability, accessibility, accommodation, acceptability, and affordability.

Availability

Availability refers to the relationship between the amount and type of services provided by health care workers and the amount and type of services required by the population in need. The goal is to have the best possible match between the services provided and those needed. For example, a community with a large elderly population should have more geriatric services than a community with a younger demographic.

Accessibility

Another barrier to utilizing health care services is accessibility, such as geographic factors; thus, the second dimension examines the accessibility of health care services. Accessibility describes the relationship between the location and supply of health care providers and services (e.g., therapy clinics) and the location and transportation resources of the population (i.e., potential patients). Health services tend to be located in population centers that are large enough to support them. People

Table 2–1. Penchansky and Thomas Access Factors

Availability: the amount and type of services provided in relation to the population's need.

Accessibility: the location and supply of health care services in relation to the population's location and transportation resources.

Accommodation: the organization and appropriateness of health care services, as well as the population's ability to use those services.

Acceptability: the attitude between health care providers and the population toward one another.

Affordability: the price of health care services in relation to the population's ability to pay.

Source: R. Penchansky and J. W. Thomas, (1981). The concept of access: Definition and relationship to consumer satisfaction. *Medical Care* 19, 2(1981): 127–40.

living outside of these centers, such as sparsely populated rural areas, may not have access to the full range of health care services, regardless of their ability to afford those services. People who must travel great distances to reach the care that is needed may postpone or go without needed medical services. Practically, this means that though services are available, they are not accessible to the individuals in need. Rural communities across the country are some of the most at risk in having less than ideal access to health care services. Even in urban areas, there are barriers to the accessibility of health services, including human-made barriers (e.g., freeway patterns) and natural barriers (e.g., rivers).

Accomodation

The third dimension, accommodation, addresses three related issues: (1) the manner in which health care providers, services, and facilities are organized; (2) the population's ability to use these providers, services, and facilities; and (3) the population's opinion of the appropriateness of the providers, services, and facilities. Accommodation is affected by temporal factors that can create barriers which may keep care-seekers from accessing health care providers and services. Among these barriers are, for example, the potential mismatch between the schedules of providers and patients that results from inflexible working hours, the ability to attain childcare, or a host of other factors. These issues need to be considered when organizing health care services so that they are "accommodating" to potential patients.

Acceptability

The fourth dimension, acceptability, examines the attitudes and perceptions that health service providers and the population have toward one another. For example, cultural differences, including language barriers, differing values on health, or conflicting customs or beliefs, may exist. All of these differences may prevent an individual from reaping the full benefits of available health care services, even though the care may be available, accessible, accommodating, and affordable.

Affordability

The final dimension, affordability, is concerned with the price of health care services or the ability of the population to pay. Financial access to health care services is closely tied to health insurance and the ability to obtain insurance coverage. (Health insurance is addressed more fully in Chapters 5 and 6.) However, as has been discussed, health insurance coverage or one's ability to afford medical care is not the only factor to consider in examining access to health care services. Health insurance, by itself, does not guarantee access to care; for example, the necessary health care provider or therapy clinic may not be available where the patient lives. Additionally, patients may need a referral from a primary care physician to seek specialized services.

As Penchansky and Thomas's conceptualization demonstrates, there are many factors that may affect the ability to access health care services. All of these dimensions (i.e., availability, accessibility, accommodation, acceptability, and affordability), along with the predisposing factors of potential patients (e.g., age, sex, and occupation), need to be considered to fully understand the degree of access that defined populations have to health care services. Policymakers and health care practitioners must account for the many dimensions of access as they plan for the delivery of health care. However, it is difficult to determine which barrier is most important. Each person may have his or her own unique barriers to overcome; thus, the most problematic barrier to receiving care varies across individuals.

Though barriers vary across individuals, as a whole our country's biggest access-related problem is the affordability of health care services (Vistnes and Zuvekas 1999). Adequate health insurance is essential to overcome the affordability barrier and gain access to appropriate and timely medical care. Though health insurance, as has been argued, is only one of the dimensions of access, it is an important part of the financing and delivery of health care services in this country; the next section takes a closer look at this barrier.

ACCESS AND HEALTH INSURANCE

One key factor in making health care services accessible is health insurance coverage. The affordability of health care services is one of the greatest barriers we face as a nation with regard to access to the health care system (Stoddard 1994). It is one of the main reasons that almost every presidential administration has introduced some sort of health care reform. Access to, and the affordability of, health care services continues to be an issue that policymakers and private citizens must address.

Financial access to health care services is assured mostly by means of securing some form of health care insurance. Over the years, health insurance has provided the means for individuals to access the health care system and for health care providers to collect payment for services rendered. For most Americans under 65 years old, health insurance is obtained through their employer or the employer of a family member (Clemans-Cope, Garrett, and Hoffman 2006). In 2005, 62 percent of nonelderly Americans (those below 65 years old), belonged to employer-based health plans (Fronstin 2007). While the majority of nonelderly persons are covered through private insurance, Medicare provides coverage for people over 65, and Medicaid pays for services for those eligible to receive funds from the Temporary Assistance to Needy Families or the Supplemental Security Income program (SSI). The specifics of health insurance are discussed in Chapter 5; the focus of this section is the growing problem of the **uninsured** and how it relates to accessing health care services.

Characteristics of the Uninsured

The number of individuals without health insurance has increased steadily over time (see Figure 2–1 ■), despite government efforts to plug the gaps in insurance

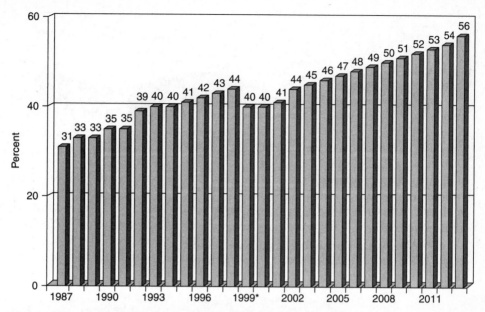

Figure 2–1. The Number of Uninsured (in Millions) by Year
*1999–2005 estimates reflect the results of follow-up verification questions and implementation of Census 2000-based population controls.
Note: Projected estimates for 2004–2013 are for nonelderly uninsured based on T. Gilmer and R. Kronick, "It's the Premiums, Stupid: Projections of the Uninsured Through 2013," *Health Affairs* Web Exclusive, April 5, 2005.
Source: The Commonwealth Fund 2006; Data calculated from U.S. Census Bureau, March CPS Surveys 1988 to 2006.

coverage through various programs (Kuttner 1999). According to the Commonwealth Fund, the total number of nonelderly uninsured persons in 2005 was approximately 47 million (The Commonwealth Fund 2007).

The 47 million figure represents approximately 18 percent of the nonelderly population in 2005, an increase of 1.3 million over the last year, and an increase of 7 million since 2000. While the ranks of the uninsured continue to grow, the demographics and factors that place people at risk for being uninsured go relatively unchanged. The Kaiser Commission on Medicaid and the Uninsured (KCMU) reported a number of factors that contribute to the risk of being uninsured (KCMU 2006):

- Adults more than children are likely to be uninsured (see Figure 2–2 ■). Low-income children qualify for Medicaid or SCHIP, but adults qualify only for Medicaid if they are disabled, are pregnant, or have dependent children.
- More than 60 percent of the uninsured adults did not attend college.
- Minorities are more likely to be uninsured than white Americans. Disparities in the number of uninsured are not tied solely to income.

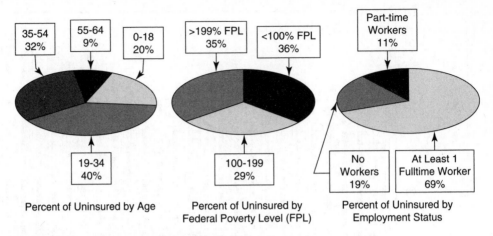

Figure 2–2. **Characteristics of the Uninsured**
Source: Kaiser Commission on Medicaid and the Uninsured 2006.

- The poor and the near-poor are at the greatest risk of being uninsured (see Figure 2–2 ■). This is due, in large part, to the high cost of health insurance. Of the nation's uninsured, two-thirds of them are classified as poor or near-poor. (Note: poor is defined as less than 100 percent of the federal poverty level—e.g., for a family of four, the federal poverty level is $19,971.)
- Most uninsured work (see Figure 2–2 ■). Four out of five uninsured come from working families.

Health Status of the Uninsured

Discussions of health care reform are often centered on the attainment of a sense of equity with regard to the delivery and accessibility of health care services (Seiden 1994). Whether or not an individual has health insurance makes a difference when and where people get the medical care they need. Currently, a lack of insurance coverage results in large discrepancies between the health care services available to the insured and the uninsured. The amount and type of health care services that people who are uninsured can afford and obtain are severely limited. The consequences of having limited access to needed health care services can be severe.

One reason that the uninsured do not get timely needed care is the lack of a regular place to receive care. As shown in Figure 2–3 ■, over 40 percent do not have a regular place to go for advice or consultation (KCMU 2006). About 20 percent of the uninsured report that their regular source of care is the emergency room, compared with only 3 percent of those with insurance (KCMU 2003). The lack of a regular provider is likely the main reason that those without health insurance are three times more likely to report problems with getting needed medical care. Other reasons

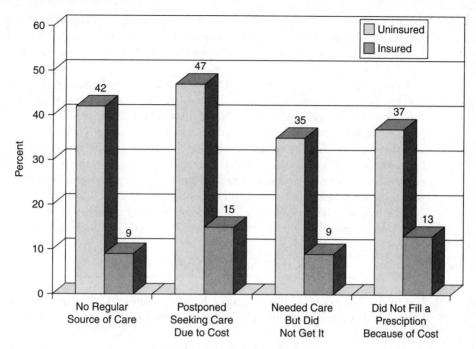

Figure 2–3. Barriers to Accessing Health Care Services
Source: Kaiser Commission on Medicaid and the Uninsured.

for not getting needed care include the cost associated with that care. High costs also prohibit some persons without insurance from filling needed prescriptions as part of a physician's care plan (see Figure 2–3 ■). The postponement of seeking care can have catastrophic consequences. For example, Braveman, Schaaf, Egerter, Bennett, and Schecter (1994) found that uninsured patients with appendicitis were more likely to have their appendix rupture due to delaying surgical intervention than were insured patients.

In addition to postponing needed care, the uninsured are less likely to receive timely preventive care that may have an impact on their health status (Franks, Clancey, and Gold 1993). The KCMU reports (2006) that those with insurance are significantly more likely to have had recent mammograms and colon and cervical cancer screenings. Thus, uninsured individuals with cancer are diagnosed in later stages of disease, which usually results in poorer outcomes. This is just one example of how the lack of health insurance adversely affects the health of individuals, at least in part, because of inadequate access to health care services.

The Working Uninsured

So why are there so many uninsured, and why has the number of uninsured continued to increase over the years? There are multiple factors to consider in examining the increasing trend of uninsured persons. Two of these factors are the declining trend of employer-based insurance benefits and the rising premium costs for those who have insurance through their employer, as well as for those who buy health insurance individually.

Health insurance in the United States is tied to employment (Kuttner 1999), but past studies have shown that the number of Americans with employer-based health care insurance has decreased over the last 10 years (Hoffman 1998). A 2006 Kaiser report on the uninsured indicates that this trend is continuing. There are many reasons that there are working uninsured, including a reduction in employer-sponsored insurance. Many of the reasons can be tied to one of the following two issues: the high cost of health care services and resulting insurance premiums, as well as increases in employees' contributions to their health benefits (see Figures 2–4 ■ and 2–5 ■).

Employers, especially smaller employers, are sensitive to changes in health care premiums. With the continued growth rate of health insurance premiums,

Active Learning Exercise

On the Internet, go to the Kaiser Family Foundation at http://www.kff.org and read more about the uninsured. How would you address this issue on a practice level?

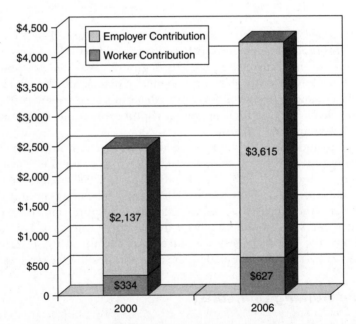

Figure 2–4.   Employer and Worker Premium Costs for Individual Coverage
Source: Kaiser Commission on Medicaid and the Uninsured.

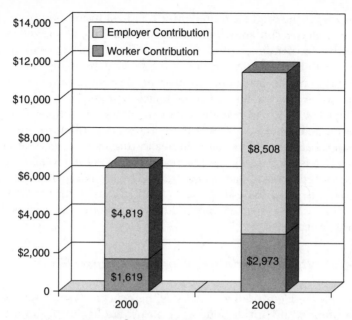

Figure 2–5.   Employer and Worker Premium Costs for Family Coverage
Source: Kaiser Commission on Medicaid and the Uninsured.

┌─ Active Learning Exercise ─────────────────

The United States lacks a national health insurance program. Some states, however, are acting to create access to health insurance for all citizens. Visit http://www.kff.org/uninsured/7494.cfm to learn about how Massachusetts has acted to create universal access to health insurance.

---

many employers either do not offer health benefits or have trouble affording their share of the health insurance premium. This results in greater financial burdens being placed on the patient/consumer. Employees must cover more and more of the health insurance premium. From 2003 to 2006, the burden has nearly doubled for both single and family coverage, until it now exceeds the annual salary of a minimum-wage worker (KCMU 2006).

COST OF HEALTH CARE

To understand why the cost of health care is such an important issue, the remainder of this chapter will summarize health care financing in the United States, including an overview of health care expenditures, where the money comes from, and where it goes. After exploring the sources of revenues and expenses, we discuss the possible reasons for the unprecedented growth in health care spending, the role of government, and cost-containment mechanisms that have developed to slow the growth of health care spending here in the United States and internationally.

With both private and public resources developing a multitude of health care programs and health plans, the financing of medical care in the United States is very complex. The percentage of **gross domestic product** spent on health care represents millions of dollars in revenue for many businesses and industries. Thus, the provision of health care services is big business. According to the National Center for Health Statistics (2006), national health care expenditures reached $1.9 trillion in 2005. Translating this figure to a per-person expense reveals that health care spending reached a per-capita level of $6,280. This level of spending represents 16 percent of the U.S. gross domestic product (GDP). The Center for Medicare and Medicaid Services (CMS) projected that health care expenditures will reach $4 trillion by 2015 (Borger et al. 2006).

Health Care Financing: Where It Comes From

As shown in Figure 2–6 ■, in 2004, 55 percent of personal health care expenditures were funded by private sources (e.g., private health insurance and out-of-pocket costs), while public sources such as Medicare and Medicaid funded 45 percent of national health care spending (National Center for Health Statistics 2006). On the private side, private health insurance, obtained mostly through employers, accounted for 36 percent of expenditures, and out-of-pocket payments accounted for 15 percent. Out-of-pocket payments include payments for services not covered by

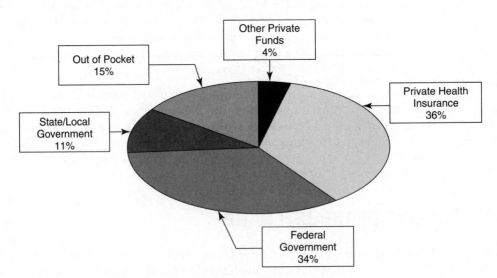

Figure 2–6.   Personal Health Care Expenditures by Source of Funds
Source: National Center for Health Statistics, 2006.

private insurance, as well as co-payments, co-insurance, and deductibles (see Chapter 5 for definitions).

Americans spent $658.5 billion for private health care insurance in 2004, representing an increase of 8.6 percent over the previous year (Borger et al. 2006). Borger et al. also report that Medicare spending for health care in 2004 grew to $309 billion, an increase of 8.9 percent over the previous year. Medicaid spending also rose from the preceding year to $173.1 billion, an increase from 2003 of 6.1 percent.

Health Care Financing: Where It Goes

Figure 2–7 ■ shows where health care expenditures went in 2004. Hospital care is the largest single component of health care spending, representing 36 percent of personal health care expenditures. The next-largest component of expenditures is physician services, which account for 26 percent of the national expenditures. The remaining expenditures break down as follows: 12 percent for prescription drugs, 7 percent for nursing home care, and 18 percent for other health care expenditures, which included visits to nonphysician providers, medical supplies, and other health services (National Center for Health Statistics 2006).

Of the two largest health care expenditures, hospitals accounted for $570.8 billion in 2004 and physicians $399.9 billion (Borger et al. 2006). Borger et al. expect that hospital spending will continue to grow at more than two percentage points higher than the GDP; however, it is projected that prescription drugs will exhibit a relative slowdown in spending. In 2004, prescription drugs accounted for

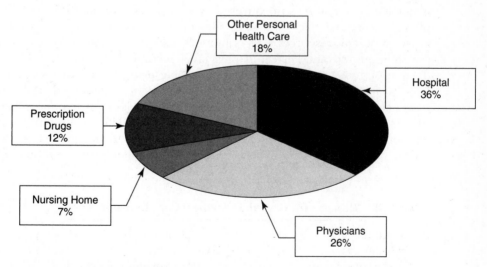

Figure 2–7. Personal Health Care Expenditures by Type of Expense
Source: National Center for Health Statistics, 2006.

$188.5 billion in expenditures, which translated to a growth of 8.2 percent over 2003. This growth rate was 2 to 10 percentage points lower than in preceding years (Borger et al. 2006). Reasons for the slowdown in prescription drug expenditures include the expiration of patents and the subsequent prescription-to-nonprescription conversions, a slowdown in new drug approvals, and higher cost-sharing for patients/consumers. However, it is expected that 2005 drug expenditure growth will outpace the growth in overall health care expenditures and growth in the economy (Hoffman et al. 2006).

The Growth of Health Care Expenditures

As noted earlier, the health care expenditure in the United States is significant and it has had almost uninterrupted growth over the past few decades. Since 1970, the average rate of health care spending has grown at an annual rate of 9.9 percent, or 2.5 percentage points faster than the GDP (KCMU 2006). The Centers for Medicare and Medicaid Services have estimated that health care expenditures will rise to over $4 trillion in 2015 (Borger et al. 2006). Reasons influencing this growth in expenditures include a complex interaction of economic factors, demographic changes, and system factors (see Table 2–2 ■).

Economic factors relating to the growth in health care spending include inflation, market structure, and insurance. Most experts would agree that, of all the potential reasons, inflation (both general and for medical care) is the major driving force behind the increases in health care expenditures. Health care markets are unique and different from other economic markets, such as commodity markets (Folland, Goodman, and Stano 1997). "Perfect" markets balance supply and demand at a price that is competitively determined by buyers and sellers in a marketplace. The marketplace has many informed buyers and sellers who exchange known economic resources. Buyers and sellers are free to enter and exit the market as conditions warrant. Perfect markets create competition that allows for the production of goods and services at an affordable price. Health care markets differ from perfect markets, and access to health care services is not uniform; thus, price is not always competitively determined, but rather is regulated and fixed. Consumers are often at an information disadvantage in making health care purchasing decisions; therefore, it is difficult for consumers to evaluate their purchases. Providers are often prevented by regulation, licensure, and tradition from entering high-cost

Table 2–2.   Reasons for Growth in Medical Care Expenditures

A. Economic	B. Demographic Change
1. Inflation	C. System
2. Market structure	1. Provider behavior
3. Insurance	2. Technology

markets in order to offer a comparable service at a lower cost. Finally, health care insurance has a unique effect on health care markets.

The role of health insurance is a major contributor to the growth in health care expenditures (Peden and Freeland 1995; Fuchs 1990). The protective role of health care insurance has acted to insulate consumers from the true costs of their health care purchases. Because of this, some observers cite the market failure of health care insurance as a major cause of expenditure growth. In sum, inflation, market structure, and health insurance have prevented the forces of competition from working to restrain the growth of health care costs.

Demographic effects also play a role. The elderly population (i.e., those over 64) continues to grow very rapidly. For example, 36.8 million persons in 2005 were 65 or over, an increase of 3.2 million, or 9.4 percent, from 1994 (U.S. Department of Health and Human Services 2007). The elderly population, due to the increase in the incidence of sickness with age, accounts for a large portion of health care expenditures. Indeed, persons 65 and over have many more contacts with their health care provider. For example, the National Center for Health Statistics (2006) shows that elderly males have one-and-a-half to two times as many physician office or hospital outpatient visits than those 55 to 64 years old, and the gap between younger cohorts is even greater. Thus, we must prepare ourselves for the influence of an aging population on both the cost and utilization of health care services.

Many factors affect growth in health care costs, including administrative bureaucracy, provider behaviors, the lack of a well-coordinated care system that may lead to unsafe duplicative or conflicting care plans, and the American affinity for high-technology health care (Davis et al. 2007). For example, Davis et al. point out that the complexities associated with duplicative, uncoordinated requirements and administrative costs for providers lead to high overall administrative costs, including the proportion of insurance premiums that are used to cover those costs. Indeed, according to the Commonwealth Fund National Scorecard (2006) on U.S. Health System Performance, the United States spends a higher percentage than any other country, and almost three times as much as Canada, on health administration and insurance.

Inefficiency is not only a result of complex administrative systems, but also a product of provider behavior. Some of the abuse is a result of physicians practicing "defensive medicine" in order to protect themselves from costly legal actions. The practice of defensive medicine is an expenditure-increasing activity, and some analysts believe that major savings would be produced if it could be stopped (Fuchs 1990). Again, others report that malpractice reform would only result in savings of $8 million annually, a small fraction of the total health care expenditures (Schwartz and Mendelson 1994). As we will discuss shortly, incentives in payment mechanisms also have powerful effects on provider utilization of health care services and overall costs.

Finally, the American fascination with high-technology health care has resulted in the identification and treatment of more disorders (Sultz and Young 1999). The costs of delivering this technology are associated with higher overall costs to the system.

PAYMENT MECHANISMS AND HEALTH CARE EXPENDITURES

Efforts to contain health care costs have led to various payment mechanisms designed to control health care spending. The intent of theses payment mechanisms is to slow the growth of health care expenditures. This section briefly explains the various payment mechanisms for health care providers and the incentives that each of these mechanisms has created. Specifically, four major payment structures are discussed in this section: (1) fee-for-service, (2) case-based, (3) capitation, and (4) global budgeting. All four of these payment systems are currently used in the U.S. health care system (Reinhardt 1993). Their basic features are summarized in Table 2–3 ■.

After World War II, the increase in health insurance and the introduction of Medicare and Medicaid, in 1965, created a formal payment system for health care providers. At this time, the health care industry was much smaller and relatively inexpensive. While hospitals were paid either on a per-day or a per-stay basis, the primary payment mechanism for physicians was known as **fee-for-service** (FFS). This approach entailed charging the patient a separate fee for each service provided by the physician. If the patient had health care insurance, the insurer paid the fee either in full or at least in part. Some of the FFS charges depended on the physician's specialty and geographic region. Thus, variation existed in the charges for certain services across physicians. For this reason, some payers began to institute a more uniform payment system that was still fee-for-service, but based on usual, customary, and reasonable charges for a given area. As occupational therapy and physical therapy services grew with the overall system, a similar payment structure was utilized.

This payment mechanism created an incentive for providers to add additional days or tests. For example, physicians added a test that would have results that were interesting but not essential. Similarly, hospitals were inclined to keep a patient an extra day "just to be sure" it was safe and the patient was ready to leave the hospital. Occupational therapy and physical therapy services were viewed as an extension of medical care and thus had similar incentives. In this payment system, the patient (or insurer) bears all of the financial risk while the provider has no risk at stake. In cases when patients have health insurance, FFS drives up expenditures. Patients are

Table 2–3. Characteristics/Incentives of Payment Mechanisms

Payment Mechanism	Characteristics	Incentive on Risk/Costs
Fee-for-service	Provider paid for each procedure rendered	Highest utilization/costs All risk borne by payer
Case-based rate	Provider paid for each episode of care	Shared risk with payer
Capitation	Provider paid flat rate	All risk borne by provider
Global budgeting	Flat, all-inclusive budget	Known, capped costs

not fiscally responsible because their insurance is handling all payment claims. Providers have no incentive to limit procedures or provide unnecessary care. Several observers have cited the inflationary effect of this type of payment structure (Reinhardt 1994).

As the shortcomings of the fee-for-service payment mechanism were exposed, alternative payment structures began to emerge. One of these changes was the enactment by Medicare in 1983 of a change from a fee-for-service payment system for hospitals to **case-based payment**. This reimbursement system shifted payment from a retrospective reimbursement system to a prospective payment system (see Chapter 7). Reimbursement was predetermined primarily on the basis of the patient's diagnosis. This diagnostic-related group (DRG) payment system provided one payment for all services relating to a given diagnosis, instead of paying separately for all the different services used in treating the patient. The DRG payment schedule included adjustments based on the teaching status of the hospital, its geographic location, and outlier cases (i.e., patients whose treatments significantly exceeded the norm in cost). The incentive created by DRG payments was for hospitals to use resources more efficiently and avoid unnecessary procedures in treating patients. Today, prospective payment systems are a major part of financing health care services in the public and private sectors. Essentially, prospective payment systems put providers on a budget in regard to which to expend resources (deliver care). Case-based payment is very commonly experienced by therapists providing care in institutional settings (e.g., hospitals, nursing homes, and home health agencies).

The third payment mechanism, the flat fee per patient per month, a feature of some types of health maintenance organizations, is a form of managed care (see Chapter 6). This payment mechanism is known commonly as **capitation**. In it, providers are paid a monthly fee for each patient enrolled in their practice. If the cost of treating a patient is less than the capitation, greater profits are realized; however, if a patient's care is more than the monthly capitation, the health care provider loses money. This system creates an incentive for the provider to keep the patient well to avoid costly care and thus keep most of the capitation as profit. The incentives in a capitated payment system are opposite of those in a fee-for-service environment. In addition, the financial risk to the provider of greater utilization of service than anticipated is also much higher.

Global budgeting, the fourth payment mechanism, is used primarily for hospitals, especially in Canada. Provinces provide a predetermined amount to a hospital to cover all of its operational expenses. In the United States, the Indian Health Service uses a global budgeting mechanism.

ACCESS AND COST: A THERAPIST PERSPECTIVE

Even when an individual has adequate health care insurance, access to health care practitioners may be limited. Historically, physicians have controlled access to physical and occupational therapy services. As will be discussed in Chapters 5 and 6, many insurers require that the insured see a primary care doctor before visiting a

specialist, including physical and occupational therapists. The primary care physician acts as a gatekeeper who must refer patients to more specialized care.

However, this situation is changing as licensure laws increasingly recognize
the ability of the public to access therapy services without a physician referral. In
states throughout the United States, both physical and occupational therapists are
working from a legislative standpoint to improve **direct access** to their services.
Thus, patients would be able to bypass their primary care physician and go directly
to a therapist for evaluation and treatment. Providing patients with direct access to
their services has been a goal of physical and occupational therapists for some time.

The American Occupational Therapy Association's (AOTA's) current statement on this issue asserts that referrals are not required for the provision of occupational therapy services. However, the AOTA maintains that occupational therapists
must be aware of and adhere to the requirements of third-party payers, such as
managed care organizations (American Occupational Therapy Association 2000).
Thirty-seven states have no physician-referral requirements for occupational therapy (Smith 2000). Nine states (Delaware, Illinois, Louisiana, New Hampshire, New
York, North Dakota, Pennsylvania, Texas, and Washington) permit an evaluation,
but no treatment, without physician referral. Nevada permits evaluation and treatment in non-medical settings. Alabama, Delaware, and Kansas permit evaluation
and treatment in educational settings only.

Direct access to physical therapy services has been a major professional objective for the last two decades. Since regulation of health care providers is a state issue,
this process has been long and arduous. Currently, 43 states permit direct access to
physical therapy in some form. Another six states (Connecticut, Kansas, Hawaii,
Michigan, Missouri, and Oklahoma) and the District of Columbia restrict direct access to a physical therapy evaluation (APTA 2006). Two states (Alabama and Indi-
ana) prohibit patient contact with a physical therapist without a physician referral.

Effects of Direct Access on Therapy Practice

The research evidence indicates that 9 to12 percent of a physical therapist's practice may be by direct access. These studies are dated, but provide some insight into the extent of direct access to physical therapy. In a study of 1,580 patients with lower back pain treated by 208 health care providers in North Carolina, Mielenz et al. (1997) reported that 12.6 percent of the patients received physical therapy through direct access. Additionally, one-third of responding physical therapists in Massachusetts used direct access, which accounted for 8.8 percent of their practice (Crout, Tweedie, and Miller 1998). In an early study of direct access to physical therapy, Domholdt and Durchholz (1992) reported that 45 percent of physical therapists utilized direct access, which accounted for 10.3 percent of their practice. A report by Snow et al. (2001) found that three in four persons would go to a physical therapist by direct access, but two in three persons had no knowledge that they were permitted to do so.

More recent work has focused on the clinical decision-making ability of physical therapists related to direct access. Jette et al. (2006) found that physical therapists made correct decisions 87 percent of the time for musculoskeletal conditions, 88 percent of the time for noncritical medical conditions, and 79 percent of the time for critical medical conditions. Correct decision-making percentages were higher for physical therapists who were certified orthopedic specialists. Childs et al. (2005) found that experienced physical therapists had better knowledge than medical students, physician interns, and medical residents in managing musculoskeletal conditions. Physical therapists in military settings have been found to have the requisite knowledge to be effective in a direct access environment (Childs et al. 2007).

A common argument against direct access to physical therapy services alleges that it is unsafe and that the cost and usage of therapy services both increase when there is no physician referral. The evidence fails to demonstrate that direct access to physical therapy increases cost or utilization rates (Mitchell and deLissovy 1997). Sandstrom (2007) found no difference in physical therapist malpractice suits in states that permitted direct access versus states where it was prohibited. Moore et al. (2005) found that military personnel being treated through direct access were at "minimal risk for gross negligent care."

CONCLUSION

Access to health care services is a complicated issue, including cost as well as noncost barriers. Many interacting factors create an environment that promotes or blocks access to appropriate health care providers. Devising a health care system that will distribute a finite set of resources in a way that is acceptable to health care professionals, employers, and consumers is a never-ending challenge for health care policymakers. Add to this challenge concerns about patient safety, quality of care, and improved quality of life, and the problem becomes more complex and compelling. Approaches to ensuring appropriate access to, and financing of, health care services will continually change. In the near future, the health care industry's response to various calls for reform, as well as other market forces, will dictate how the United States pays for its health care. Therapists must understand the many factors that influence access and health expenditure if they are to better help their patients navigate the barriers that make obtaining needed care more difficult. Direct access to therapy services provides an opportunity for physical therapists and occupational therapists to demonstrate the safe and effective application of therapy care that can improve access and lower the overall costs of health care.

CHAPTER REVIEW QUESTIONS

1. Recall the three foundational policy principles that define health policy.
2. Define predisposing factors, need factors, and enabling factors.
3. Define each of Penchansky and Thomas's five dimensions of access.
4. What is the relationship between health insurance and access to health care services?
5. Define the characteristics of the uninsured.
6. Describe the effect of direct access to therapy services on the cost and quality of health care.
7. Identify the percentage of U.S. health care spending that comes from public sources and private sources.
8. What is the largest single category of U.S. health care spending? The next-largest category?
9. What category of U.S. health care spending had the greatest rate of inflation in the late 1990s?
10. Identify three reasons for rising health care costs in the United States.
11. Define fee-for-service, flat fee per medical case, flat fee per person, and global budgeting. What is the effect of each of these payment systems on health care costs?
12. Define prospective and retrospective payment systems and their role in health care cost containment.
13. Review how health care is paid for in Canada, Sweden, and Great Britain. How do these systems differ from the systems that finance health care in the United States?

CHAPTER DISCUSSION QUESTIONS

1. The development of a marketing plan for a therapy practice will benefit from a consideration of the principles of access. Discuss how you could use Penchansky and Thomas's model of access to determine whether to open a therapy practice.
2. Discuss how the unique American policy decision to support both private and public health insurance affects access to health care.

3. Is direct access to occupational and physical therapy essential? Do you think it will increase access for the population? Explain your answer.
4. The United States is the only major industrialized democracy without a system of national health care insurance. How would the development and implementation of national health care insurance in the United States affect the cost of health care?
5. It is estimated that more costs of health care may be transferred to the consumer from the employer/government in the form of higher premiums, deductibles, and co-payments. What would the effect of these changes be on the growth of the costs of health care? On occupational therapists and physical therapists?
6. Discuss the incentives of fee-for-service and capitated payment systems on the cost of health care. How do these systems promote or inhibit access to care?
7. Americans spend more money on specialized, high-technology medical care than people in other countries do. This decision may affect the availability of resources for other worthwhile social goals (e.g., education, transportation). What effect do you believe this policy decision may have on persons with disabilities or with other forms of medically stable, chronic diseases?

REFERENCES

American Occupational Therapy Association (AOTA). 2000. Statement of occupational therapy referral (Approved 1994). AOTA FAX-on Request, FAX No. 907.

American Physical Therapy Association. A Summary of Direct Access Language in State Physical Therapy Practice Acts. Direct Access to Physical Therapy Laws. August 2006. http://www.apta.org/AM/Template.cfm?Section=Top_Issues2&TEMPLATE=/CM/ContentDisplay.cfm&CONTENTID=37168 (accessed July 10, 2007).

Anzick, M. 1993. Demographics and employment shifts: Implications for benefits and economic security. *EBRI Issue Brief* No. 140. Washington DC: Employee Benefit Research Institute.

Barton, P. B. 1999. *Understanding the U.S. health services system.* Chicago: Health Administration Press.

Borger, C., S. Smith, C. Truffer, S. Keehan, A. Sisko, J. Poisal, and M.E. Clemens. M.E. 2006. Health spending projections through 2015: Changes on the horizon. *Health Affairs Web Exclusives* 25 (2): w61–73.

Braveman, P., V.M. Schaaf, S. Egerter, T. Bennett, and W. Schecter. 1994. Insurance related differences in the risk of ruptured appendix. *N Engl J Med* 331(7): 444–49.

Childs, J. D., J.M. Whitman, M.L. Pugia, P.S. Sizer, T.W. Flynn Jr., and A. Delitto. 2007. Knowledge in managing musculoskeletal conditions and educational preparation of physical therapists in the uniformed services. *Mil Med* 172(4): 440–445.

Childs, J.D., J.M. Whitman, P.S. Sizer, M.L. Pugia, T.W. Flynn, and A. Delitto. 2005. A description of physical therapists' knowledge in managing musculoskeletal conditions. *BMC Musculoskelet Disord* 6: 32.

Clemans-Cope, L., B. Garrett, and C. Hoffman. 2006. Changes in Employees' Health Insurance coverage, 2001-2005. Kaiser Commission on Medicaid and the Uninsured, Issue Paper (Report # 7570).

Crout, K. L., J. H. Tweedie, and D. J. Miller. 1998. Physical therapists' opinions and practice regarding direct access. *Phys Ther* 78(1): 52–61.

Davis, K., C. Schoen, S. Guterman, T. Shih, S.C. Schoenbaum, and W. Ilana. 2007. Slowing the growth of U.S. health care expenditures: What are the options?. The Commonwealth Fund. http://www.cmf.org/publications/publications_show.htm?doc_id=449510 (accessed June 2007).

Domholdt, E., and A. G. Durchholz. 1992. Direct access use by experienced therapists in states with direct access. *Phys Ther* (8): 569–74.

Folland, S., A. C. Goodman, and M. Stano. 1997. *The economics of health and health care.* 2nd ed. Upper Saddle River NJ: Prentice Hall.

Franks, P., C. M. Clancey, and M. R. Gold. 1993. Health insurance and mortality. *JAMA* 270(6): 737–41.

Fronstin, P. 2007. *Employment-based Health Benefits: Access and Coverage, 1988–2005.* Washington DC: Employment Benefit Research Institute (Issue Brief No. 303).

Fuchs, V. 1990. The health sector's share of the gross national product. *Science* 247(4942): 534–38.

Fuchs, V. R. 1993. National health insurance revisited. In *Debating health care reform: A primer from Health Affairs,* ed. J. K. Iglehart. Bethesda MD: Project Hope. 81–91.

Hoffman, C. 1998. *Uninsured in America: A chart book.* Kaiser Commission on Medicaid and the Uninsured. *http://www.kff.org.*

Hoffman, J.M., N.D. Shah, L.C. Vermeulen, R.J. Hunkler, and K.M. Hont. 2006. Projecting future drug expenditures—2005. *Am J Health-Sys Pharm* 62: 149–167.

Jette, D.U., K. Ardleigh, K. Chandler, and L. McShea. 2006. Decision-making ability of physical therapists: Physical therapy intervention or medical referral. *Phys Ther* 86(12): 1619–1629.

KCMU. 2003. *Access to Care for the Uninsured.* Kaiser Commission on Medicaid and the Uninsured. Report # 41442.

KCMU. 2006. *The Uninsured: A Primer.* Kaiser Commission on Medicaid and the Uninsured Report #7451-02.

Kuttner, R. 1999. The American health care system: Health insurance coverage. *N Engl J Med* 340(2): 163–68.

Mielenz, T. J., T.S. Carey, D.A. Dyrek, B.A. Harris, J.M. Garrett, and J.D. Darter. 1997. Physical therapy utilization by patients with acute low back pain. *Phys Ther* (10): 1040–51.

Mitchell, J. M., and G. deLissovy. 1997. A comparison of resource use and cost in direct access versus physician referral episodes of physical therapy. *Phys Ther* 77(1): 10–18.

Moore, J.H., D.J. McMillian, M.D. Rosenthal, and M.D. Weishaar. 2005. Risk determination for patients with direct access to physical therapy in military health care facilities. *J Orthop Sports Phys Ther* 35(10): 674–78.

National Center for Health Statistics. 2006. Characteristics on Trends in the Health of Americans. Hyattsville, MD.

Peden, E. A., and M. S. Freeland. 1995. A historical analysis of medical spending growth, 1960–1993. *Health Affairs* 14(2): 235–47.

Penchansky, R., and J. W. Thomas. 1981. The concept of access: Definition and relationship to consumer satisfaction. *Med Care* 19(2): 127–140.

Reinhardt, U. E. 1993. Reorganizing the financial flows in American health care. *Health Affairs* 12: 172–93.

————.1994. Planning the nation's workforce: Let the market in. *Inquiry* 31(3): 250–63.

Sandstrom, R. 2007. Malpractice by physical therapists: Descriptive analysis of reports in the National Practitioner Data Bank Public Use Data File, 1991–2004. *Journal of Allied Health* 36: 201–208.

Schwartz, W. B., and D. M. Mendelson. 1994. Eliminating waste and inefficiency can do little to contain costs. *Health Affairs* 13(1): 224–38.

Seiden, D. J. 1994. Health care ethics. In *Health care delivery in the United States,* ed. A. R. Kovner. New York: Springer. 486–531

Sered, S., and Fernandopulle. 2005. *Profiles of the uninsured: Uninsured Americans tell their stories.* http://www.cmwf.org/General/General_show.htm?doc_id=256036 (accessed June 2007).

Smith, K. 2000. Direct access important to profession's future. AOTA. http://www.aota.org/Pubs/OTP/Columns/CapitalBriefing/2000/cb-052200.aspx (accessed July 10, 2007).

Snow, B.L., E. Shamus, and C. Hill. 2001. Physical therapy as primary health care: Public perceptions. *J Allied Health* 30(1): 35–38.

Spillman, B. C. 1992. The impact of being uninsured on utilization of basic health care services. *Inquiry* 29(4): 457–66.

Stoddard, J. J., R. F. St. Peter, and P. W. Newacheck. 1994. Health insurance status and ambulatory care for children. *N Engl J Med* 330(20): 1421–25.

Sultz, H. A., and K. M. Young. 1999. *Health care USA: Understanding its organization and delivery,* 2d ed. Gaithersburg, MD: Aspen Publishers.

The Commonwealth Fund. 2007. *Looking Back, Moving Forward: Access to Health Care.* http://www.commonwealthfund.org/chartcartcharts/chartcartcharts_show.htm?doc_id=472707 (accessed June 2006).

U.S. Department of Health and Human Services. 2007. A Statistical Profile of Older Americans Aged 65+. U.S. Department of Health and Human Services, Administration on Aging (accessed May 19, 2008).

Vistnes, J.P., and S.H. Zuvekas. 1999. *Health insurance status of the civilian noninstitutionalized population: 1997.* MEPS Reseach Findings No. 8. AHRQ Pub. No. 99–0030. Rockville MD: Agency for Health Care Research and Quality.

Woolhander, S., and D. Himmelstein. 1991. The deteriorating administrative efficiency of the U.S. health care system. *N Engl J Med* 324(18): 1253–58.

3

Quality of Health Care

CHAPTER OBJECTIVES

At the conclusion of this chapter, the reader will be able to:

1. Compare and contrast the population- and personal-based conceptualizations of health care quality.
2. Describe the following basic components of a quality health care system:
   a. Adequate structure
   b. Effective processes
      1. Evidence-based practice
   c. Satisfactory outcomes
3. Review the mechanisms and provide examples of measuring and reporting on the quality of the health care system, using:
   a. Peer review
   b. Accreditation
   c. Report cards
4. Discuss the legal foundations for quality in the health care system:
   a. Professional regulation
   b. Patient rights
   c. Medical negligence
5. Identify future developments to improve health care system quality and address health disparities.

KEY WORDS: Accreditation, Clinical Practice Guideline, Evidence-based Practice, Health Disparities, Interpersonal Excellence, Medical Negligence, Outcomes, Patient Privacy, Patient Safety, Pay for Performance, Peer Review, Process, Quality Improvement, Professional Regulation, Standards, Structure, Technical Excellence

Case Example

Molly Smith, OTR, is the manager of rehabilitation services at Community Hospital. She is being asked by her administrator to provide information to support the continuance of an arthritis education program in her department. She knows that patients and therapists are reporting

satisfaction with the service, but she needs more information. After researching the alternatives, she decides to discuss with her staff the identification and implementation of a standard health status survey for persons with arthritis as the best method to gather good information about both the need for the program and improvements that patients are making in the program.

Case Example Focus Question:

1. Consider and explain how the use of evidence can support new clinical programs. Why is evidence important?

INTRODUCTION

Quality is the third foundational principle of health policy. As already explained, health policy establishes access to, and finances, the health care system. People and society want access to, and are willing to pay only for, a high-quality health care system. In this chapter, we will explore the meaning of quality health care. Recent studies have pointed out serious deficiencies in the health care system, such as the high rate of medical error (Committee on Quality of Health Care in America 1999). Depending on one's perspective, Americans either are receiving the highest-quality health care in the world or are not getting an adequate return on quality from the most expensive health care system in the world. We will also discuss the basic components of a quality personal health care system: structure, process, and outcomes. We will introduce methods to measure the quality of each of these components. Finally, we will review the basic foundation of quality: the legal rights of patients to be protected and informed when interacting with the health care system.

PERSPECTIVES ON HEALTH CARE QUALITY

There are two fundamental paradigms with which to analyze the quality of health care services in the United States: one is personal based and the other population based. Each of these perspectives is influenced by the structure of the current system, contemporary social expectations, and legal mandates to ensure quality health care. The personal-based perspective focuses on the patient–provider relationship and the organization, delivery, and outcome of the services patients receive. It is the perspective used most commonly by physical therapists, occupational therapists, and other providers. The population-based perspective analyzes health care quality by examining the experiences and health status of populations and subgroups. The roots of the population-based perspective of health care quality can be traced to the universalism philosophy (see Chapter 1). A definition of quality from this perspective includes not only medical care, but also socioeconomic status and the community environment. Table 3–1 ■ compares and contrasts the population- and personal-based concepts of quality.

For patients with chronic diseases and disabilities, the quality of their health entails much more than medical care. The population-based quality perspective is

Table 3–1. Population-Based vs. Personal-Based Concepts of Health Care Quality

	Population-Based	*Personal-Based*
Theoretical Model	Public health	Medical
Key Components	Quality of life/health status	Patient–provider interaction
	Function	Structure, process, outcome
	Satisfaction	Satisfaction
How to measure?	Survey, interview	Peer review, accreditation
	Community-based	Within the health care system

increasingly being used to understand the quality of life of persons with disabilities living in community environments. A plethora of measures of quality of life for persons experiencing disablement exist, including both general and disability-specific measures of health status. General measures of health status—e.g., the Medical Outcomes Study SF-36 (Ware and Sherbourne 1992)—can compare the health status of a person experiencing disablement with that of the age-matched general population. Disease-specific measures (e.g., the Arthritis Impact Measurement Scales 2) are often more sensitive and specific to health status in these specific populations, but have limited ability to define quality of life in comparison to that of the general population. As we will discuss later, these measures also provide a method for assessing the outcomes of physical therapy and occupational therapy and demonstrating the effectiveness of the care involved.

A personal-based perspective is common to the administration and practice of physical therapy or occupational therapy services. The Institute of Medicine (1990) defines quality of health care as "the degree to which health services for individuals and populations increase the likelihood of desired health outcomes and are consistent with current professional knowledge." In contrast to population-based perspectives, this definition focuses on services: how they are delivered and what their result is. To further illustrate this perspective, Table 3–2 ■ lists "seven pillars of quality"

Table 3–2. Seven Pillars of Quality Health Care

A. Efficacy—the best care provided under the best circumstances.

B. Effectiveness—the best care provided under ordinary, everyday circumstances.

C. Efficiency—care that considers the relationship of cost to the amount of improvement in health.

D. Optimality—care that is the best value between cost and amount of improvement in health.

E. Acceptability—care that is accessible and meets patient preferences.

F. Legitimacy—care that meets societal expectations of optimal services.

G. Equity—care that is fair and just for all people.

Source: Donabedian, A. (1990). "The seven pillars of quality." *Arch Path Lab Med* 114 (11): 1115–8.

┌─ **Active Learning Exercise** ─────────────────────────────┐

Reflect upon an occasion when you or a family member received health care.
Did the experience meet your expectations for quality? Why or why not?

as defined by Avedis Donabedian (1990), a seminal thinker on the quality of the
health care system. As can be observed from the table, different conceptualizations
of the meaning of quality health care exist. In any event, accountability for the quality of a health care service is important: Providers must measure and meet minimal
standards for the quality of the care they dispense. (We will discuss more about how
providers measure, assure, and improve the quality of health care, including therapy services, later in this chapter.)

   Both of these perspectives on quality health care are affected by the legal
mandates to ensure high-quality health care services. The basis for governmental
actions is the expectation that providers have a responsibility to provide the best
care for the patients they serve. It is important to understand the legal requirements for health care quality as the "floor," or minimum societal expectation, for
health care quality. Legal mandates focus on public safety. For example, the tort system of law provides a legal recourse for people to address medical errors. Provider-
caused medical errors and negligent practices are harms that are remediated in the
courts. Licensure and other forms of regulation ensure a base level of provider
capability to serve the public and protect it from harmful practices. The law also
establishes fundamental rights for patients in their interactions with the system.

   In the next section, we will introduce and explore another Donabedian model
for understanding the quality of personal health care: a model whose components
are structure, process, and outcomes.

STRUCTURE, PROCESS, AND OUTCOMES

In 1966, Avedis Donabedian put forth a template that is widely accepted today as
the basis for understanding the framework of quality in the health care system (see
Figure 3–1 ■). This template has three components: **structure**, **process**, and **outcomes**.

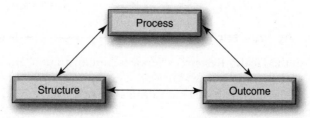

Figure 3–1. Donabedian Quality of Health Care Framework

Table 3–3.   Features of Structure, Process, and Outcomes

	Structure	*Process*	*Outcome*
Key components	Physical facilities Human resources	Technical excellence Interpersonal excellence	Results
How measured?	Access to care Professional regulation	Standards Peer review	Survey Interview

Structure comprises the permanent features of the health care system—hospitals and the various health care providers. Process is the method of delivery of care. Outcomes are the results of the health care encounter. Over the years, the definition and measurement of quality have developed steadily from an initial focus on structure, to how health care is delivered (process), to outcomes. Today, outcomes (e.g., medical error rates and functional outcomes) are very important to the examination of the quality of health care in America. Let us consider each of the three components of health care quality separately. The basic features of structure, process, and outcome are displayed in Table 3–3 ■.

Structure

Structure is the basic foundation of the health care system. It comprises the services and the organization of the health care system and, as such, is closely related to the health policy principle of access. A quality system has to have the physical and human resources with which to deliver services at locations that can be accessed by the public it serves. If a location or region lacks the facilities or the types of providers to provide appropriate care, it is defined as "medically underserved"; in other words, it lacks a proper structure to meet the needs of the population it serves. The Health Resources Services Administration (2007) maintains a database of health professional shortage areas and provides grant funding to alleviate structural problems of this kind. Health care systems with these problems are typically in rural areas or poor districts of urban areas. Besides impaired access, regulation of providers, whether they be therapists or long-term care facilities, is the basis for the determination of adequate structural quality.

> ### — Active Learning Exercise —
>
> Visit the Health Resources Services Administration, Bureau of Health Professions Data Warehouse at its website: http://hpsafind.hrsa.gov/. Look up your home county. Is it a Health Professional Shortage Area or Medically Underserved Area?

Process

Process is the method by which health care is delivered. It has two components: technical excellence and interpersonal excellence (Donabedian 1988). Technical excellence comprises the ability of the health care provider to make informed decisions, as well as the skill of the health care provider to improve the patient's situation. In essence, a quality health care intervention should shorten the length of time of a disabling condition, reduce its severity, or both. The measurement of technical excellence requires the utilization of accepted intervention protocols and a mechanism of review to determine the appropriateness of the actual intervention.

Today, the emphasis in health care quality is on **evidence-based practice**, defined as the "integration of the best research evidence with clinical experience and patient values" (Sackett, Strauss, and Richardson 2000). The goal of this emphasis is for clinicians to ascertain, interpret, and utilize the best evidence in making treatment decisions. A number of studies of occupational and physical therapists indicate that, while therapists recognize the importance of evidence-based practice, the implementation of evidence-based practice into their work has been more limited. Dysart and Tomlin (2002) found that lack of time, high costs, weak research analysis skills, and a higher value placement on experience versus research limited the incorporation of evidence-based practice into the work of occupational therapists. Similarly, Maher, Sherrington, Elkins, Herbert, and Moseley (2004) found that access to evidence, problems with interpreting evidence, and other "organizational barriers" limited the implementation of evidence-based practice for physical therapists. Bridges, Bierema, and Valentin (2007) found that the desire for learning, the highest degree held, and practicality were positively associated with use of evidence-based practice. Bennett, McKenna, Hoffmann, Tooth, McCluskey, and Strong (2007) found that a discipline-specific online database improved the ability of occupational therapists to access evidence. Evidence-based practice knowledge and skills have been demonstrated to improve with the education of health professionals, but behavior change "may take months, even years" (McCluskey and Lovarini 2005).

Technical excellence is determined by measuring provider performance against a set of **standards**—statements that describe either minimal or optimal actions that providers should take in a clinical situation. Standards form the basis for

---

Active Learning Exercise

Visit the Physiotherapy Evidence Database (PEDro) at http://www.pedro.fhs. usyd.du.au/index.html or APTA's Hooked on Evidence website at http://www. hookedonevidence.com/ to learn about an evidence-based database for physical therapists. Go to OT Search to learn about a similar database for occupational therapy evidence-based practice: http://otsearch.aota.org/

the **accreditation** process. Standards are also incorporated into procedural documents called **clinical practice guidelines**, which are "systematically developed statements to assist practitioner and patient decisions about appropriate health care for specific clinical circumstances" (Institute of Medicine 1990). When based on the professional literature, clinical practice guidelines are an example of evidence-based practice. An increasing number of guidelines have been developed in the last decade in response to the demonstrated variation in medical care practice across the country. In addition, many individual providers (including physical therapists and occupational therapists) have developed practice guidelines in order to standardize practice, improve outcomes, lower costs, and reduce the risk of negligent activity.

Peer review is the primary mechanism for measuring provider performance against standards or a clinical practice guideline. The Institute of Medicine (1990) has defined medical review criteria as "systematically developed statements that can be used to assess the appropriateness of specific health care decisions, services and outcomes." Peer review usually evaluates the activities of the provider by close examination and consideration of the documentation. It is widely used by providers and payers to determine the appropriateness of the care given. Quality-assurance and quality-improvement programs are standard managerial procedures used by therapists to measure and report clinical quality internally and to accrediting agencies.

Interpersonal excellence relates to how care is provided and considers the humanistic features of the process (Donabedian 1988). Patient satisfaction measurement is the form of process assessment most commonly used to determine interpersonal excellence. Measurement of interpersonal excellence is used by both providers and health plans.

Outcomes

Outcomes are a "technology of patient experience" (Ellwood 1988). As the results of the patient's care, outcomes are an important measure of the quality of the health care system. They are typically measured by examining the health status of the person or, in the case of a person with a disability, the status of disablement. Generic health status measures are commonly used to measure quality of life. A variety of disease-specific measures are available to assess health status for specific populations. Both types of measures are used to measure outcomes. As accountability for system performance has increased, the measurement and reporting of outcomes has become more important.

Generic Health Status Measures Generic health status assessment is one type of patient outcomes measurement. Tools have been designed to measure health status, quality of life, and global health outcomes. Generic health status surveys are especially valuable when a clinician wants to monitor the health status of an individual or a population. These surveys typically measure overall health status across physical, psychological, and social domains to provide a more complete picture of health. Another advantage to certain generic health status measures is norm referencing and, in some cases, age-matched referencing. This feature allows a comparison of results with the average health of the population. The Medical Outcome Study–Short Form (SF-36), developed by Ware and Sherbourne (1992), is a well-known global health status measure. The SF-36 is a quick norm-referenced survey of eight domains of physical, social, emotional, and mental health status. It is widely used as a measure of outcomes for many types of medical pathologies.

Disease- Specific Outcome Measures Many diseases have outcome measures to assess health status and patient outcomes for persons who experience those diseases. These measures are advantageous in that they assess specific features of the condition and are usually more sensitive to detecting an improvement or a change in condition than a generic health status survey is. An example of a disease-specific outcome measure is the Arthritis Impact Measurement Scales 2, which measures the health status of persons with arthritis in physical, emotional, and social domains (Meenan, Gertman, and Mason 1980).

Therapy-Specific Outcome Measures Improved functioning and a lowered need for external-care assistance is a critical outcome in the care of persons with temporary or permanent disablements. Contemporary outcomes measurement in rehabilitation settings includes patient-reported measures of health status, a report on interpersonal excellence, clinical measures of disablement, and a descriptive report of all patients served by a provider (Dobrzykowski 1997). A number of outcome measurement and reporting systems have been developed in the last 20 years.

The Focus on Therapeutic Outcomes (FOTO) tool, a commercially available outcomes management system, measures disablement in outpatient orthopedic settings (FOTO 2007). Studies of the FOTO database have demonstrated the effectiveness of outpatient orthopedic rehabilitation procedures (Dobrzykowski and Nance 1997; Amato, Dobrzykowski, and Nance 1997). In medical rehabilitation, the Uniform Data System for Medical Rehabilitation (1997) and its outcome measurement tool, the Functional Independence Measure (FIM™), is the standard for functional-limitations outcomes assessment. In 2006, APTA introduced the Outpatient

---

Active Learning Exercise

Visit the Medicare consumer website at http://www.medicare.gov. On the home page, find the link to Compare Home Health Agencies in Your Area. Click on this link, enter your zip code, and then compare occupational therapy or physical therapy services for the home health agencies in your area. How useful did you find this information? Would it influence your purchasing decision?

Physical Therapy Improvement in Movement Assessment Log (OPTIMAL) as an outcome reporting system.

Report Cards   Report cards are intended to increase consumer awareness of the quality of the health care they are purchasing and receiving. Werner and Asch (2005) stated that the intent of report cards is to promote the preferential selection of good physicians and to motivate physicians to compete on quality. Wicks and Meyer (1999) identify five features of a useful report card system for quality reporting: interested consumers, understandable report cards, a focus on outcomes and high-priority quality areas, utilization of accurate measures, and a reward system to encourage provider accountability based on the results of the report card. The adoption by Medicare of the use of report cards to inform the public of the quality of hospitals, nursing homes, and home health agencies has increased attention on provider report cards. Public report cards have been associated with reduced mortality rates for cardiac surgery (Epstein 2006). Their overall effect, however, has been modest, with some reports of greater usage when patients are dissatisfied with or changing health plans (Schultz, Thiede-Call, Feldman, and Christianson 2001; Braun, Kind, Fowles, and Suarez 2002).

ACCREDITATION

Accreditation is the primary method by which institutional providers measure their structure, process, and outcomes against consensus quality standards. Most individual providers—e.g., private therapy clinics—are not accredited. Payer review of provider documentation is the dominant method for determining the quality of individual practitioner performance. Accreditation is a voluntary process by which an institutional provider allows a focused survey of its organization and operations using the accrediting body's standards. If the institution meets the accrediting body's standards, it receives a public proclamation of its quality until the next accreditation is required. We will discuss three major accreditation organizations that are of interest to occupational therapists and physical therapists: the Joint Commission on the Accreditation of Health Care Organizations, the Commission on the Accreditation of Rehabilitation Facilities, and the National Committee on Quality Assurance.

Joint Commission on the Accreditation of Healthcare Organizations

The Joint Commission on the Accreditation of Healthcare Organizations (JCAHO) is the oldest accrediting body of health care organizations in the United States (JCAHO 2007). Originally established in 1951 to accredit hospitals, JCAHO now accredits a full array of health care organizations, including skilled nursing facilities, home health agencies, and behavioral health organizations. JCAHO has developed performance standards for the structure, organization, and processes of the institutions it accredits. Surveys are conducted by teams of JCAHO employees who conduct on-site reviews and interview key leaders and workers. JCAHO uses the ORYX program to demonstrate an outcomes management system. JCAHO maintains an online report card of its accredited organizations at http://www.qualitycheck.org.

A major initiative of JCAHO has been the development and assessment of provider performance related to **patient safety** and **quality improvement**. In November 1999, the Institute of Medicine released *To Err Is Human: Building a Safer Health System*, a major report on the quality of health care in the United States. This report found that up to 98,000 deaths annually in the United States could be attributed to medical error. The report attributed more deaths to medical error than to highway accidents, breast cancer, or AIDS. Falls have been identified as one of the most common forms of adverse events experienced by elderly patients (Thomas and Brennan 2000; Rothschild, Bates, and Leape 2000). Most of these errors were attributed to the design of the health care system and not to individual provider practices (Leape 1997; Casarett and Helms 1999). Mu, Lohman, and Scheirton (2006) found that most errors committed by occupational therapists were related to interventions, especially treatments or supervision of patients.

In 2001, the Institute of Medicine released *Crossing the Quality Chasm: A New Health System for the 21st Century*. This report advocates a redesign of the health care system to bolster the clinical information infrastructure, encourages the use of evidence-based practice by clinicians, and calls for the inclusion of clinical quality indicators, as well as cost-efficiency measures in determining the system's functioning. In response, JCAHO has implemented the ORYX system and the National Patient Safety Goal initiative (see Table 3–4 ■) to focus hospital attention on quality and safety improvement.

Commission on Accreditation of Rehabilitation Facilities

The Commission on the Accreditation of Rehabilitation Facilities (CARF) was created in the late 1960s to perform institutional quality-review assessment for organizations that serve persons with disabilities (CARF 2000). CARF accredits organizations that serve persons with physical and behavioral disabilities. Like JCAHO, CARF utilizes performance standards to determine quality, but unlike JCAHO, it utilizes part-time surveyors recruited from the clinical fields to conduct the surveys. The CARF accreditation process emphasizes patients' rights and a provider commitment to quality improvement.

Table 3–4. 2007 JCAHO National Patient Safety Goals

- Improve the accuracy of patient identification.
- Improve the effectiveness of communication among caregivers.
- Improve the safety of using medications.
- Reduce the risk of infections associated with health care.
- Accurately and completely reconcile medications across the continuum of care.
- Reduce the risk of patient harm resulting from falls.
- Reduce the risk of influenza and pneumococcal disease in institutionalized older adults.
- Reduce the risk of surgical fires.
- Implement applicable National Patient Safety Goals and associated requirements by components and practitioner sites.
- Encourage patients active involvement in their own care as a patient-safety strategy.
- Prevent decubitus ulcers associated with health care.
- Identify safety risks inherent in an organization's population.

Source: Facts About the 2007 National Patient Safety Goals. http://www.jointcommission.org/PatientSafety/NationalPatientSafetyGoals/07_npsg_facts.htm (accessed January 30, 2007).

National Committee on Quality Assurance

The National Committee on Quality Assurance (NCQA) was formed in the 1990s by business, labor, and the insurance industry as a body to accredit quality in health plans—specifically, forms of managed care (NCQA 2007). NCQA assesses health plans in regard to access and service, provider qualifications, wellness and prevention activities, and care for people who have chronic diseases and illnesses. NCQA utilizes a focused survey of health plans to make its accreditation decisions.

LEGAL ISSUES AND QUALITY

For certain health care quality and safety issues, the government has set mandatory minimum standards for medical care and has established mechanisms to enforce these standards. These issues include **professional regulation, patient privacy**, and **medical negligence**.

The purpose of professional regulation is to protect the public from harm by poorly prepared practitioners. Professional regulation can take one of three forms: registration, certification, or licensure. Registration, the least rigorous process, is the voluntary registration of an individual with an association of practitioners. Certification is the process whereby a state or national board attests that an individual has met the minimum educational standards of the board. The National Board for Certification in Occupational Therapy is a certification body for occupational therapists (NBCOT 2007). Licensure is the most stringent form of professional regulation.

It codifies into state law the scope of practice, educational qualifications, testing requirements, and disciplinary procedures for a profession. All 50 states require physical therapists to be licensed. Licensure laws vary from state to state. A model state practice act for physical therapy has been presented by the Federation of State Boards of Physical Therapy (see *www.fsbpt.org* for more information). As of 2007, 47 states require occupational therapists to be licensed (AOTA 2007). As with physical therapy, laws vary from state to state. A model practice act for occupational therapy has been developed by the American Occupational Therapy Association (see http://www.aota.org/members/area4/docs/MPA2006.pdf). This act is often used to inform state licensure practice acts. The regulation of physical therapist assistants and occupational therapy assistants varies from state to state. It is very important for therapists and therapist assistants to understand their state's statutes that regulate assistant practice.

Informed consent and patient confidentiality during health care interactions are fundamental patient rights that have emerged in the law over the last half-century. Annas (1998) has identified five core patient rights in health care: the right to information, the right to privacy and dignity, the right to refuse treatment, the right to emergency care, and the right to an advocate. Occupational therapists and physical therapists are legally required to obtain informed consent prior to treatment. This means that the patient needs to be provided with information in order to decide whether to accept or refuse treatment. Specifically, the therapist needs to inform the patient of the type of procedures to be employed, any risks or hazards involved, the anticipated outcome of the intervention, whether alternatives to the treatment exist, and the consequences of not receiving treatment. Two other forms of informed consent are an advanced directive and a durable power of attorney. An advanced directive is a legal document that details what treatment a patient does or does not wish to be given when the patient is no longer able to make a decision about such matters. Examples of an advanced directive are a living will and a "do not resuscitate" order in a hospital setting. A durable power of attorney is a legal document that designates another person to make health care decisions if the patient becomes unable to do so.

In 2003, new privacy standards for the protection of "individually identifiable" health information went into effect (U.S. Department of Health and Human Services 2003). These federal regulations apply provisions of the 1996 Health Insurance Portability and Accountability Act (HIPAA). Providers are required to identify and track the flow of personal health care information in their practices and systems, and take the necessary steps not to disclose information for nontreatment, nonpayment purposes. In general, patient consent (authorization) is not required when personal health information is used for treatment, payment, and routine health care operations (e.g., the education of students). Other uses, however, require patient authorization for release of information. Examples of other uses include the marketing and business relationships a practice may have with other providers (except insurance companies). In addition, providers are required to disclose the minimum necessary information to achieve the business objective. The regulations provide for specific consumer rights to their personal health information and a record of how it has been disclosed. Therapists must take specific steps to prevent the oral release of personal health information, as well as its technical release (e.g., via a computer screen in a waiting area). Civil and criminal penalties for unauthorized disclosure have been defined in the regulations.

Remediation for medical error or negligence is achieved through civil court action. An action by a therapist that produces a wrong (called a tort) resulting in injury is termed medical negligence or malpractice. The law provides for relief from this wrong by permitting the injured party to sue the provider for damages caused by the action. Medical negligence is the failure by a provider to perform those duties and functions which would be done by a similarly trained provider in the same situation. The person suing the provider must demonstrate that the actions of the provider caused the harm and that damages or injuries were suffered by the patient. Standards of care, accreditation policies, organizational policies and procedures, clinical practice guidelines, expert opinion, and professional publications are all key measuring sticks to determine the ability and actions of the provider accused of medical negligence. Good patient-communication skills, insurance, and legal representation are necessary for adequate protection of the therapist in a medical negligence situation (Scott 1991). The incidence of malpractice by physical therapists and occupational therapists is quite low. Sandstrom (2007) found that the incidence of physical therapist malpractice was 2.5 cases per 10,000 therapists. A typical physical therapist malpractice settlement was treatment related and occurred in an urban state by a physical therapist age 30 to 50 for an amount between $10,000 and $15,000.

THE FUTURE OF HEALTH CARE QUALITY

In *Crossing the Quality Chasm*, the Institute of Medicine (2001) identified six areas in need of improvement in the United States health care system: safety, effectiveness, patient-centeredness, timeliness, efficiency, and equitability. Among the recommendations for achieving progress in these areas is to increase accountability and transparency of the system, promote evidence-based practice, increase the use of information technology, and align payment policies with quality initiatives. As we have discussed in this chapter, several of these recommendations have already been initiated and significant progress has been made. The public now has Internet access to basic quality report cards on organizational providers (e.g., hospitals, nursing homes, and home health agencies). Evidence-based clinical practice guidelines are widely available for many conditions. **Pay for performance** is emerging as a strategy to reward providers who meet basic quality expectations (see also Chapter 6). Public policies such as the Tax Relief and Health Care Act of 2006, which includes a quality measures reporting system, address pay for performance (AOTA 2007). As a first step toward implementing pay for performance, the federal agency called the Centers for Medicare and Medicaid Services (CMS) is rewarding physicians with a 1.5 percent bonus if they report data on the quality of their care (Pear 2006). CMS will continue to look at quality measures and outcomes as possible alternatives to other forms of Medicare payments (Dan Jones, personal communication December 20, 2006), and other insurers will pay close attention to these changes. Physical and occupational therapists can expect changes to occur that affect all areas of health care, likely including therapy practice.

A second major challenge for the health care system will be to make progress in the health status of all Americans and to decrease and eliminate **health disparities**. A health disparity is "a significant disparity in the overall rate of disease incidence, prevalence, morbidity, mortality or survival rate" between population groups (NIH 2001, p. 3). Braveman (2006) has defined a health disparity as the "difference in which disadvantaged social groups—such as the poor, racial/ethnic minorities, women, or other groups who have persistently experienced social disadvantage or discrimination—systematically experience worse health or greater health risks than more advantaged social groups. 'Social advantage' refers to one's relative position in a social hierarchy determined by wealth, power, and/or prestige" (p. 167).

Examples of health disparities include those based on racial disparities, age disparities, and disparities experienced by persons with disabilities. African-Americans experience greater rates of morbidity and mortality in several disorders, including cardiovascular disease, cancer, diabetes, and disability (Siminoff and Ross 2005; Oliver and Muntaner 2005; Centers for Disease Control and Prevention 2005). It has been demonstrated that children with juvenile arthritis (Brunner et al. 2006), children with intellectual disabilities (Krahn, Hammond, and Turner 2006; Haverkamp, Scandline, and Roth 2004), and children from socially disadvantaged backgrounds (Bauman, Silver, and Stein 2006) experience more health problems than other children. Finally, a study by Nosek et al. (2006) found that women with disabilities experience an average of 14.6 secondary conditions, compared with 75 percent of their community-based sample, which reported about 10 conditions.

Strategies are needed to comprehensively address these differences in health status. Michaud, Murry, and Bloom (2001) identified occupational hazards and physical inactivity as being among the major causes of disability and illness worldwide. Occupational and physical therapists have important contributions to make to address these issues (see Public Health section in Chapter 11).

CONCLUSION

In this chapter, we have reviewed the fundamentals of determining and measuring quality in the health care system. Figure 3–2 ■ depicts a "quality pyramid" describing the components of quality in the U.S. health care system. At its base are the fundamental rights patients have to be informed and involved in decision-making and to have health conditions be treated with privacy and respect. The next three levels of the pyramid define components of quality for the personal health care system. Structure is the fixed physical and human resource investment in health care quality. Process is the delivery of health care by this structure. Outcomes are the newest level of health care quality to be emphasized—the results of the intervention. The final

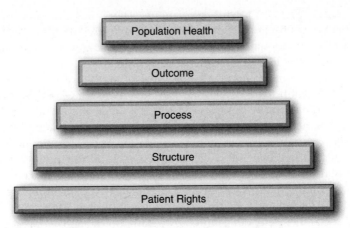

Figure 3–2.   The Quality Pyramid

level is population health. High-quality population health will be the final achievement of the U.S. health care system if it is to truly become the best in the world.

In the first three chapters of this book, we have introduced and discussed the fundamental principles of health policy: access, cost, and quality. An ideal system would provide excellent access to high-quality services at an affordable cost. For many middle- and upper-income Americans, the elderly, and certain segments of the poor, this statement is a reality today. For many socially disadvantaged Americans, that statement is not fulfilled. Future policymaking will, hopefully, maintain the characteristics of an ideal system and extend its reach to all Americans.

CHAPTER REVIEW QUESTIONS

1. Review and discuss the evidence pertaining to the quality of the U.S. health care system.
2. Define quality from the population-based and personal-based perspectives.
3. Define the legal foundation for quality in the health care system as it pertains to:
   a. provider regulation
   b. patient privacy
   c. medical negligence
4. What are the features of each component of Donabedian's model of health care quality?
   a. structure
   b. process
   c. outcome
5. How is each component of Donabedian's model of quality measured?
   a. structure
   b. process
   c. outcome

6. What is the purpose of accreditation?
7. Compare and contrast the organizations that conduct accreditation functions in the health care system.

CHAPTER DISCUSSION QUESTIONS

1. A concern about utilizing the population-based perspective in determining the quality of health care is that providers do not have the resources or responsibility to affect concerns outside the health care system. Do you agree with this position? Why or why not?

2. One reason cited for the high rate of medical error in the U.S. health care system is the risk to providers of legal suits due to medical negligence. This risk acts as a barrier to the reporting and analysis of medical error. What effect do you believe this situation may have on medical error? How would you reconcile the competing claims of providers who are fearful of repercussions for openly discussing their errors with the demands of some patients to recover, through the courts, for damages received at the hands of providers?

3. Report cards are one method for reducing the information barrier between provider and patient in making medical care decisions. From your perspective, what are the positives and negatives of report cards in relation to health care quality? Would you use one to make a health care purchasing decision? Under what circumstances? What would you like to know about the quality of your health care provider?

REFERENCES

Amato, A., E. Dobrzykowski, and T. Nance. 1997. The effect of timely onset of rehabilitation on outcomes of outpatient orthopedic practice. *J Rehabil Outcomes Meas* 1(3): 32–38.

American Occupational Therapy Association. 2007. Medicare Quality Measures for Occupational Therapy Coming Soon. http://www.aota.org/nonmembers/area1/links/link22.asp (accessed April 9, 2007).

American Physical Therapy Association. Introduction to OPTIMAL. http://www.apta.org/AM/Template.cfm?Section=Research&CONTENTID=36589&TEMPLATE=/CM/ContentDisplay.cfm (accessed February 1, 2007).

Annas, G. J. 1998. A national bill of patient rights. *New Engl J Med* 338(10): 695–99.

Bauman, L.F., E.F Silver, and R.E. Stein. 2006. Cumulative social disadvantage and child health. *Pediatrics* 117(4): 1321–28.

Bennett, S., K. McKenna, T. Hoffmann, L. Tooth, A. McCluskey, and J. Strong. 2007. The value of an evidence database for occupational therapists: An international online survey. *Int J Med Inform* 76(7): 507–13.

Braun, B.L., E.A. Kind, J.B. Fowles, and W.G. Suarez. 2002. Consumer response to a report card comparing healthcare systems. *Am J Manag Care* 8(6): 522–28.

Braveman, P. 2006. Health disparities and health equity: Concepts and measurement. *Ann Rev Public Health* 27: 167–194.

Bridges, P.H., L.L. Bierema, and T. Valentin. 2007. The propensity to adopt evidence-based practice among physical thrapists. *BMC Health Serv Res* 7: 103.

Brunner, H.I., J. Taylor, M.T. Britto, M.S. Corcoran, S.L. Kramer, P.G. Melson, U.R. Kotagal, T.B. Graham, and M.H. Passo. 2006. Differences in disease outcomes between Medicaid and privately insured children: Possible health disparities in juvenile rheumatoid arthritis. *Arthritis Rheum* 55(3): 378–84.

Casarett, D., and C. Helms. 1999. Systems errors vs. physicians' errors: Finding the balance in medical education. *Acad Med* 74(1): 19–22.

Centers for Disease Control and Prevention. 2005. Health disparities experienced by black and African Americans—United States. *MMWR Morb Mortal Wkly Rep.* 54(1): 1–3.

Commission on the Accreditation of Rehabilitation Facilities. 2008. http://www.carf.org/ (accessed May 20, 2008).

Dobrzykowski, E. 1997. The methodology of outcomes measurement. *J Rehabil Outcomes Meas* 1(1): 8–17.

_____ and T. Nance. 1997. The Focus on Therapeutic Outcomes (FOTO) outpatient orthopedic rehabilitation database: Results of 1994–1996. *J Rehabil Outcomes Meas* 1(1): 56–60.

Donabedian, A. 1966. Evaluating the quality of medical care. *Milbank Q* 44: 166–203.

_____. 1988. The quality of care: How can it be assessed? *JAMA* 260(12): 1743–48.

_____. 1990. The seven pillars of quality. *Arch Pathol Lab Med* 114(11): 1115–18.

Dysart, A.M., and G.S. Tomlin. 2002. Factors related to evidence-based practice among U.S. occupational therapy clinicians. *Am J Occup Ther* 56(3): 275–84.

Ellwood, P. 1988. Shattuck Lecture. Outcomes management: A technology of patient experience. *New Engl J Med* 318(23): 1549–56.

Epstein. A.J. 2006. Do cardiac surgery report cards reduce mortality? Assessing the evidence. *Med Care Res Rev* 63(4): 403–26.

Field, M. J., and K.N. Lohr, eds. *Guidelines for Clinical Practice: From Development to Use.* Washington DC: National Academy Press.

Focus on Therapeutic Outcomes, Inc. 2007. Outcomes Data Collection Options. http://www.fotoinc.com/products.htm (accessed February 7, 2007).

Guide for the Uniform Data Set for Medical Rehabilitation (including the F. I.M. instrument). 1997. Version 5.1, Buffalo NY: State University of New York at Buffalo.

Havercamp, S.M., D. Scandline, and M. Roth. 2004. Health disparities among adults with developmental disabilities, adults with other disabilities, and adults not reporting disability in North Carolina. *Public Health Rep* 119(4): 418–26.

Health Resources Services Administration. Health Professional Shortage Areas. http://hpsafind.hrsa.gov (accessed February 1, 2007).

Institute of Medicine. 1990. *Clinical practice guidelines: Directions for a new program.* Washington DC: National Academy Press.

Institute of Medicine. 1999. *To err is human: Building a safer health system.* Washington DC: National Academy Press.

Institute of Medicine. 2001. *Crossing the quality chasm: A new health system for the 21st century.* Washington DC: National Academy Press.

Joint Commission on the Accreditation of Healthcare Organizations. 2007. About Accreditation. http://www.jointcommission.org/GeneralPublic/About_Accreditation.htm (accessed February 1, 2007).

Krahn, G.L., L. Hammond, and A. Turner. 2006. A cascade of disparities: Health and health care access for people with intellectual disabilities. *Ment Retard Dev Disabil Res Rev* 12(1): 70–82.

Leape, L. L. 1997. A systems analysis approach to medical error. *J Eval Clin Pract* 3(3): 213–22.

Maher, G.C., C. Sherrington, M. Elkins, R.D. Herbert, and A.M. Moseley 2004. Challenges for evidence-based physical therapy: Accessing and interpreting high-quality evidence on therapy. *Phys Ther* 84(7): 644–54.

McCluskey, A., and M. Lovarini. 2005. Providing education on evidence-based practice improved knowledge but did not change behaviour: A before and after study. *BMC Med Educ* 5: 40.

Meenan, R.F., P.M. Gertman, and J.H. Mason. 1980. Measuring health status in arthritis. The arthritis impact measurement scales. *Arthritis Rheum* 23(2): 146–52.

Michaud, C.M., C.J. Murray, and B.R. Bloom. 2001. Burden of disease-implications for future research. *JAMA* 285(5): 535–39.

Mu, K., H. Lohman, and L. Scheirton. 2006. Occupational therapy practice errors in physical rehabilitation and geriatric settings. A national survey study. *Am J Occup Ther* 60(3): 288– 97.

National Board for Certification in Occupational Therapy. About Us. http://www.nbcot.org/webarticles/anmviewer.asp?a=45&z=12 (accessed February 1, 2007).

National Center for Minority Health and Health Disparities. Annual Report on Health Disparities Research – Fiscal Year 2001. http://ncmhd.nih.gov/our_programs/strategic/AnnRptHealthDisp.asp (accessed February 1, 2007).

National Committee for Quality Assurance. About NCQA. http://www.ncqa.org/about/about.htm (accessed February 1, 2007).

Nosek, M.A., R.B. Hughes, N.J. Petersen, H.B. Taylor, S. Robinson-Whelen, M. Byrne, and R. Morgan. 2006. Secondary conditions in a community-based sample of women with physical disabilities over a 1-year period. *Arch Phys Med Rehabil* 87(3): 320–27.

Oliver, M.N., and C. Muntaner. 2005. Researching health inequities among African Americans: The imperative to understand social class. *Int J Health Serv* 35(3): 485–98.

Pear, R. 2006. Medicare in a different tack links doctors' pay to practices. *New York Times*, December 12, A1, A18.

Rothschild, J. M., D. W. Bates, and L. L. Leape. 2000. Preventable medical injuries in older patients. *Arch Intern Med* 160(18): 2717–28.

Sackett, D.L., S.E. Strauss, and W.S. Richardson. 2000. *Evidence Based Medicine: How to Practice and Teach EBM* 2nd edition. Edinburgh Scotland, Churchill Livingstone.

Sandstrom, R. 2007. Characteristics of medical malpractice by physical therapists: Results of the National Practitioner Data Bank, 1991–2004. *J Allied Health* 36(4): 193–200.

Schultz, J., K. Thiede-Call, R. Feldman, and J. Christianson. 2001. Do employees use report cards to assess health care provider systems? *Health Serv Res* 36(3): 509–30.

Scott, R.W. 1991. The legal standard of care. *Clin Management* 11(2): 10–11.

Siminoff, L.A., and L. Ross. 2005. Access and equity to cancer care in the USA: A review and assessment. *Postgrad Med J* 81(961): 674–79.

Thomas, E.J., and T.A. Brennan. 2000. Incidence and types of preventable adverse events in elderly patients: Population-based review of medical records. *BMJ* 320(7237): 741–44.

United States Department of Health and Human Services. Office for Civil Rights. Medical privacy: National standards to protect the privacy of personal health information. http://www.hhs.gov/ocr/hipaa/finalreg.html (accessed January 6, 2003).

Ware, J. E., and C. D. Sherbourne. 1992. The MOS 36-item short-form health survey (SF-36) I. Conceptual framework and item selection. *Med Care* 30(6): 473–83.

Werner, R.M., and D.A. Asch. 2005. The unintended consequences of publicly reporting quality information. *JAMA* 293(10): 1239–1244.

Wicks, E.K., and J.A. Meyer. 1999. Making report cards work. *Health Affairs* 18(2): 152–55.

4

Public Policies Addressing
Social Disablement

CHAPTER OBJECTIVES

At the conclusion of this chapter, the reader will be able to:

1. Discuss different societal perspectives about disabilities.
2. Describe the focus of key public policies for people with disabilities.
3. Explain how therapists can access each of the public policies about disabilities.
4. Apply concepts in this chapter to a case study or active learning exercise.

KEY WORDS: Assistive Technology, Barriers, Empowerment, Inclusion, Independent Living, Related Services, Vocational Rehabilitation, Office on Aging

ABBREVIATIONS FOR PUBLIC POLICIES DISCUSSED IN THIS CHAPTER:

ADA: Americans with Disablities Act

ATA: Assistive Technology Act

DDA: Developmental Disabilities Act

FHA: Fair Housing Act

IDEA: Individuals with Disabilities Education Act

OAA: Older American Act

SSA: Social Security Act

WIA: Workforce Investment Act

RA: Rehabilitation Act

Case Example

Richard is a pleasant, outgoing 12-year-old boy with mild cerebral palsy. He has normal intelligence but has some motor deficits. Because of the Individuals with Disabilities Act (IDEA), Richard has benefited from additional services provided by the school system. When Richard entered school in kindergarten, he was placed in a special classroom with five other children, but by third grade he was mainstreamed into a regular classroom. Over the years, Richard has received services from both occupational and physical therapists. Richard would not have been able to be mainstreamed into the regular classroom setting without the help of the therapists. Richard has benefited immensely from the IDEA. If he had been born prior to the enactment of the law, he likely would not have even attended school. Yet Richard has needs beyond the classroom environment that are not addressed by the IDEA. He needs a better wheelchair and other low-tech assistive technology to assist him with doing his activities of daily living (ADL) at home. Richard also would benefit from receiving training and computer software to assist him with using his computer at home. His family has minimal financial resources, as his father is currently unemployed.

Richard's astute therapists recognize that many of his needs can be helped by public policy and other community resources beyond the IDEA, so they do their research. In his state, Richard can receive a new electric wheelchair funded by Medicaid. His low-tech ADL needs can be provided by a community-based church lending service. His computer software training can be provided by the State Assistive Technology Project. People from Richard's State Assistive Technology Project are even able to assess his home and school for suggested modifications. They can offer Richard's family the opportunity to buy adaptive equipment, including the computer software, at a discounted cost. So, because of all these resources from various public policies and the help of his therapists, Richard is able to have an optimal quality of life.

Case Example Focus Question:

1. What effect does the Individuals with Disabilities Education Act and the Assistive Technology Act have on Richard's experience of disablement?

INTRODUCTION

In Chapter 1, we introduced the social disability model as an important paradigm with which to understand disablement. The social disability model defines disablement as a sociopolitical experience that is created as the result of the marginalization of people with disabling conditions by the policies, social structures, and attitudes of the nondisabled population. The source of the disablement experience is not in the individual, but rather in the community. In this chapter, we will focus on public policies that have been developed to address the isolation of, and discrimination against, people with disabling conditions—people like Richard in the case study.

U.S. citizens have historically held different perspectives about people with disabilities. For example, at the beginning of the 20th century it was considered humane to place people with disabilities in institutions to be protected from society. Our current perspective is to encourage people with disabilities to be included in societal, school, work, and living activities. In current terminology, this philosophy is called **inclusion**, integration, or mainstreaming. It is written into many policies and approaches. For example, the American Physical Therapy Association House of

Delegates position on Americans with disabilities states, "People with disabilities share the same rights as all other individuals to have access to and opportunities for full economic, social and personal development. The American Physical Therapy Association (APTA) shall advocate for full inclusion for people with disabilities in all aspects of community life and within the profession of physical therapy" (APTA 2007, 11). The American Occupational Therapy Association (AOTA) has developed several position papers related to disability and inclusion (AOTA 1992a; AOTA 1993b; AOTA 1993b; AOTA 1995; AOTA 2000; Hansen and Hinojosa 2004).

Thoughtful readers may question the different perspectives about disabilities that have been adapted from the beginning of the 20th century until now. However, societal perspectives are never right or wrong; rather, they reflect the beliefs and knowledge of what people thought was the best approach at the time. For example, in the United States a paradigm shift about disabilities occurred between 1968 and 1988. Several factors contributed to this different perspective. People with disabilities were living longer. There was more community exposure to people with disabilities. Disability organizations that advocated for the rights of people with disabilities emerged. In addition, a disability rights movement and an independent-living philosophy were strong contributing factors. The disability movement considered the civil rights of the "minority" group of people with disabilities (Bristo 1996). The independent-living philosophy was based on self-rule and self-help, and political and economic rights (Bristo 1996). Therefore, a paradigm shift occurred, from viewing people with disabilities solely from a medical perspective to an inclusion model. With the medical model, people with disabilities were perceived as "sick" or "impaired" and needing a cure. The newer perspectives incorporated people with disabilities into a community-based model emphasizing inclusion. Thus, disability began to be seen as a larger societal problem requiring societal intervention, and this perspective is reflected in many of the recent disability laws, including the Americans with Disabilities Act (ADA) (Bristo 1997). Table 4–1 ■ describes the paradigm switch from a medical model perspective to the current perspective.

The perspectives of a society about important issues like disability are supported by policy, for public policy is the codification of the shared values of a society (McClain 1996), and policies develop when society does not deal appropriately with a perceived issue. Policies about disabilities can also be viewed as regulatory and allocative tools mandated by the government (McGregor 2001). Therefore, it is relevant for therapists to become aware of the different policies about disabilities, how they are regulated and allocated, and the values influencing them. Therapists commonly work with some, but not all, of society's health care–related policies. For example, therapists working in school systems provide services to children through the Individuals with Disabilities Education Act (IDEA). IDEA supports the education of children and youths with disabilities. However, therapists may not be as familiar with the Developmental Disabilities Act (DDA) or the Rehabilitation Act (RA). Yet these acts offer services that help similar clients, and therapists can educate both people with disabilities and their caregivers about the benefits of these bills.

The public policies presented in this chapter will be divided into three main sections based on the people they serve and the societal values they represent. In

Table 4–1.   Contrast of Paradigms

	Old Paradigms	*New Paradigms*
Definition of disability	The individual is limited by his/her impairment or condition	The individual with an impairment requires an accommodation to perform functions required to carry out life activities
Strategy to address disability	Fix the individual, correct the deficit	Remove barriers, create access through accommodation and universal design, promote wellness and health
Method of addressing disability	Provision of medical, vocational, or psychological rehabilitation services	Provision of supports (e.g., assistive technology, personal assistance services, job coach)
Source of intervention	Professionals, clinicians, and other rehabilitation service providers	Peers, mainstream service providers, consumer information services
Entitlements	Eligibility for benefits based on severity of impairment	Eligibility for accommodations seen as a civil right
Role of disabled individual	Object of intervention, patient, beneficiary, research subject	Consumer or customer, empowered peer, research participant, decision-maker
Domain of disability	A medical "problem"	A socioenvironmental issue involving accessibility, accommodations, and equity

Adapted by Betty Jo Berland from materials prepared for the NIDDR's Long-Range Plan by Gerben DeJong and Bonnie O'Day and reprinted with permission from NIDRR, Washington DC (NIDDR 2000).

the first section, policies representing two specific age groups—youths and older adults in our society—are presented and discussed. The second section represents civil rights policies that focus on people who work and live in our society, and includes an examination of the Americans with Disabilities Act and federal income replacement or supplementation programs through the Social Security Administration. The third section represents a policy related to technology, which helps people of all ages with disabilities, and a policy that helps people with disabilities obtain fair housing. We will consider the following public policy acts: the ADA, the **Assistive Technology** Act (AT), Developmental Disabilities Act (DDA), Fair Housing Act (FHA), Individuals with Disabilities Act (IDEA), Older American Act (OAA), Social Security (SS), and Work Investment Act (WIA). The premise behind these policies correlates well with the therapy profession's belief in the value and dignity of people with disabilities and the recognition of a need for a quality of life. Table 4–2 ■ overviews the prime focus of each of these laws. The chapter presents the main considerations about each and how the laws are relevant to helping therapy clients.

Table 4–2.   Focus of Disability Policies

Disability Policy	Focus
Americans with Disabilities Act (ADA)	A major civil rights act that provides protection not only in employment, but in transportation and public accommodations, in telecommunications, and with state and local governments, for people with disabilities. Expanded coverage to areas not previously covered by other federal disability acts.
Assistive Technology Act (ATA)	Supports state programs for public-awareness programming to increase access to technology.
Developmental Disability Act (DDA)	Services those with mental retardation and other developmental disabilities. Provides protection and advocacy. Promotes "independence, productivity, integration and inclusion into the community."
Fair Housing Act	The Federal act that prohibits housing discrimination, includes discrimination against people with disabilities.
Older Americans Act	A Federal, state, tribal, and local collaboration for "organizing, coordinating and providing community-based services and opportunities for older Americans and their families" (AOA, n.d. β2).
Workforce Investment Act (WIA)/ Rehabilitation Act (RA)	Helps people with disabilities maximize their employment abilities and independent living abilities, and supports inclusion in society.

Administration on Aging (AOA) (n.d.). Fact Sheets: Older Americans Act. Retrieved on October 28, 2007 from http://www.aoa.gov/press/fact/alpha/fact_oaa.asp. L. F. Rothstein, *Disability and the Law* (1992); K. Jacobs, Work assessments and programming (1996).

PUBLIC POLICIES SUPPORTING YOUTHS AND OLDER ADULTS

Public policy supports the societal value of helping the future of our youths and children. Historically, Americans have also valued helping older adults with many public policies. In this section, we will discuss the Individuals with Disabilities Education Act, the Developmental Disabilities Act, and the Older Americans Act.

The Individuals with Disabilities Education Act (IDEA)

IDEA is rooted in earlier legislation enacted in 1975 called the Education for Handicapped Act (EHA), or P.L. 99-142 (NICHCY 2000). This legislation resulted from the strong advocacy efforts of groups, such as the National Association for Retarded Citizens (The Arc), interested in children with disabilities receiving better educational opportunities. Prior to EHA, many children with disabilities did not get an education, and families had to find their own means for educational services (Bristo 1996; Mellard 2000). IDEA and its predecessor, EHA, are considered to be landmark legislative acts that have helped the integration of disabled youths into American society (Bristo 1997; Mellard 2000). IDEA supports special education in the **least-restrictive environment** (LRE) for children and youths, from birth though age 21. IDEA enables children with disabilities to receive **a free and appropriate public education (FAPE)** (NICHCY 2000).

Approximately every five years, IDEA gets amended. The purpose of amending this or any law is to focus on achieving the original goals of the act and to make sure that the bill reflects current issues. The current IDEA has four parts, with therapy defined as a **related service** in Part B (Assistance to States for Education of All Children with Disabilities). Part B addresses special education and related services for preschool through school-age children who have disabilities. Under Part B, guidelines are discussed for an individualized education program (IEP). The IEP, which is completed by a team, is essentially the individual student's plan for meeting identified goals. Examples of other regulations addressed in Part B are free and appropriate public education, nonacademic services, hearing aid checks, methods of ensuring services, and personnel qualifications. With the 2004 revisions, clarifications that influence the provision of therapy were made in many of these areas (AOTA 2006, September 27).

Occupational therapy and physical therapy are defined as a primary service in Part C, the section that addresses primarily children, from birth though 36 months, with disabilities and their families. Under Part C, an Individualized Family Service Plan (IFSP) is developed. This plan, which identifies the services that a child will receive, is done in conjunction with the child's parent(s). It is important to note that, while Part C addresses the needs of young children, Part B's changes include early intervening services for children in kindergarten through 12th grade enrolled in regular classrooms who need additional support. With the 2004 revisions, related services can be included to assist students receiving early intervening services with education (AOTA 2006). The AOTA website has more specific information about other changes in Part B and Part C that affect therapy (www.aota.org).

Amendments involve the political process and compromises between the political parties within the Senate and Congress. Several bills have been introduced to provide full funding for the IDEA (e.g., the Full Funding for IDEA Now Act H.R.526.IH), but to date, these bills have not passed. Regulations implement the policies set forth in the law. With the 2004 amended IDEA, regulations focused on aligning the bill with the No Child Left Behind Law (NCLB, P.L. 107-10; AOTA n.d). It is not unusual for related bills to have similar language or to align together on the basis of the political climate and attitudes of the time. Anytime a major bill is amended, coalitions lobby for issues that are important to their members. Examples of coalitions involved with IDEA are the National Education Association, the American Association of School Administrators, and professional organizations such as American Occupational Therapy Association and the American Physical Therapy Association.

The current IDEA has accomplished many of its original goals. Most children with disabilities are now educated in their neighborhood schools and are mainstreamed into regular classrooms. Most children are enrolled in postsecondary education, and there has been an improvement in high school graduation rates and employment rates (U.S. Department of Education 2005).

IDEA and Therapy

IDEA supports services for children with mental retardation, hearing impairments (including deafness), speech or language impairments, visual impairments (including blindness), serious emotional disturbances, orthopedic impairments, autism, traumatic brain injury, other health impairments, or specific learning disabilities (P.L. 108-446, Section 602 3A i). The 2004 amendment's changes included adding homeless children with disabilities who are wards of the state (P.L. 108-446, Section 612, 3; 634, 1).

Under IDEA, Part B, therapists provide related services. Related services are interventions needed to help children benefit from their programs of special education. Therefore, therapy is not perceived as, nor should it be, a medically based intervention. Thus, therapists trained in traditional medical settings will need to adapt to a different therapy focus. Physical and occupational therapy services can follow children as long as the Individualized Education Program (IEP) process determines a need for intervention.

All children followed by this law receive an IEP. With the 2004 amendments to the IDEA law, short-term objectives are no longer mandated to meet the child's annual IEP goal and are required only for a very small percentage of children who have the most significant cognitive disabilities. However, parents can still request that their child's IEP include short-term objectives. Progress in meeting the child's annual goals is still documented, and there is periodical reporting of progress in meeting the annual IEP goals (AFB, n.d.; FAPE 2004). Therapists and others, including parents, participate in the IEP process, which is therefore based on collaborative planning designed to integrate parent and school personnel (Muhlenhaupt 2000). With the 2004 changes, some IEP team members can be excused, with parent and school district permission, from attending an IEP meeting if their area of expertise is not discussed (AFB n.d.; FAPE 2004). There are very clear guidelines that therapists must follow to address the required areas of an IEP. However, again the focus for therapy services is that the student needs services related to occupational therapy or physical therapy.

As mentioned earlier, therapists also follow young children from birth through 36 months and support their families as a primary service under Part C of IDEA. These young children are treated in their natural context or their typical environment, which can be the home, day care, or even a playground (Opp 2007, July 25). Thus, the setting for therapy need not be the school system, as it is in Part B. Like

Part B, Part C has a plan of care, which is called the Individualized Family Service Plan (IFSP). Parents guide the priorities of this plan. State regulations determine whether the family needs to co-pay for services or whether there can be a health insurance subsidy (Opp 2007, July 25).

Therapists need to keep abreast of legislative changes related to IDEA and how they affect therapy. They need to learn how IDEA is regulated in their state and in their school system. They need to take a proactive stance before and when the act is reauthorized, especially since so much of school-based practice is defined and largely funded by this act. Table I in the appendix provides a concise history of IDEA. In Chapter 11, we will further describe the system created by this law: special education.

The Developmental Disabilities Act (DDA)

In the United States, there has been a long history of people with developmental disabilities (mental retardation) not getting adequate services. However, it was only in the 1960s, during President Kennedy's administration, that treatment of people with mental retardation became a high-priority societal concern. This concern corresponded with an overall societal interest in civil rights. During this period, the societal view of mental retardation changed from its being congenitally caused to a view in which it was seen as resulting from a societal problem related to poverty, prenatal care, and other social influences (Hightower-Vandamm 1979).

The legislative roots of the modern-day Developmental Disabilities Act were established in 1963 with two federal laws: P.L. 88-156 was aimed at helping higher-risk mothers, and P.L. 88-164 provided federal funds for building facilities for people with mental retardation (Hightower-Vandamm 1979). Although these legislative acts were important beginnings, they were very limited in their scope of coverage, as they addressed the physical institutions and not programming. Furthermore, the two laws covered only people with mental retardation and disregarded those with other developmental disabilities. Therefore, by 1970, a new law, P.L. 91-517, expanded the definitions for conditions covered by the law and began to focus on community-based coverage. The focus on community-based care reflects the societal value of integration and deinstitutionalization of persons with mental disabilities. P.L. 91-517 provided the foundation for some parts of today's modern law, such as establishing a state-designated agency responsible for planning programs. However, the act still limited coverage to the disabilities of cerebral palsy, epilepsy, and mental retardation (Hightower-Vandamm 1979). Although it mentioned "other neurological conditions," the act did not clearly define them for adequate coverage. It was not until the current law was enacted in 1975 and amended several times afterwards that the definitions for disabilities were expanded. Under the modern law, the term "mental retardation" was replaced with "developmental disabilities." It is important to mention that in 1975 the climate was right for enactment of the current law, as other federal acts helping people with disabilities were being enacted at the same time. These other public policies included the RA and the EHA. The 1960s and 1970s were an important and creative period for the disability rights movement.

The intent of the DDA was to promote independent living, productivity, and community integration, as well as to provide protection and advocacy for persons with developmental disabilities (Graney 2000; Rothstein 1992). Since 1975, there have been a number of reauthorizations, and behind each of them is the advocacy of coalitions to help people with various conditions. For example, the Arc, a group strongly associated with the DDA, has advocated for better conditions for people with developmental disabilities in institutional and educational environments (National Council on Disabilities 1997). (See Appendix Table II for a concise history of policies related to the DDA.)

The current Developmental Disabilities Act, authorized between 2000 and 2007, is divided into several titles. Title I has four parts, which include (1) state councils on developmental disabilities, (2) protection and advocacy systems, (3) university-affiliated programs, and (4) projects of national significance. States have some discretion under the law to design their own systems for the councils, protection and advocacy agencies, and university-affiliated programs. As a result, these programs have different forms in the various states (Gordon 2000). The state councils help advocate for people with developmental disabilities (Graney 2000). State councils have four purposes: consumer **empowerment**, systems change, obtaining resources for people with developmental disabilities and their family members, and promoting community inclusion (NADDC 2000). The protection and advocacy agencies mediate and handle legal situations for people with developmental disabilities. The university-affiliated programs provide interdisciplinary education and training for professionals, conduct applied research, and provide training and technological assistance for people with disabilities, their families, and others. The projects of national significance involve research, evaluation, and demonstration projects (Graney 2000).

Title II of the DDA provides support to families with children who have disabilities. Examples of family support are respite care and subsidies to families (Title II, section 202). Title III is a limited scholarship program for staff assisting individuals with developmental disabilities.

The DDA and Therapy

In 2005, there were approixmately 4.5 million individuals with developmental disabilities in the United States (U.S. Department of Health and Human Services n.d.). Many of these people can benefit from public policies, such as the DDA. The intent of the DDA was to manage the arrangement of services and advocacy efforts on behalf of those with developmental disabilities and not to provide direct services (Graney 2000). Therefore, most therapists are not directly involved with the act, and it does not reimburse therapy services. The DDA has much the same philosophical intent as therapy services, namely, helping people achieve maximal independence and potential (Gordon 2000). Nevertheless, over the years, the American Occupational Therapy Association has taken an active role in lobbying for the different amendments (Boyd et al. 1996). Therapists working in university-affiliated programs are directly affected by the DDA.

The Older Americans Act (OAA)

The Older Americans Act (OAA) was enacted originally in 1965, along with other programs that support older Americans, such as Medicare and Medicaid. (Medicare and Medicaid are discussed in Chapters 7 and 8; for a history of this law, go to Table III of the Appendix.) The purpose of the OAA, a federal, state, tribal, and local collaboration (AOA 2006), is to enhance the quality of life for older Americans. This is reflected by its 10 broad objectives, outlined in Title I (Takamura 2001) and summarized in Table 4–3 ■. The OAA created many benefits for older Americans, including the Administration on Aging, state grants for programs and services, and research and training (AOA n.d.). The current OAA includes a national aging services network of "56 state units on aging, 655 area agencies on aging, 243 tribal organizations, 29,000 community-based organizations, and over 500,000 volunteers" (AOA 2006, March 9). These different divisions oversee programs for older adults. State programs funded by the OAA provide a variety of services for older adults, including housing, nutrition, health, employment, retirement, health promotion, protection, and advocacy services, as well as other social and community services (AOA n.d). Therapists should consider referring patients/residents that they work with to their local office on aging, to state units, or to one of the tribal organizations for many beneficial services. (See Table III in the Appendix for a concise history of this act.) Therapists often observe the positive impact of the act on the patients they serve. For example, in home health environments, some of the patients that they follow may be receiving "Meals on Wheels." Some therapists have received grants from their OAA for programming (T. Nanof, Personal communication, November 6, 2007).

Table 4–3. Summary of the Objectives of the Older Americans Act

- Adequate income for older adults in retirement
- The best mental and physical health for all older adults
- Suitable housing considering special needs and costs
- Full restorative services for long-term care and a variety of community-based services to support older adults
- Nondiscriminatory employment
- "Retirement in health, honor, and dignity"(p. 2)
- Participation in meaningful activities
- Adequate community services and resources
- Benefits from research
- "Freedom, independence, and the free exercise of individual initiative in planning and managing their own lives"(p. 2)

Adapted from The Center for Social Gerontology, Unofficial compilation –by Title. http://www.tcsg.org/law/2006OAATitleI.pdf (accessed October 27, 2007).

Active Learning Exercise

As you read descriptions about the Developmental Disabilities Act and the Older Americans Act, think critically of ways that you could use these laws to help patients/clients. In addition, go to your state's website to research local services, such as your area Office on Aging.

WORK-RELATED POLICY ACTS

Case Example

Maria: A therapist who worked in a program financed by her state vocational rehabilitation program

> *Maria was trained to work as an occupational therapist in traditional practice. Her first position was at an acute care hospital, where she specialized with orthopedic patients. Maria enjoyed the position, but felt that she wanted to do more with her skills, talents, and interests. Her dream was to reach out to Hispanic people who had work injuries. Therefore, she started researching opportunities and found that therapists can become case managers and that some therapists are involved in work programs. Maria found another therapist to be a mentor and then assumed a position as a case manager helping Hispanic people who had been injured on the job at a work-training program financed by the state's vocational rehabilitation program.*

Maintaining or promoting the ability of people to work is a strong value associated with self-worth, status (Baker and Jacobs 2003), and a sense of productivity that has consistently been part of American society. People with disabilities want to be productive working members of our society (National Council on Disabilities 2004) (see Chapter 1). Presidential initiatives, such as the New Freedom Initiative, and tax incentives to remove architectural barriers for businesses that employ people with disabilities encourage these values (National Council on Disabilities 2004). Therefore, it is not surprising that a large number of public policies are related to maintaining the abilities to work or to encouraging people with disabilities to work. Examples of these public policies are the Workforce Investment Act (Rehabilitation Act), the Americans with Disabilities Act, and the Work Incentive Improvement Act of 1999. This section overviews these public policies. We will also discuss the Social Security programs that provide vital income support for persons with disabilities who cannot work.

The Workforce Investment Act (WIA) (Rehabilitation Act, [RA])

The current Workforce Investment Act, previously known as the Rehabilitation Act, has a long history based on the strong American value of promoting productive work among members of our society. (A history of these laws since 1970 is summa-rized in Tables IV and V of the Appendix.) Public policy, even at the beginning of the 20th century, was related to this value. Both the Workers' Compensation law and the Rehabilitation Act (RA) have roots at the beginning of the 20th century (see Chapter 6 for more about workers' compensation). Modern disability policies can be traced to the 1970s. Therapists, however, may not be as familiar with the WIA, which also helps clients with work-related concerns and promotes the civil rights of people with disabilities.

Parts of the Rehabilitation Act became a foundation for the subsequent Amer-icans with Disabilities Act. Section 501 established "a federal interagency committee on employees who are individuals with disabilities" (Tucker 1994, 48). A key part of section 501 is the requirement that federal agencies have an affirmative action plan for the employment of people with disabilities. Section 503 requires nondiscrimina-tion on the basis of disability and puts an affirmative action plan in place for federal agencies that contract for $10,000 or more. Section 504 prohibits discrimination in employment, education, architectural accessibility, and health, welfare, and social services for recipients of federal financial assistance (Tucker 1994). Section 504 was landmark legislation, for it was the first civil rights declaration for people with dis-abilities (Bristo 1997; Tucker 1994). For the "first time in federal legislation discrim-ination was defined as the failure to provide a reasonable accommodation to a qualified person with a disability" (L.M. Conyers, 2002 as cited by Conyers and Ahrens, 2003, 59). With the elevation of this law to a civil rights act, people with dis-abilities were allowed a legal means of advocating for their rights. Because of the controversies over this regulation, people in the disabilities movement attained in-creased public visibility (Bristo 1997).

The Workforce Investment Act and Therapy

The Workforce Investment Act helps people with disabilities by providing many beneficial services. Section 103 of the act (Workforce Investment Act of 1998, 105-220, § 404) lists many services, including, but not limited to, training programs and centers, vocational rehabilitation services, prosthetic and orthotic services, di-agnosis and treatment for mental and emotional disorders, and transportation services. Section 103 also mentions visual services and reading services for people who are blind and interpreter services for people who are deaf. In addition, Sec-tion 103 lists technical and consultation assistance for individuals seeking self-em-ployment, establishing a small business, or needing assistance on the job. This act also provides consultative and technical assistance to educational programs to help students with disabilities make the transition to postschool activities and employ-ment (see Section 103 of the act for a full listing of the available services covered).

Neither physical therapy nor occupational therapy has been strongly involved with the modern act. However, therapy can become involved in helping people im-prove their functioning and become more independent with self-care in order to engage in employment (Dunn 2000). Vocational rehabilitation specialists work primarily with people who have disabilities and need these services. The 1998 amendments more clearly defined the Rehabilitation Act as an employment program, which results in even less involvement from therapists. The amendments specify that therapy can become involved only if therapy services cannot be funded by another source (Dunn 2000). Thus, if Medicaid (see Chapter 9) covers rehabilitation services for a person, the RA would not reimburse for rehabilitation. In addition, the Rehabilitation Act is a state–federal program, with states responsible for the delivery of services according to a state plan, and state agency programs vary widely in focus (Dunn 2000). Therapists wishing to provide services funded by this law will need to be familiar with community-based models vs. medical-based models and should communicate with their state agencies.

Work Incentives Improvement Act of 1999 (P.L. 106-170) and Ticket to Work and Self-Sufficiency Program

The Work Incentives Improvement Act of 1999 (P.L. 106-170) provides another opportunity for therapists to work with disabled persons to facilitate their return to work. This act includes a voluntary nationwide program (TTW and Self-Sufficiency Program) to "increase opportunities for SSA disability beneficiaries aged 18 to 65 to obtain employment, vocational rehabilitation, and support services, ultimately to replace their SSA benefits with benefits from work" (National Council on Disabilities 2004, 86). The Work Incentives Improvement Act of 1999 helps clients eliminate some of the *disincentives* to finding work, such as losing federal subsidized health insurance of Medicaid and Medicare, with the *incentive* of continual coverage at work. It also provides exceptions for further review of disability (National Council on Disabilities 2004).

The Future of Work-Related Public Policies

It is obvious that progress has been made through public policies to meet the need for people with disabilities to work and be engaged in society. Yet there continues to be room for improvement. According to a report from the U.S. Census Bureau, approximately 11.8 million adults, or 6 percent of the population, have a medical condition that "makes it difficult to find a job or remain employed" (U.S. Census Bureau 2006, 1). Overall, people with disabilities have lower employment rates than the nondisabled American population (56 percent of adults with disabilities are employed, versus 88 percent of the nondisabled population). People who have more severe disabilities experience even lower employment rates (43 percent) (U.S. Census Bureau 2006). Some ideas suggested by the National Council on Disabilities (2004) to help more people with disabilities obtain employment are for increased usage of technology, increased awareness from employers about disabilities, and hiring people with disabilities within governmental agencies. Other suggestions are for providing more funding and removing barriers to finding work, such as the loss of health insurance, for people with disabilities.

The Americans with Disabilities Act (ADA)

The most broadly reforming civil rights act, helping disabled people of all ages, is the Americans with Disabilities Act (ADA) of 1990. The ADA is a federal antidiscrimination law guaranteeing equal opportunity, and not just equal treatment, for those with disabilities (Wells 2000). Previous acts, such as the Civil Rights Act of 1964, the RA, and the EHA, established the climate for the development of the ADA (Bristo 1997; Wells 2000). The Civil Rights Act of 1964 was the first federal act to consider discrimination in public places and tie the promise of nondiscrimination to the receipt of federal funds (Wells 2000). The ADA expanded some of the premises of the RA, especially section 504 (Rothstein 1992). The perspective of inclusion under the EHA helped influence public opinion about the ADA (Bristo 1997).

The Americans with Disabilities Act was revolutionary in many ways. One was its use of language. The act changed the verbiage of public policy from "handicapped" people to people "who have disabilities" (Rothstein 1992). This "people first" language reflected a change in societal values toward empowerment and respect for people with disabilities. Another unique aspect was the focus on the abilities and aptitudes of people with disabilities, with an emphasis on societal inclusion (Bowman 1992). Thus, the ADA considered work, along with other related societal areas, as a way to help keep people with disabilities working and included in the larger fabric of society. For example, the act dealt with the dilemma of people who might be able to work at a job but not successfully access the transportation system to get there or not be able to get to the actual jobsite in a facility. The act made public areas accessible even for disabled persons who were not working. Therefore, the inclusion of public transportation and architectural accessibility in the ADA reflects the law's broad perspective. As stated, a primary purpose of the ADA is to help people with disabilities be employed and have the same advantages as others who are not disabled (Goren 1999). To qualify as having a disability, the person must "[have a] physical or mental impairment that substantially limits one or more major life activities, [have] a history or record of such an impairment, or [be] perceived by others as having such an impairment" (*www.pueblo.gsa* 2000).

The ADA has four titles. Title I deals with employment and requires employers who have 15 or more employees to provide equal employment opportunities to qualified individuals with disabilities. This title also mentions protection against discrimination in hiring, promotion, and pay. It provides restrictions on questions about disabilities before the job is offered. In addition, Title I requires that employers make "reasonable accommodations" to allow the person to work, unless there is "undue hardship." Title II covers state and local governments. It requires that people with disabilities be provided with equal opportunity to benefit from such services as public education, employment, transportation, health care, social services, courts, voting, and town meetings. Title II also requires that governments follow architectural standards in the construction and renovation of buildings. In addition, Title II requires reasonable modification of policies and procedures to avoid discrimination against those who have disabilities. Another part of Title II is the provision of coverage for public transportation so that there is no discrimination against people with disabilities in using the services. Title III covers public accommodations—businesses such as retail stores, hotels, and restaurants. Public accommodations must comply with standards and requirements in terms of architecture and access. Title IV covers telephone accessibility for people with hearing and speech disabilities. It requires telephone companies to enable people with hearing and speech disabilities to use special adaptive phones, such as telecommunications devices for the deaf (TDDs) (AOTA 1993b; *www.pueblo.gsa* 2000).

Massive public policy like the ADA does not solve all of society's problems, but does provide a framework for improvement. Still, in spite of improvement in many areas of life for people with disabilities, issues remain that are related to the ADA. Examples of workplace issues are the exclusion of people with disabilities from the social life on the job, the existence of interpersonal problems in the workplace, and stereotyping people with disabilities (Gupta 2006). People who have severe mental health conditions experience discrimination in the workplace because of having the two labels of a mental illness and a disability (Conyers and Ahrens 2003). However, people with disabilities who experience discrimination can voice their concerns through the Equal Employment Opportunity Commission (EEOC), which implements the parts of the ADA dealing with employment discrimination (The U.S. Equal Employment Opportunity Commission n.d; Gupta 2006). In many communities, cost issues exist related to the adjustment of the physical environments for accessibility. Finding reliable, reasonable, and accessible transportation is still a problem in some communities (National Council on Disabilities 2004).

Therapy and the ADA

With the emphasis on maximizing functioning in ADL and performance skills, an awareness of activity demands and client factors, and a thorough consideration of all aspects of a person's contextual environment, therapists can help people with disabilities who are affected by the ADA (AOTA 2000). In different ways, the Americans with Disabilities Act has an impact on therapists and involves therapy with the law (AOTA 2000). From a manager's perspective, the ADA influences hiring decisions. Direct questions concerning a disability cannot be asked of a person during an interview. The manager should be interested in whether the qualified person can perform the "essential functions" of a job in the therapy department. As discussed, the ADA requires employers to make "reasonable accommodations" to allow the qualified person to work, as long as these accommodations do not entail "undue hardship." Therefore, managers of therapy departments may be involved in the process of implementing reasonable accommodations.

A unique way for therapists to get involved with the ADA is as consultants (Hanebrink and Parent-Brown 2000; Fontana 1999). Therapists have the skills to be ADA consultants. However, it is important that therapists have a strong knowledge base about the law in order to implement it in practice. It is helpful to review the law, attend training seminars, network with ADA advocacy organizations, and read relevant newsletters (Fontana 1999). Hanebrink and Parent-Brown (2000) also suggest that therapists can increase their knowledge base by participating on local private and government committees for people with disabilities and by attending continuing education courses. Simply networking with people involved in implementing the act may be very beneficial.

With a knowledge base about the ADA, therapists can consult about legislation and architectural codes, assist local government agencies, and provide suggestions for reasonable accommodations (AOTA 2000). Consulting with human resource departments may involve doing jobsite analysis and writing job descriptions (Wells 2000). Jobsite analyses and job descriptions describe the important job functions and help to identify reasonable accommodations (Grupa, Gelpi, and Sain 2005). In addition, through performing work assessments, therapists can address ergonomic adaptations (Stockdell and Crawford 1992) and adaptive equipment needs so that the person can work in a safe environment (Gupta 2006). Perhaps therapists can provide expert-witness testimony (Hanebrink and Parent-Brown 2000) as well. Therapists may also choose to conduct research for intervention strategies and related programs (Bowman 1992). Suggested avenues of consultation include government agencies, public transportation and communication bodies, businesses, and the individuals who have disabilities (Hanebrink and Parent-Brown, 2000). Furthermore, therapists may consider working as a team with architects, engineers, and others to help meet the requirements of the ADA (Wells 2000).

The ADA is so broad that it can help people of all ages and with many types of disabilities. For example, many of the adaptations can help elders remain part of society. Especially as society ages, worksite adaptations may help elders who choose to remain working (McGinty, Bachelder, and Hilton 1994). Adaptations can be made to help children and adolescents with disabilities remain in appropriate environments (Kalscheur 1992). Some suggested areas for interventions to meet ADA requirements with youths are play, sports, education, gathering places, and entertainment environments (Kalscheur 1992). Therapists may also help qualified disabled students in higher education (Bowman and Marzouk 1992). Furthermore, an occupational therapist with a strong background in mental health may become involved with making reasonable accommodations for those with mental health diagnoses. With mental health interventions, the focus may be on the psychosocial aspects of employment, such as communication skills, time management, multitasking, concentration, and self-efficacy (Crest and Stifle 1992).

Finally, the National Institute on Disability and Rehabilitation Research (NIDRR) "has established ten regional centers to provide information, training, and technical assistance to employers, people with disabilities, and other entities with responsibilities under the ADA" (My Company 2007, 1). These centers may provide resources that therapists can use to help their clients access employment, public services, public living situations, and communications (My Company 2007).

Social Security Income Programs

The federal Social Security program offers two disability benefit packages: Social Security Disability Income (SSDI) and Supplemental Security Income (SSI). Each of these programs provides important income protection and supplementation for persons with disabilities. They provide a benefit "floor" for the workforce to prevent a person with a disability from becoming financially destitute. This program is vitally important for those persons experiencing severe and persistent disablement where work is not possible.

SSDI provides a monthly income for a person who is considered to be permanently disabled (i.e., has a qualifying medical condition that is expected to last at least one year or to result in death) (Social Security Administration 2007). To qualify, a person has to meet a "recent-work test" and a "duration-of-work test." The recent-work test requires the person to have worked at least half of the time in the recent past (which varies by the person's age). The duration-of-work test requires a person to have worked a minimum number of years. If the person meets these tests, then medical information is ascertained and a state disability determination office decides whether or not the person qualifies for SSDI on the basis of the following questions:

- Are you working? If your monthly income exceeds the limit, you do not qualify.
- Is your medical condition severe? Your ability to do "basic work activities—walking, sitting and remembering" must be impaired for at least one year.
- Is your medical condition on the List of Impairments? A list of approved conditions is maintained by the state disability determination office.
- Can you do the work you did before? If not, you do not qualify.
- Can you do any other type of work? If you can do other work, you do not qualify.

Persons who qualify are eligible for a monthly Social Security check based on their "annual lifetime earnings." After two years of permanent Social Security disability, a person qualifies for health insurance through Medicare. In short, this amount of income is dependent upon the income received when one was working. Spouses and unmarried children are also eligible for benefits in some cases. To encourage people on SSDI to return to the workforce, the government has instituted a "Ticket to Work" program that provides vouchers for persons on SSDI for vocational training and counseling.

Supplemental Security Income (SSI) provides income protection for persons who are elderly, blind, or experiencing a disability and also are low income or have meager financial assets (Social Security Administration 2007b). Income limits vary from state to state and include all forms of income (e.g., Social Security payments, pensions, insurance benefits). Financial assets must be less than $2,000 ($3,000 for a married couple), excluding a house, car, burial account, and small life insurance policies. Persons who meet these criteria receive an additional monthly income and in many states, may qualify for Medicaid.

┌─ **Active Learning Exercise** ──────────────────────────────────┐

Go to the U.S. Department of Housing and Urban Development website,
http://www.hud.gov/groups/disabilities.cfm, and review the material on
helping people with disabilities with their housing needs. Consider a scenario
for which you might access this site or recommend a person with a disability to
access this site.

└──┘

┌─ **Active Learning Exercise** ──────────────────────────────────┐

Recent changes in the Social Security disability programs are encouraging persons to return to work without having their important benefits revoked. Visit
http://www.ssa.gov/pubs/10095.html and read about these initiatives. What
are the incentives in this program, and how do they reflect societal values discussed in Chapter 1?

└──┘

Housing Programs for Persons with Disabilities

Occupational and physical therapists work in a community with people who have disabilities. Being an advocate may involve educating people with disabilities about public policies related to housing. A key law is the Fair Housing Act of 1968, amended in
1988 to include discrimination in housing based on disability. Therapists should also
consider the ADA, as it includes information about accessibility guidelines for buildings and other facilities.

TECHNOLOGY AND PERSONS WITH DISABLING CONDITIONS

Therapists recognize the importance of technology in enhancing their client's independence. They use a variety of low-tech devices, such as long-handled reachers,
as well as high-tech devices, such as electric wheelchairs and even computer technology, as part of their practice. Society, too, has recognized the need for promoting the usage of technology for people with disabilities to maximize their
independence. This recognition came with the Assistive Technology Act of 1998,
one of the most recent bills aimed at helping people with disabilities.

The Assistive Technology Act of 1998

The Assistive Technology Act (ATA) became law in 1998. It promotes the usage of
technology to improve the functioning, independence, and quality of life of persons with disabilities. The ATA reflects the rapidly changing and increasingly sophisticated development of technology for people with disabilities. Many of these

changes came about after World War II, when advancing technology for health care became a societal value (Lenker 2000). As Bristo (2000) states, "for people with disabilities . . . technology changes the most ordinary of life activities from impossible to possible."

The intent of the original act was "systems change," to be initiated by state technology-assistance programs. The focus was on advocacy for and modeling of changes in systems that would increase access to and funding of assistive technology. Amendments in 1994 increased the focus on advocacy as a strategy for systems change. The 1998 act shifted the focus to system-capacity building. This shift, while not removing the responsibility to conduct systems-change activities, appears to allow for activities that would enhance or expand the delivery of assistive technology services (as well as the development of new assistive technology and alternative financing systems) (Schultz 2000).

The Assistive Technology Act of 2004

The 2004 amendments accomplished many changes, which made state programs more consistent, ensuring the likelihood that persons with disabilities could make informed decisions about assistive technology through equipment demonstrations and loans. These amendments allow people with disabilities to acquire assistive technology through reutilization and alternative financing programs (Mark Schultz, personal communication, February 5, 2000). (See Table VI in the Appendix for a brief history of the Assistive Technology Act and its amendments.)

Therapists and the ATA

The original purpose of the ATA was for education and awareness rather than for the provision and funding of technology. However, recent changes in the ATA allows for clients to access and acquire assistive technology. As defined by the 2004 act, assistive technology is "Any item, piece of equipment, or product system, whether acquired commercially, modified, or customized, that is used to increase, maintain, or improve functional capabilities of individuals with disabilities" (PL 108-364, section 3, #4). The utilization of resources provided by this act helps therapists understand current assistive technology, especially because technology is such a rapidly developing area. Therapists may refer their clients to state centers established by this law, in order to familiarize them with the most current technology available. People in state centers also can encourage client access to technology, provide technological assistance and education throughout the state, and possibly provide loaner equipment programs (Brachtesende 2003). In addition, the act may help therapy clients through funded research for the development of new technology. At the state level, therapists may become involved with educational programs about assistive technology.

Yet, in spite of federal legislation, such as the ATA, access to assistive technology for therapy clients can remain a challenge, as few insurance companies in the

┌─ **Active Learning Exercise** ─────────────────────────────────────┐

Find the assistive technology project for your state on the World Wide Web.

    a. Identify its location(s) and what services the project provides. Remember that there is some leeway on how services are provided from state to state.

    b. Next, find an assistive technology site for another state website, and compare and contrast services offered by your state with those offered by the other state.

    c. (For practicing therapists) Think about the clients from your current case load in order to determine whether any can be helped by the assistive technology project in your state.

    d. Tour an assistive technology project site and find out options for technology that may help your clients.

└──┘

traditional medical system cover many devices (Brachtesende 2003). Therefore, therapists should examine all community options to obtain this essential equipment. Suggested community options include the state agencies for assistive technology; local drug stores; local community lending closets, often through churches; local health-related organizations, such as the Arthritis Foundation; local chapters for disability organizations, such as Easter Seals; and community-service organizations, such as Lions Clubs (Brachtesende 2003). Therapists interested in assistive technology should also become aware of and network with the Rehabilitation Engineering and Assistive Technology Society of America (RESNA). The purpose of this interdisciplinary organization is "to improve the potential of people with disabilities to achieve their goals through the use of technology." RESNA is involved in "promoting research, development, education, advocacy and provision of technology; and by supporting the people engaged in these activities" (RESNA).

WORKING WITH POLICIES ADDRESSING SOCIAL DISABLEMENT

As therapy practice moves more into the community, it will be beneficial to become aware of policies that address social disablement. Even if therapists do not receive direct reimbursement from some of the relevant acts, they can advise many of their patients by becoming familiar with the various programs that are out there.

    Therapists can learn how to access and work with these policies through networking and advocacy skills. Therapists must recognize that disability policies are laws that can be changed by legislative systems on both the federal and state level. As with any law, the revision of a policy involves the identification of the pertinent issues, the design of the policy, public support, and legislative decision-making (McGregor 2001). The brief historical analysis of the different policies presented in this chapter show that these laws have gone through many changes over time. Some of the amendments have improved access to and coverage of therapy, such as the amendments to the IDEA. Other amendments have tightened therapy coverage, such as the amendments to the Workforce Investment Act. Prior to each amendment, therapists should advocate for their concerns on the state and national level (see Chapter 12 for a discussion of advocacy).

It is also beneficial for therapists to understand the philosophy and priorities of the state agencies that institute these policies. Each state program institutes policies a little differently. It takes networking to find out a given state's priorities regarding disability policies. Networking will also help locate special-interest groups that may influence these policies. State agencies often have grant funding for research, and therapists might choose to access that funding. Furthermore, therapists must understand that the federal laws are superseded by any state statutes that provide greater protection for people with disabilities (Wells 2000).

In addition, it is important to be aware that, for any federal law with state mandates, there is a constant tension between federal and state control, especially related to funding issues. Johansson (2000, 1) reflected that there has been "a 'shift' in developing policy and programs from the federal government to the states. This offers opportunities for innovation, but it also introduces 'new tensions and complexities' into the process of securing benefits." Thus, funding controversies are an economic certainty (Reed 1992).

Therapists must also be aware of trends in public policy related to disability. For example, all of these acts profess to hold the philosophy of inclusion or integration of a person with a disability into the "least restrictive environment" in society and an enhancement of his or her functioning. This paradigm switch has increased the quality of life and participation of people with disabilities in our society, which has been well illustrated with the exemplars of IDEA and ADA. All of these laws have similar definitions of disability, with the exception of IDEA (Turner 1996), and specific requirements that a person must meet in order to qualify (Rothstein 1992). With amendments, some policies may adapt parts of other policies. For example, several policies have adapted protection and advocacy boards. Trends will change, and, as discussed at the beginning of the chapter, views about disability will also change.

Finally, even though federal laws are available to help people with disabilities, there remain many barriers, controversies, and room for improvement with all of these acts. Several plausible explanations exist for these problems. First, the history of legislation for people with disabilities has not been a planned effort, but rather a piecemeal attempt to deal with their concerns (Bowman 1992). Thus, many of the policies that have been discussed overlap in some areas and have become similar over the years. Also, services for different disabilities can be piecemeal. For example, someone with a developmental disability might benefit from services from the DDA, the IDEA, the ATA, and perhaps Medicaid and Medicare. Yet if state resources are unfamiliar, an individual might miss receiving beneficial services. Second, public policy can be very incremental and may involve multiple levels of federal and state bureaucracy (McGregor 2001). It is the bureaucrats who actually institute the policies, and interpretations can vary. As Bristo (1997, 25) states, "The customer with disabilities seeking services faces a maze of programs, requirements

— Active Learning Exercise —

Interview a contact person (either in person, on the phone, or by e-mail) from a state agency funded by public policy that helps people with disabilities. Determine how the selected agency could help your clients. Prepare a minimum of two to three questions to ask. Examples of state agencies are Vocational Rehabilitation Projects and Assistive Technology Projects.

Sample Questions:

What types of clients does your organization work with?

What does your organization do?

What type of referrals to your organization would be appropriate from therapy?

Are there services that therapy can access to help clients?

and bureaucratic obstacles." Furthermore, decisions regarding the provision of services continue to be made by bureaucrats rather than by people with disabilities, thus promoting dependence (Bristo 1997). Third, because public policies are federal laws, compromises are made during the debates in the House and Senate (Reed 1992). These compromises often deal with the funding aspects of the policies. IDEA, for example, has never been fully funded and is currently funded at approximately 17 percent of federally authorized levels (T. Nanof, personal communication, November 6, 2007). Fourth, the written language and regulations of the acts may also include limitations (Nosek 1992). For example, the terminology "essential functions of the job and reasonable accommodation" is not clearly defined in the ADA and can be interpreted in many ways (Gupta, Gelpi, and Sain 2005). Fifth, even though these policies are in effect, people in society may not understand the issues related to the provision of services for disabilities (Wells 2000). For example, people who are minorities and have a disability may encounter dual discrimination and have trouble obtaining services (Wells 2000). Even members of Congress may present a barrier because of a lack of understanding of, and a failure to support, disability policies (Bristo 1996). Last, the real power of all these laws is how they are actually implemented in reality and not on paper (Nosek 1992). For even with such policies, people with disabilities are older, more impoverished, and less educated than those without disabilities (Bristo 1996). Thus, the end analysis of all these policies is how they really help the disabled members of our society.

CONCLUSION

Numerous public policies have been enacted in the last 35 years to address social disability by reducing social barriers and empowering persons with disabling conditions. We have discussed the history, purpose, and effectiveness of many of these policies.

Social disability that affects children, youths, and persons with disabling conditions who work, as well as restrictions on access to assistive technology, have been reduced by these government actions. Together, such policies have created a more inclusive society.

CHAPTER REVIEW QUESTIONS

1. Define "inclusion," "mainstreaming," "barriers," and "empowerment."
2. Review the history and purpose of the following disablement-related laws:
   a. Individuals with Disabilities Education Act
   b. Developmental Disabilities Act
   c. Older Americans Act
   d. Workforce Investment Act
   e. Americans with Disabilities Act
   f. Social Security income programs
   g. Assistive Technology Act

   Who is eligible for services? What types of services are provided? How are physical and occupational therapists involved in delivering services to eligible populations?

CHAPTER DISCUSSION QUESTIONS

1. Reflect on the paradigm switch in the 20th century regarding views about disability. What were the different values influencing disability prior to the 1960s and after the 1960s?
2. Briefly describe the focus of policies discussed in this chapter. What are some of the similarities and differences between the different disability policies?
3. Discuss why it is beneficial for therapists to know about policies (such as the DDA and the ATA) even though they do not provide direct services through these laws.

INTERNET RESOURCES

http://www.adata.org/ADA Technical Assistance Program: Enhances public consciousness, technical assistance, training, materials, and referrals throughout the country.
http://fedlaw.gsa.gov/ Contains the full texts of the federal disability laws.
http://www.igc.apc.org/ Provides information on DDA programs.
http://naric.com/ Provides information on each state's assistive technology program.
http://www.igc.apc.org/ Developmental disabilities council information.
http://www.ed.gov/policy/speced/guid/idea/idea2004.html/ U.S. Department of Education, IDEA information
http://idea.ed.gov/ OSEP, Building the Legacy of IDEA
http://www.ideapartnership.org IDEA Partnership Project
http://www.resna.org/ Rehabilitation Engineering and Assistive Technology Society of America

REFERENCES

AFB (n.d.). Summary of Key Sections of the Individuals with Disabilities Education Improvement Act (IDEA) of 2004 Public Law 108–446: 2005. Josephine L. Taylor Leadership Institute National Education Program. http://www.afb.org/Section.asp?SectionID=58&TopicID=264&DocumentID=2768 (accessed February 12, 2007).

American Occupational Therapy Association. (2002). Occupational therapy practice framework: Domain and process. *Am J Occup Ther* 56: 609–39.

American Occupational Therapy Association. 1992*a*. Occupational therapy services in work practice. *Am J Occup Ther* 46: 1086–88.

_____. 1993*b*. The role of occupational therapy in the independent living movement. *Am J Occup Ther* 47: 1079–80.

_____. 1995. Occupational therapy: A profession in support of full inclusion. *Am J Occup Ther* 50: 855.

_____. 2000. Occupational therapy: and the Americans with Disabilities Act (ADA). *Am J Occup Ther* 54: 622–25.

AOTA (n.d). The New IDEA 2004: Section-by-section analysis of Part B regulations as they relate to occupational therapy. http://www.aota.org/nonmembers/area21/links/link08.asp (accessed February 5, 2007).

AOTA. 2006. The new IDEA: Summary of the Individuals with Disabilities Education Improvement Act of 2004 (P.L. 108-446). http://www.aota.org/nonmembers/area21/docs/IDEAanalysis.pdf (accessed February 5, 2007).

AOTA. 2006, September 27. Section-by-section analysis of IDEA 2004 Part B regulations. http://www.aota.org/Practitioners/Advocacy/Federal/Issues/IDEA/Id04/Regs/36304.aspx (accessed October 30, 2007).

American Office on Aging. 2006, March 9. Choices for freedom: Modernizing the Older Americans Act. http://www.aoa.gov/about/legbudg/oaa/Choices_for_Independence_White_Paper_3_9_2006.doc (accessed October 27, 2007).

American Office on Aging (n.d.) Older American Act: Overview. http://www.aoa.dhhs.gov/about/legbudg/oaa/legbudg_oaa.asp (accessed October 27, 2007).

American Physical Therapy Association. 2007. *House of delegates policies,* p. 11. http://www.apta.org (accessed February 5, 2007).

Baker, N. A., and K. Jacobs. 2003. The nature of working in the United States: An occupational therapy perspective. *Work* 20: 53–51.

Bachelder, J. M., and C. List-Hilton. 1994. Implications of the Americans with Disabilities Act of 1990 for elderly people. *Am J Occup Ther* 48: 73–81.

Berland, B. J., and K. D. Seelman. 2000. "Introduction and Background," in *Overview of NIDRR's Long Range Plan.* http://www.ncddr.org/rpp/lrp_ov.html

Bowman, O. J. 1992. Americans have a shared vision: Occupational therapists can create the future reality. *Am J Occup Ther* 46(5): 391–96.

_____ and D. K. Marzouk. 1992a. Implementing the Americans with Disabilities Act of 1990 in higher education. *Am J Occup Ther* 46(6): 521–33.

_____ and _____. 1992b. Using the Americans with Disabilities Act of 1990 to empower university students with disabilities. *Am J Occup Ther* 46(5): 450–56.

Boyd, K., C. DeMarco, K. Figetakis, S. Robinson, S. Sullivan, J. Young, C. Custard, M. DiCarlo, M. Laners, K. Serfas, and K. Vigil. 1996. Developmental Disabilities Act. Unpublished ms., Creighton University, Omaha, Nebraska.

Brachtesende, A. 2003, May. Helping clients obtain funding for assistive technology. *OT Practice* 5 (8): 18–21.

Bristo, M. 1996. *Achieving Independence: The Challenge for the 21st Century.* Washington DC: National Council on Disabilities.

————. 1997. *Equality of Opportunity: The Making of the Americans with Disabilities Act.* Washington DC: National Council on Disability.

————. 1999. *Lift Every Voice: Modernizing Disability Policies and Programs to Serve a Diverse Nation.* Washington DC: National Council on Disabilities.

Conyers, L. M., and C. Ahrens. 2003. Using the Americans with Disabilities Act to the advantage of people with severe and persistent mental illness: What rehabilitation counselors need to know. *Work* 21: 57–68.

Crest, P. A., and V. C. Stifle. 1992. The Americans with Disabilities Act of 1990 and employees with mental impairments: Personal efficacy and the environment. *Am J Occup Ther* 46(5): 434–43.

DeJong, G., and B. O'Day. 2000. Contrast of Paradigms: "Old" paradigms vs "new" paradigms. *www.ncddr.org* (accessed November 21, 2007).

Dunn, D. 2000, November. Personal communication.

FAPE (n.d.). IDEA 2004 Summary. http://www.fape.org/idea/2004/summary.htm (accessed February 12, 2005)

Fontana, P. 1999, December 20. Pushing the envelope: entering the industrial arena. *OT Practice,* 4(12): 20–22.

Gordon, M. 2000, November. Personal communication.

Goren, W. D. 1999. *Understanding the Americans with Disabilities Act: An Overview for Lawyers.* Chicago: General Practice, Solo and Small Firm Section, American Bar Association, ABA Publishing Co.

Graney, P. J. 2000. RS20194: Developmental Disabilities Act: 106th Congress legislation. Washington DC: Domestic Policy Division. Congressional Research Service, Library of Congress.

Gupta, J. 2006. Workplace accommodations. Challenges and opportunities. *OT Practice* 11(11): 14.

Gupta, J., T. Gelpi, and S. Sain. 2005. Reasonable accommodations and essential job functions in academic and practice settings. *OT Practice* 10 (15): CEI-CE 8.

Hanebrink, S., and B. Parent-Brown. 2000. ADA consulting opportunities. *OT Practice* 5(17): 12–16.

Hansen, R. H., and J. Hinojosa. 2004. *Nondiscrimination and Inclusion Position Paper American Occupational Therapy Association, Inc.* Occupational Therapy's Commitment to Nondiscrimination and Inclusion. http://www.aota.org/members/area2/links/link40.asp?PLACE=/members/area2/links/link40.asp (accessed February 5, 2007).

Hightower-Vandamm, M. D. 1979. Developmental Disabilities Act: An historical perspective, part 1. *Am J Occup Ther* 33(6), 355–59.

Individuals with Disabilities Education Act of 2004, Pub. L. No. 108-446. http://frwebgate.access.gpo.gov/cgi-bin/getdoc.cgi?dbname=108_cong_public_laws&docid=f:publ446.108.pdf (accessed May 25, 2008).

Jacobs, K. 1996. "Work assessments and programming," in *Willard and Spackman's occupational therapy,* eds. H. L. Hopkins and H. D. Smith, 226–48, 8th ed. Philadelphia: J. B. Lippincott.

Johansson, C. 2000a, November. Disability advocates say more could be done. AOT
———. 2000, January 31. Health Care News: Top 10 emerging practice areas to watch in
    the new millennium. *OT Practice, 5*(3), 7–8.
———. 2000c. Work incentives bill signed. AOTA. http://www.aota.org (accessed No-
    vember 2007).
Kalscheur, J. A. 1992. Benefits of the Americans with Disabilities Act of 1990 for children
    and adolescents with disabilities. *Am J Occup Ther* 46(5): 419–27.
Kelley, M. 2000, November. Personal communication.
Larkin, V. M., R. J. Alston, R. A. Middleton, and K.B. Wison. 2003. Underrepresented
    ethnically and racially diverse aging populations with disabilities: Trends and rec-
    ommendations. *J Rehab* 69(2): 26–31.
Lenker, J. A. 2000. Certification in assistive technology. *OT Practice* 5(16): 12–16.
LD Online (n.d.). IDEA 2004. http://www.ldonline.org/features/idea2004 (accessed
    February 12, 2007).
Marshall, E.M. 1985. Looking back. *Am J Occup Ther* 39(5): 297–300.
McClain, J. 1996, January. Personal communication.
McGregor, D. 2001. "Health policy," in *Delivering Health Care in America: A Systems Ap-
    proach,* eds. L. Shi and D. A. Singh. Gaithersburg, MD: Aspen.
Mellard, E. 2000. "Impact of federal policy on services for children and families in
    early intervention programs and public schools," in *Best Practice Occupational
    Therapy: In Community Service with Children and Families,* ed. W. Dunn. Thorofare,
    NJ: Slack, Inc.
Muhlenhaupt, M. 2000. OT services under IDEA 97: Decision-making challenges. *OT
    Practice* 5(24): 10–16.
My Company, Administrator. 2007, February 7. ADA and its centers. http://www.otinfo.
    org/index.php?option=com_content&task=view&id=15&Itemid=1. (accessed Feb-
    ruary 13, 2005).
NADDC. 2000. National Association of Developmental Disabilities Council. http://www.
    igc.apc.org
National Information Center for Children and Youth with Disabilities (NICHCY). Janu-
    ary 2000. *NICHY News Digest 21 (2nd ed.),* 1–35. http://www.nichcy.org/pubs/
    newsdig/nd2ltxt.htm (accessed December 5, 2000).
Nosek, M. A. 1992. The Americans with Disabilities Act of 1990: Will it work? *Am J Occup
    Ther* 46(5): 466–67.
Opp, A. 2007, July 25. Occupational therapy in early intervention: Helping children suc-
    ceed. AOTA. http://www.aota.org/News/Consumer/40021.aspx (accessed Octo-
    ber 30, 2007).
Perinchief, J. 1996. "Service management," in *Willard and Spackman's Occupational Ther-
    apy,* eds. H. L. Hopkins and H. D. Smith, 375–93. Philadelphia: J. B. Lippincott.
PL 108-364. http://www.resna.org/taproject/library/laws/pl108-364.rtf (accessed Feb-
    ruary 16, 2007).
Redick, A. G., L. Mclean, and C. Brown. 2000. Consumer empowerment through occu-
    pational therapy: The Americans with Disabilities Act Title III. *Am J Occup Ther*
    54(2): 207–213.
Reed, K. L. 1993. The beginnings of occupational therapy, in *Willard and Spackman's oc-
    cupational therapy,* 8th ed., eds. H. L. Hopkins and H. D. Smith. Philadelphia: J. B.
    Lippincott.

_____. 1996. "The beginnings of occupational therapy," in *Willard and Spackman's occupational therapy,* eds. H. L. Hopkins and H. D. Smith, 26–39. Philadelphia: J. B. Lippincott.

RESNA. 2000. Rehabilitation Engineering and Assistive Technology Society of North America Internet site: RESNA Government Affairs. http://www.resna.org

RESNA. (n.d.). Mission statement. http://www.resna.org/AboutRESNA/Mission/Mission.html (accessed February 16, 2007).

Reyes-Akinbileje, B. 1999. CRS Report for Congress: Technology assistance for people with disabilities: Summary of P.L. 100–407 and P.L. 103–218. Washington DC: Congressional Research Service, Library of Congress.

Rothstein, L. F. 1992. *Disability and the Law.* Colorado Springs, CO: McGraw-Hill.

Schultz, M. 2000, December. Personal communication.

Social Security Administration. 2007. *Disability Benefits.* SSA Publication No. 05-10029. http://www.ssa.gov/pubs/10029.html#part2 (accessed May 9, 2007).

Social Security Administration. 2007b. *Supplemental Security Income.* SSA Publication No. 05-11000. http://www.ssa.gov/pubs/11000.html (accessed May 9, 2007).

Stockdell, M., and M. S. Crawford. An industrial model for assisting employers to comply with the Americans with Disabilities Act of 1990. *Am J Occup Ther* 46(5): 427–33.

Tomlin, G. 2000. The history of P & A programs. http://boots.law.ua.edu/

Tucker, B. P. 1994. *Federal disability law.* St. Paul, MN: West Publishing Co.

U.S. Census Bureau. 2006, July, 16. Facts for features: Americans with Disabilities Act: July 26. (accessed February 13, 2007).

U.S. Department of Health and Human Services. n.d.. Administration on Developmental Disabilities Fact Sheet. http://www.census.gov/Press-Release/www/releases/archives/facts_for_features_special_editions/006841.htmlhttp://www.acf.hhs.gov/programs/add/Factsheet.html (accessed February 11, 2007).

The U.S. Equal Employment Opportunity Commission (n.d). Disability discrimination. http://www.eeoc.gov/types/ada.html (accessed February 13, 2007).

Wells, S.A. 2000. The Americans with Disabilities Act of 1990: Equalizing opportunities. *OT Practice* 5(6): CE1–8.

Workforce Investment Act of 1998, Pub. L. No. 105–220, § 404, 112 Stat. 936, 1148–49 (codified as amended at 29 U.S.C. § 723 Supp. IV 1998).

5
Fundamentals of Insurance

CHAPTER OBJECTIVES

At the conclusion of this chapter, the reader will be able to:

1. Discuss the social purpose and organization of health care insurance.
2. Define and relate the basic features of an insurance contract.
3. Describe insurance contracts using three methods of classification.
   a. By Sponsorship
      1. private insurance
      2. self-insurance
      3. direct contracting
   b. By Method of Cost Sharing
      1. indemnity
      2. service benefit plans
   c. By Covered Events/Services
      1. long-term care insurance
      2. workers' compensation
      3. casualty insurance
4. Discuss the rationale for the regulation of health care insurance markets.

KEY WORDS: Actuarial Analysis, Assignment of Benefits, Beneficiary, Community Rating, Cost Limits, Moral Hazard, Premium, Risk, Underwriting

Case Example

Melissa is a certified hand therapist and has decided to develop a business plan for a private hand therapy practice. She has developed a good working relationship with local physicians who are interested in helping her by referring patients in need of therapy. As part of her business plan, Melissa needs to identify her sources of funding for her practice. She knows through experience that most of her current patients have either employment-based health care insurance or workers' compensation insurance that pays for therapy. She networks with other providers in the community and identifies the major insurance companies in the area. She contacts them and learns of their interest in her as a provider. She also learns that policyholders of their plans have different out-of-pocket costs they are responsible for, depending on the insurer and type of insurance. She also learns that, depending on the insurance company and the type of insurance plan, she will be paid using different methods of payment. Some insurance plans will pay her for each procedure she completes; other insurance plans will pay her per-patient visit, irrespective of the procedures she performs. She also realizes that each company has different paperwork to be completed. The complexity of the insurance system surprises her, but she recognizes that she will need to understand it in order to be successful in her private practice.

Case Example Focus Question:

1. What effect does the insurance/reimbursement system have on the business of private therapy practice?

INTRODUCTION

Insurance is a financial mechanism that shares and disperses the risk of financial loss due to the occurrence of an adverse event within a population. Insurance performs an important social function by improving the financial stability of individuals and organizations. Individuals and organizations pay a fee (premium) to create a pool of resources that will provide income or service benefits to holders (beneficiaries) of an insurance contract (policy). A beneficiary who experiences an adverse event covered by the contract is eligible to receive benefits. Since insurance funds the majority of therapy services, physical therapists and occupational therapists need to understand the form and structure of insurance in order to meet contractual obligations for the reimbursement of their care.

In this chapter, we will introduce the social function of insurance, the basics of an insurance contract, a classification system of insurance contracts, and how insurance is regulated. Chapter 7 is devoted to the most common form of health care insurance today: managed care. Chapters 8 and 9 will discuss the largest social insurance programs in the world: Medicare and Medicaid. We begin the chapter with an explanation of the social purpose and organization of health care insurance.

WHY HAVE HEALTH CARE INSURANCE?

Purpose of Insurance

Insurance performs an important social purpose in protecting individuals and organizations against unforeseen and severe financial loss. For many employees, health care insurance is an important part of a work-related benefit package. Without insurance, many ill or injured persons would be forced into liquidation of assets and bankruptcy to pay for the costs of medical illness and disability.

Insurance is a set of two contracts. One contract is between the insurance company and the contract holder. This agreement defines a set of benefits that the contract holder is entitled to if an event occurs that is covered by the contract. The second contract is between the insurance company and the provider of the health care service. This agreement defines the payment structure and amount that will be reimbursed when contract holders use their insurance. In both cases, an important function of insurance is to manage the risk of an adverse event.

Risk and Insurance

The basic purpose of insurance is to share and disperse the negative consequences of an adverse event. Health care insurance prevents any one individual or group of individuals from suffering serious financial hardship or poor health due to an illness or injury. To prevent this from occurring, individuals come together to form a **risk** pool that collects a fee (**premium**) from each member (**beneficiary**) which can be disbursed to individuals who actually incur an event covered by the contract. The purchase of insurance does not guarantee that one will receive benefits equal to the amount of money contributed to the pool. In fact, if all the beneficiaries received benefits equal to or greater than the amount they contributed, the risk pool would be financially bankrupt. Implicit to the concept of insurance is the sharing of risk. Insurance exists to provide "peace of mind," in that the individual will receive benefits in case of the occurrence of an adverse event. Those without insurance are placed at risk of significant loss of financial resources and/or health.

Insurance also provides a stable source of funds for health care providers, including therapists. The money in the risk pool is available to pay for services when persons do not have the personal resources to pay. In this case, the risk of the provider not being paid is kept relatively low, in contrast to the situation of care provision to the person without insurance. Insurance companies are required to maintain adequate reserves to pay for claims that are made against the risk pool. This requirement helps to maintain a stable health care system.

ORGANIZATION AND ADMINISTRATION OF HEALTH CARE INSURANCE

The organization and administration of an insurance program is performed by private companies and by the government. Private insurance companies are regulated by state governments that, at a minimum, require insurance plans to maintain adequate financial reserves to cover the needs of the risk pool. The United States, unlike most industrialized countries, does not provide universal medical care coverage for its citizens. As a consequence, health care insurance in the United States is a dualistic mix of public and private insurers (see Chapter 1). This public–private system results in both the freedom of individuals to purchase an insurance contract as well as the reality that a large segment of the population is without any health care insurance coverage at all (see Chapter 2).

Actuarial Adjustment and Insurance

In order for insurance to be a stable source of funding for therapy and medical care, the collected premiums must cover the benefits to pool members, cover the administrative expenses of the insurance plan, and, in the case of private insurers, generate a profit. The premium fee is determined by a process called **actuarial analysis**. Actuarial analysis commonly considers demographic factors (e.g., age, gender, medical history), past medical care utilization rates, and known cost data to make statistical decisions about future utilization and costs. An actuarial adjustment determines the premium fee on the basis of the information included in the actuarial analysis. For example, people over the age of 65 would pay a greater amount for medical care insurance than individuals in their early twenties. Actuarial adjustment provides for equity in cost sharing based on the likely need for benefits. Performed improperly, actuarial methods can result in excessive profits or losses for the insurer and can affect the availability and affordability of health care insurance to the public.

Moral Hazard and Insurance

Moral hazard is an insurance problem that can be caused by both the beneficiary and the insurer. Moral hazard is financially irresponsible behavior regarding insurance. Individuals create moral hazard by choosing not to purchase health care insurance when they have the capability to do so or by utilizing unnecessary medical care services covered by the insurance. People who choose not to purchase health care insurance shift the costs of their unpaid medical care to people who pay into the risk pool. People who overutilize services raise the costs of health care for all insured individuals.

Insurance companies commit moral hazard through the process of actuarial analysis or actuarial adjustment. Favorable selection results from an actuarial process that preferentially identifies people with anticipated low health care costs, an approach that will result in lower beneficiary premiums and higher insurer profits. Favorable selection also creates a pool of individuals with higher health care costs who may not be able to obtain affordable insurance. Individuals in this pool are affected by adverse selection.

By the mid-1990s, the problems of rising insurance costs and moral hazard made it increasingly difficult for people to obtain or maintain health care insurance. To address the problem caused by insurance moral hazard, some states attempted to mandate a form of actuarial adjustment called **community rating**. Community rating requires insurance companies to set a premium fee based, not on individual experience, but on the experience of everyone in a given city, county, or other geographic area. Individuals with high costs and low costs are included in the geographic region. However, community rating has been less than successful. Premium rate increases to cover all persons, both the healthy and the sick, resulted in many people withdrawing from the insurance plans. In effect, community rating caused adverse selection.

BASICS OF AN INSURANCE CONTRACT

A medical care insurance contract with a beneficiary defines eligibility for benefits, what events and services are covered by the plan, what the cost limits of the insurance plan are, and how coordination of benefits will occur (see Table 5–1 ■). Insurance contracts with providers define the mechanisms and circumstances of payment for services (see Table 5–2 on page. 93). It is important to understand that an insurance contract does not pay for all of the services that can be requested by a beneficiary or delivered by a provider. For example, most insurance contracts exclude payment for luxury or experimental services. Insurance contracts do not tell providers what to do—insurance contracts inform the beneficiary and the provider about what services are covered and how much of the cost of care will be paid for by the insurance company. Insurance contracts only provide benefits to eligible beneficiaries for covered events and covered services.

Eligibility

Eligibility is established on the basis of criteria set by the sponsor of the insurance plan. The United States lacks a comprehensive single source for health care insurance that

Table 5–1. Basic Features of an Insurance Contract

A. Eligibility
 1. Established by the sponsor of the plan.
B. Covered Events
 1. Medical problem diagnosed by a credentialed physician.
 2. Contract is responsible for event precipitating the illness or injury (e.g., workers' compensation insurance is responsible for work-related illness or injury).
 3. Excludes illness or injury caused by war or by riot, as well as self-inflicted illness or injury.
C. Covered Services
 1. Stated in contract
  a. Reasonable and necessary
  b. Acceptable medical practice
 2. Excludes experimental and certain elective procedures (e.g., cosmetic surgery).
D. Beneficiary Cost Limits
 1. Plan limits: lifetime, overall limit, annual, out-of-pocket limit.
 2. First-dollar coverage: deductible or co-payment.
 3. Co-insurance: shared percentage-based reimbursement between insurer and beneficiary up to out-of-pocket limit.
 4. Limits on utilization: preauthorization, day-dollar-visit limits, provider selection, documentation or expectation for improvement.
E. Coordination of Benefits
 1. Primary and secondary insurance: "Birthday" rule for children.

is open for enrollment by all Americans. Instead, the United States has a mix of programs that determine eligibility in terms of the motivation of the sponsor and the willingness of the beneficiary to participate. For example, employment-based coverage is offered only to employees of a given business or members of a given labor union. Eligibility can be further restricted by previous or anticipated utilization of health care services. The process of **underwriting** determines whether an individual's personal characteristics (e.g., age, medical history) qualify the person to purchase the insurance. Strict application of underwriting rules resulted in problems with insurance portability in the mid-1990s. (We will discuss this issue later.) An insurance contract defines who is eligible to join the risk pool and contribute premiums.

Covered Events

Covered events are usually medical illnesses or injuries that have been diagnosed by a credentialed physician. The credentialing process is an insurance procedure which verifies that the provider has met minimum qualifications for the relevant area of practice. Typically, an insurance contract will not list events that are covered, but rather events that are excluded from coverage under the contract. Events due to war, civil disturbance, or self-inflicted injuries are usually not covered. Some insurance contracts exclude preventive health services. It is important to note that the type of insurance must match the covered event. For example, if a person is injured on the job, insurance will be provided by workers' compensation insurance, not an employer-sponsored group health insurance plan.

Covered Services

Once insurance eligibility is established and a covered event has occurred, a beneficiary or a provider is eligible to receive benefits for covered services from the plan. Benefits may be financial remuneration for expenses incurred due to a covered event or, more commonly, the services themselves. Services typically include physician care, hospital stays, outpatient care, rehabilitation therapy, behavioral health care, short-term nursing facility stays, and prescription drug benefits. At a minimum, services need to be "reasonable and necessary" to treat the covered event. In general, services should contribute to the recovery of the patient and meet locally acceptable standards of patient care. "Reasonable and necessary" and "acceptable" are determined by an internal review process (utilization review) performed by the insurer.

Cost Limits

Finally, an insurance contract will establish rules that limit the cost of services to the insurance plan. For the beneficiary, this occurs through plan limits, "first dollar coverage" limits, coinsurance, and limits on utilization of care. Insurance contracts between the insurance plan and providers will limit costs to the plan by means of fee schedules, case rates, and capitation. These limits define how the insurance plan will pay for professional services.

Beneficiary Cost Limits

Insurance contracts will establish two types of plan limits: an overall plan limit and an out-of-pocket limit. The overall plan limit is the maximum dollar amount the plan will pay over the lifetime of a covered member. An out-of-pocket limit is the maximum amount a beneficiary is responsible for paying during a plan year.

Second, an insurance contract will define when plan coverage begins. It is typically calculated on an annual basis by plan year. This first-dollar-coverage limit will vary by type of health care insurance plan. For example, a deductible is the amount of money to be paid out of pocket by the beneficiary before any reimbursement by the insurance company. In this form of insurance cost limit, the beneficiary is responsible for all covered costs during the plan year, up to a set amount of money (e.g., $250). Another example of a first-dollar-coverage limit is a **co-payment**, a flat fee (e.g., $20) paid by the beneficiary each time a health care service is utilized. This form of first-dollar-coverage limit is common to the health maintenance organization (HMO) form of managed care.

A third form of cost limit in insurance contracts is co-insurance. It is used in indemnity plans and some forms of managed care to share a percentage of costs between the beneficiary and the insurance plan, until the out-of-pocket limit is reached. For example, a "70–30" co-insurance means that the insurance plan is responsible for 70 percent of the costs and the beneficiary for 30 percent, after the deductible is paid and before the out-of-pocket limit is reached. Once the out-of-pocket limit is reached, the insurance contract will typically pay all remaining costs for the plan year, up to the overall plan limit.

A fourth form of cost limit in insurance contracts is limit on the utilization of covered services. Physical therapy and occupational therapy services typically require preauthorization by physician referral and, in some cases, by the insurer. Therapy services may have day, dollar, or visit limits for the plan year. An insurance contract may limit beneficiary selection of providers to a contracted panel. A typical standard for reimbursement of occupational therapy and physical therapy services in all insurance contracts is the expectation and documentation of improvement in function or health status in order to justify the continuation of services.

Provider Cost Limits

The various types of provider cost limits are summarized in Table 5–2 ■. Provider cost limits are not typically seen by the beneficiary. They are, however, integral to the contract between the insurance company and the provider. A fee schedule is a predetermined list of procedure payments that are negotiated between the

Table 5–2. Provider Cost Limits in Health Care Insurance Contracts

A. Fee Schedules
   1. Negotiated list of payment rates by health care procedure.
B. Case Rates
   1. Per diem
      a. All-procedure-inclusive daily payment rate.
   2. Per visit
      a. All-procedure-inclusive payment rate for each visit.
   3. Per episode
      a. All-procedure-inclusive rate for a treatment episode.
C. Capitation
   1. Payment to provider based on number of members in health plan.

provider and the insurance plan. It is used in many types of insurance contracts, including managed care, service benefit plans, and social insurance. A fee schedule has low financial risk to the provider. A therapist is paid for each procedure provided to a beneficiary. As long as the cost of providing that procedure is less than the payment amount, the provider is making a profit with each procedure. Case rates are all-procedure-inclusive payments that take three forms: per diem (daily), per visit, and per episode. A per-diem rate is a flat payment for a day of services. A per-visit rate is a set amount of reimbursement for each therapy visit. A per-episode rate is a negotiated fee for an entire episode of care (i.e., multiple visits or days). Case rates "bundle" procedures together into one all-inclusive payment. The cost of providing these procedures may or may not be greater than the case-rate payment. Capitation is a form of reimbursement that pays the provider for each member of a health care insurance plan. Capitated contracts share the most financial risk with the provider. Acceptance of a flat-rate payment for a set period of time means that the provider is guaranteed a payment. This flat rate, however, is not based on actual patient visits or procedures, so, in a capitated contract, the therapist is at risk of the costs of care exceeding reimbursement.

Coordination of Benefits

Some individuals will be covered by more than one insurance contract. This is a common situation in marriages where both spouses have employment-based insurance for themselves and their dependents. In such cases, a coordination of benefits occurs. The policy held by the insured person seeking services is considered to be the primary insurance, and the other coverage is considered to be secondary insurance. For children with dual parental coverage, the "birthday rule" is commonly used. The insured parent whose birthday is the earliest in the calendar year is considered to be the primary insurer.

TYPES OF INSURANCE

Health care insurance is offered to the public through different insurance product types. One way to classify health care insurance is to determine its sponsorship (e.g., commercial insurance, social insurance, self-insurance, direct contracting). The method of cost-sharing between the insurance plan, provider, and beneficiary is another method to classify insurance. For example, indemnity insurance, service benefit plans, and managed care are different types of health care insurance. Finally, the type of services covered can classify the type of insurance (e.g., health care insurance, workers' compensation, long-term care insurance).

In the next section, we will introduce several types of insurance. The next three chapters of the book will explore the managed care and social insurance forms of health care insurance in more detail. For now, we will consider these types of health care insurance:

- By sponsorship
  - private insurance
  - self-insurance
  - direct contracting
- By method of cost sharing
  - indemnity insurance
  - service benefit plans
- By events/services covered
  - long-term-care insurance
  - workers' compensation
  - casualty insurance

It is important to understand that this classification system for health care insurance does not create mutually exclusive categories of insurance. For example, a private insurance company may sponsor an indemnity, long-term-care insurance product. The classification system will help you understand the variety of insurance products that affect the practice of physical therapy and occupational therapy. Since there are many types of health care insurance available in the market, the therapist needs to understand the specific features of each product in order to understand the eligibility, events covered, services covered, and cost limitations for the patient's episode of care.

SPONSORSHIP

Private Insurance

Private insurance is most commonly provided as a benefit of employment. Health care insurance sponsored by for-profit insurance companies is commonly termed *commercial insurance*. Individuals may purchase commercial insurance on their own or through a group plan. Group health care insurance is also sponsored by non-profit organizations (e.g., labor unions, the Blue Cross insurance plans).

Self-Insurance

About half of the policyholders of employment-based insurance are covered by employers who self-insure (Gabel et al. 2003). Self-insurance means that a company or organization chooses not to participate in a risk pool organized by an insurance company (commercial insurance) and instead establishes its own separate insurance fund internally to pay for covered events and benefits. Sponsors usually contract with a health insurance company to administer the plan. Many self-insured companies and organizations supplement this method of insurance by purchasing "stop-loss" coverage to cap their liability for claims that are higher than anticipated.

Self-insurance is most common in businesses or labor unions with at least 100 members (Garfinkel 1995; Park 1999). This method of insurance enables large organizations to manage health care insurance costs by predicting and dispersing risk in a known risk pool while simultaneously avoiding expensive marketing and administrative costs. Self-insured health care insurance plans are exempt from state regulation (ERISA exemption). As a result, this form of insurance is popular with multistate organizations that would be affected by individual state mandates and regulations.

Direct Contracting

In the late 1990s, two new forms of financing for medical care services emerged that are in competition with health care insurance: buyer-sponsored organizations and provider-service organizations. Both of these types of contract mechanisms bypass the traditional insurance company actuarial function and incorporate that process into the operations of either employer purchasers or large provider organizations. In this way, direct contracting occurs between employer purchasers of health care and health care providers.

The increasing interest and sophistication of large employers in purchasing medical care insurance products has caused some of them to form cooperatives and directly contract with providers to obtain care for their employees. This type of contracting group is called a buyer-sponsored organization. A Minneapolis and St. Paul, Minnesota, coalition of large employers has formed the Buyers Health Care Action Group to competitively bid and contract for employee health coverage with area health care providers (Christianson et al. 1999). Lyles et al. (2002) found that this program performed "reasonably well" in restraining cost growth without negatively affecting quality. Provider-sponsored organizations are structures established by health care providers to market a package of benefits directly to employers and other purchasers of health care. This new method of obtaining health care has applications for physical therapists and occupational therapists (Cohn 1999).

METHOD OF COST SHARING

Indemnity Insurance

The first health care insurance products were called indemnity insurance plans. Today, indemnity insurance plans represent a very small portion of health care insurance. Indemnity insurance reimburses a beneficiary for covered health care expenses. The provider is paid by the beneficiary, who is subsequently reimbursed by the insurance company. Indemnity insurance plans utilize plan limits, a deductible form of first-dollar coverage, and co-insurance to limit costs. "Managed" indemnity plans also include limits on the utilization of services. This insurance structure is paperwork intensive, and providers often need to wait a long time for payment. To address the problem of delayed payments, the **assignment of benefits** clause was created to permit direct payment to the provider by the insurance company. Assignment of benefits is routinely obtained from the patient on admission to a physical therapy or occupational therapy practice.

Indemnity insurance is also associated with open choice, fee-for-service reimbursement structures. Beneficiaries have the right to choose any provider who will accept their insurance plan (open choice). In this structure, patients and insurers pay the provider for the reasonable and necessary charges of care on a per-procedure basis. Indemnity insurance products supply financial incentives that provide maximum choice of provider for the beneficiary, broaden the range of services delivered, and increase the cost of health care.

Service Benefit Plans

Service benefit plans developed as a modified form of indemnity insurance. These plans originated several features common to today's health care insurance plans. First, service benefit plans established panels of providers to deliver services. A provider panel is a list of physical therapists, occupational therapists, physicians, hospitals, and other providers who contract with an insurance company to provide care. Second, service benefit plans utilize assignment of benefits and pay providers directly from the insurance company. Third, service benefit plans use a fee schedule to pay for provider services. A fee schedule establishes the payment rates for contracted services.

COVERED EVENTS/SERVICES

Long-Term-Care Insurance

The increased risk of expensive long-term care and the limitations of private health care and social insurance plans in sponsoring this coverage have spawned the development of long-term-care insurance. In 2007, the average yearly cost for nursing home care in a double room was $67,500 (New York Life Insurance Company 2006) and for assisted living care was $34,000 (Prudential Insurance Company 2006). With projections that "baby boomers" will live longer (AOA 2005) and the fact that Medicare doesn't pay for most nursing home care or for assisted living care, long-term-care insurance can be a helpful safety net. To date, about 7 million Americans have purchased long-term-care insurance policies (America's Health Insurance Plans 2004). About half of U.S. businesses now offer long-term-care insurance coverage (Davis and Leach 2002). There are three different types of long-term-care insurance policies (American Association of Retired Persons 2006): individual/group, partnership plans, and combination policies. An individual/group policy may be purchased in the commercial market or through an organization and provides only long-term-care benefits. Partnership plans are available in some states and allow persons to retain more assets if they utilize the Medicaid program long-term-care benefit (see Chapter 8). Combination policies provide long-term-care benefits with a life insurance or retirement annuity. Policies typically have a waiting period (e.g., 100 days) and a plan limit on the amount of benefits.

Long-term-care insurance provides benefits to people with physical illness, cognitive impairments, and other chronic diseases that result in impairments and functional limitations. Eligibility for benefits is based on the loss of function in activities of daily living (ADL) or the onset of a significant cognitive impairment. Six ADLs are commonly examined to determine eligibility: bathing, continence, dressing, eating, toileting, and transferring (e.g., to a wheelchair). An inability to perform at least two of these tasks without assistance will usually initiate benefits (NAIC 1999). Some plans require physician certification of benefit needs (Ali 2005)

Long-term-care insurance benefits may cover services at home or in skilled nursing facilities, assisted-living facilities, and adult day care centers. Some plans will limit coverage to home-based or facility-based care. Other plans will cover services across a continuum of postacute care (American Association of Retired Persons 2006). Services can include room and board, personal assistance, and professional care (e.g., occupational therapy, physical therapy). Typically, cost limits on benefits are established as a per-diem or per-episode rate. Case management to determine eligibility and coordinate benefits is used in long-term-care insurance plans (Scharlach et al. 2003). Costs for these benefits are more reasonable the earlier in his or her life that a person gets a plan. Long-term-care insurance has been found to be effective in preventing institutionalization and reducing stress in informal caregivers (Cohen et al. 2001).

Active Learning Exercise

Go to this MSN website to calculate your life expectancy: http://moneycentral.msn.com/investor/calcs/n_expect/main.asp

Now project into the future—Considering your life expectency and the high costs of long-term-care, would you benefit from long-term-care insurance?

Workers' Compensation

Workers' compensation insurance originated in the early part of the 20th century. It was precipitated by the increasing incidence of industrial workplace injuries, lost worker wages, worker disabilities, and workplace litigation. Health and productivity losses due to work-related injury is currently estimated at $1.2 trillion annually (Fisher 2003). The purpose of workers' compensation insurance is to protect workers, free employers from excessive litigation, and decrease the incidence of occupational injuries (Clayton 2003-04). Farming, forestry, and fishing are the industries with the highest incidence of workplace injury, and executives and managers have the lowest incidence of workers' compensation claims (Leigh et al. 2006). Stressful jobs, lack of job control, and environmentally hazardous conditions are associated with higher incidence of workers' compensation claims in men (Crimmins and Hayward 2004). The prevalence of musculoskeletal injury in this population makes workers' compensation insurance a program of importance to physical therapists and occupational therapists. Back pain is the most common workers' compensation claim (Guo et al. 1999). Disparities in access to workers' compensation for African Americans has been reported (Tait et al. 2004; Dembe 2001).

Workers' compensation insurance is an example of no-fault insurance (Kiselica et al. 2004). Employers are liable for damages due to workplace-related illness and injury, regardless of the circumstances surrounding the event. The source or severity of the injury, however, can be disputed (Hirsch 1997). Workers' compensation laws establish statutorily determined benefits for workers and also protect employers from suits over expenses related to workplace injuries. Workers' compensation laws are state specific within broad guidelines established in the federal law. Some states require employers to participate in state-operated programs. Other states permit employers to purchase workers' compensation insurance in the private market. Employers pay the full premium for workers' compensation insurance, which currently covers about 127 million American workers (Green-McKenzie, 2004). Given the extent of this system, it has been recently estimated that workers' compensation does not cover 8 billion to 23 billion dollars in annual, eligible costs (Leigh and Robbins 2004).

Workers' compensation insurance consists of three benefit programs: health care insurance, disability income replacement, and vocational rehabilitation. To be eligible for workers' compensation, an individual must be injured or acquire an illness while performing employment activities or functions (Calfee 1998). The benefits may be temporary or permanent, depending on the injury or illness. About 70 percent of claims are temporary in nature, but the most expensive claims are due to permanent disability (Hirsch 1997). The medical benefits start immediately after the injury, and are unlimited. Medical benefits are provided until "maximal medical improvement" or a return to employment has occurred (Durbin 1997).

Outpatient services are the dominant mode of medical care delivery in workers' compensation programs (Himmelstein et al. 1999). Medical benefits are paid without deductible or co-insurance to the injured employee. The choice of physician and provider is a source of contention in workers' compensation law (Himmelstein et al. 1999; LaDou 2005). Since eligibility for benefits is based on a determination that an injury or illness is work related, the ability to choose a provider to make this determination is important. Some states allow an open choice of provider by the injured employee, whereas other states permit the employer to select the physician to determine eligibility for benefits.

The Occupational Health and Safety Act of 1970 established income-replacement cash benefits and vocational rehabilitation benefits as part of a minimum workers' compensation benefit package. This program accounts for 60 percent of the costs of the workers' compensation program (Himmelstein et al. 1999). Durbin (1997) has reviewed the process that determines the amount of income replacement for a worker's compensation claim. Disability is classified into five categories:

- fatal
- permanent total
- permanent partial
- temporary total
- temporary partial

Disability benefits are paid as income replacement payments (typically 66 percent of preinjury income) during the time that the worker is not employable. Temporary benefits are paid after a three- to seven-day waiting period, until maximal medical improvement is reached or the worker has a medical release to return to work (Hirsch 1997). Permanent benefits are provided after maximal medical improvement has been attained.

A physical impairment rating and a schedule of benefits are used to determine permanent disability. Certain types of injuries are nonscheduled (e.g., injury to the visceral organs, trunk, or neck and head; claims of psychological disability). Scheduled injuries include injuries to the limbs, eyes, and ears. Each of these body parts is assigned a statutory length of time, in weeks of disablement, based on a schedule. Impairment of function is rated with the use of the American Medical Association Guides to the Evaluation of Permanent Impairment (Anderson, Cocchiarella, and AMA 2000). This percentage rating is multiplied by the schedule of weeks for payment of benefits to determine the degree of permanent disability. The resulting figure is multiplied by the preinjury wage to determine the total disability award. A significant variability in rating disability across the country has been found (Patel et al. 2003; Barth 2003–04).

Workers' compensation insurance costs have been rapidly rising. In response to this trend, 24 states had authorized or mandated workers' compensation managed-care programs by the mid-1990s (Dembe et al. 1997). In 2004, California passed a major workers' compensation reform bill intended to increase the use of evidence-based practice in the state plan (Guidotti 2006). As a result, the size of disability ratings and the amount of cash benefits have fallen by one-third (Leigh and McCurdy 2006). Fraud and abuse in the workers' compensation system is commonly alleged (Hirsch 1997; Durbin 1997). Several types of moral hazard have been described in the workers' compensation program (Hirsch 1997; Durbin 1997).

First, the generous benefit packages in workers' compensation plans provide incentives for employees to file false claims or to exaggerate symptoms. Second, the high costs of the program have given employers the incentive to aggressively manage these costs and jeopardize the medical care of persons with legitimate injuries or illnesses. Third, the presence of insurance tends to make employers more safety conscious and employees less safety conscious. Fourth, the fee-for-service reimbursement mechanism of some workers' compensation plans gives providers the incentive to overtreat conditions.

Recent trends in workers' compensation include the use of managed care and self-insurance programs to restrain the growth in costs (D'Andrea and Meyer 2004). Disability case management and utilization review are now in widespread use for workers' compensation insurance. Contracted provider networks that limit the open choice of providers are also used. A newer trend is for the development of integrated primary, secondary, and tertiary care networks in workers' compensation plans that can provide 24-hour coverage. Costs are lower in these types of systems (Baldwin et al. 2002; Green-McKenzie et al. 2002).

Casualty Insurance

Automobile or homeowner's insurance include a medical care benefit. A person must have been injured in an automobile accident or home accident to be eligible for covered benefits. Depending on the state, a determination of fault in the accident situation will establish responsibility for the payment of claims. In these cases, a legal judgement is sometimes necessary to determine who will pay for therapy services. Casualty insurance is most commonly provided using a fee-for-service reimbursement structure, although managed care principles are sometimes used to reimburse providers. These products utilize case management, utilization reviews, contracted-provider networks, and discounted fee mechanisms to control costs.

REGULATION OF INSURANCE

Insurance is useful only if it provides contracted benefits when needed at an affordable cost. The failure of insurance to meet these obligations has prompted the intervention of government into the insurance marketplace. States have the primary responsibility for regulating insurance, although the ability of states to regulate medical care insurance is affected by federal legislation. In this section, we will explore the role of the state and federal governments in regulating the insurance marketplace.

Insurance Regulation

Each state has an insurance department that licenses and regulates the activities of insurance companies doing business in the state. Klein (1995) has defined two primary areas of state insurance regulation: maintaining solvency requirements and market regulation. Insurance companies are required to be licensed in their state of incorporation and in the states where they sell insurance products. Solvency requirements mandate that insurance companies maintain capital reserves and financial strategies to cover their anticipated losses. This lessens the possibility of an insurance company facing bankruptcy due to a simultaneous increase in claims and inadequate financial reserves. Some states regulate the premiums charged by insurers, and all states monitor the marketing and eligibility determination (underwriting) practices of insurance companies.

Insurance departments also investigate consumer complaints regarding insurance. The rise of managed care and changes in health care insurance have resulted in the enactment of laws restricting insurance practices in some states. Examples of these laws include the prohibition of "gag clauses" on providers and of insurance limits on maternal stays after childbirth. The ability of states to regulate health care insurance, however, is significantly limited by federal law—specifically, the Employee Retirement Income Security Act (ERISA).

Employee Retirement Income Security Act of 1974

The Employee Retirement Income Security Act of 1974 (ERISA) is a federal statute enacted to standardize the regulation of pension and employee-benefit plans. The law establishes minimal reporting requirements on pensions and prohibits state regulation of health care self-insurance plans. ERISA prevents state regulators from establishing consumer advocacy, minimal solvency, or benefit requirements in this popular form of employment-based insurance (Polzer and Butler 1997). In addition, it protects managed care organizations from state malpractice lawsuits (Hellinger and Young 2005). It does not prevent states from regulating closed provider panels in managed care organizations (see Chapter 7) through "any willing provider" laws (Goodyear 2001). Some of these allowances provided to managed care organizations by state law have been a contributing factor to the establishment of managed care legislation (e.g. Patient Bill of Rights Acts in States)

Continuation Issues

The high cost of medical care insurance has made it increasingly difficult for some people to obtain coverage. This is especially true for those who lose employment-based coverage due to a change in life status or employment. The Consolidated Budget Reconciliation Act of 1985 (COBRA) was enacted to deal with the problem of loss of health care insurance due to change in life status or employment. The Health Insurance Portability and Accountability Act of 1996 limits the ability of insurance companies to deny coverage based on preexisting conditions.

COBRA mandates that individuals who lose employment-based health care insurance for reasons other than gross misconduct are eligible to continue coverage for 18 months at full cost to themselves. This law provides that insurance must be also offered to the spouse and dependents of employees who had family-type coverage. In the event of an employee death, a divorce, or a child no longer maintaining eligible-dependent status, the spouse or dependents can purchase coverage for up to three years. Coverage is terminated on the first occurrence of one of the following events: the end of the mandated period, the employer's discontinuation of health care insurance for all employees, or the nonpayment of premiums. COBRA has been criticized for being too expensive for both the employee (Retsinas 1998) and the employer (Fronstin 1998). Fronstin (1998) reports that 10 percent of an employer's workforce is usually eligible for COBRA continuation coverage. Only about one in four eligible employees accept such coverage. These employees tend to have higher incomes and higher medical care expenses.

In the mid-1990s, people with employment-based coverage found their employment opportunities limited by stringent restrictions on eligibility for health care insurance. New hires either were not offered health care insurance if they had certain preexisting medical conditions or had to wait for long periods before coverage would begin for these problems. As a result, people became less willing to change jobs. This portability problem was called "job lock." It was remedied by the Health Insurance Portability and Accountability Act of 1996 (HIPAA), a law that established limits on an insurance company's ability to restrict eligibility for health care insurance. HIPAA allows an insurance company to establish one 12-month waiting period for preexisting conditions (Health Insurance Association of America 2000). This waiting period is modified by the date of diagnosis of the condition and previous undisrupted medical care insurance coverage prior to the new employment situation. Like COBRA, HIPAA does not regulate premium costs. As a result, individuals with high health care costs may still not be able to obtain affordable health insurance.

CONCLUSION

In this chapter, we have discussed the structure and forms of insurance that offer reimbursement for health care services, including occupational therapy and physical therapy. Health care insurance prevents financial disaster for those who are ill or disabled and provides a source of funding for health care providers. It does not cover all the costs of health care; some services are excluded, and many services require financial participation by the beneficiary and place limits on reimbursement to the provider. Insurance contracts define eligibility, covered events, covered services, and the sharing of the costs of health care insurance. Health care insurance is

---

Active Learning Exercises

1. Look at your own insurance plan to determine how therapy services are covered.
2. Find out how workers' compensation law regulates therapy services in your state.

sponsored by many types of organizations, has different forms of cost sharing, and at times provides covered benefits only for certain events (e.g., workers' compensation insurance). Primary oversight of the health care insurance industry is performed by state governments. Several federal laws have been enacted that affect access to health care insurance.

CHAPTER REVIEW QUESTIONS

1. Define the purpose of health care insurance.
2. Define and discuss the concept of risk in health care insurance.
3. What are actuarial analysis and actuarial adjustment?
4. Define moral hazard, favorable selection, and adverse selection.
5. Define the basics of an insurance contract:
   a. Eligibility
   b. Events covered
   c. Services covered
   d. Cost limits for the beneficiary and the provider
   e. Coordination of benefits
6. Compare and contrast health care insurance contracts:
   a. By sponsorship
   b. By method of cost sharing
   c. By covered events and services
7. Define the role of state and federal governments in regulating health care insurance.

CHAPTER DISCUSSION QUESTIONS

1. Mary is a 22-year-old single woman who has just accepted an entry-level position as a physical therapist. She is provided with a pool of benefit dollars from which she can purchase a variety of benefits, including vacation, retirement plan, and health care insurance benefits. Consider and discuss the effects of a decision to purchase or decline to purchase health care insurance on Mary and the community.
2. Mr. Smith is receiving therapy services in your outpatient clinic. He has a service benefit plan with a $200 annual deductible, a $500 out-of-pocket maximum, 75–25 co-insurance, and a $1 million overall plan limit. To date, he has utilized $100 worth of covered plan benefits. Therapy charges are $500. What is the out-of-pocket cost of therapy services to Mr. Smith?
3. Consider this statement: "Insurance contracts do not tell providers what to do. Insurance contracts inform the beneficiary and provider about what services and how much of the cost of care will be paid for by the insurance company." Define and discuss the implications of this statement for the practice of occupational therapy and physical therapy.

REFERENCES

Administration on Aging. 2005. Profile of older Americans 2005. AOA. http://www.aoa. gov/PROF/Statistics/profile/2005/2005profile.pdf (accessed April 9, 2007).

Ali, N.S. 2005. Long term care insurance: buy it or not? *Geriatr Nurs* 26(4): 237–40.

America's Health Insurance Plans. 2002. Long-Term Care Insurance in America, 2002. Washington DC: AHIP.

Anderson, G.B.J., and L. Cocchiarella, eds. 2000. Guides to the Evaluation of Permanent Impairment, 5th ed. American Medical Association Press: Chicago.

Baldwin, M.L., W.G. Johnson, and S.C. Marcus, 2002. Effects of provider networks on health care costs for workers with short term injuries. *Med Care* 40(8): 686–95.

Barth, P.S. 2004. Compensating workers for permanent partial disabilities. *Soc Sec Bull* 65(4): 16–23.

Calfee, B.E. 1997. Workers compensation litigation review. Part I. *AAOHN J* 45(11): 609–11.

———. 1998. Workers compensation litigation review. Part II. *AAOHN J* 46(1): 45–46.

Christianson, J., R. Feldman, J. P. Weiner, and P. Drury. 1999. Early experience with a new model of employer group purchasing in Minnesota. *Health Affairs* 18(6): 100–14.

Clayton, A. Workers' compensation: A background for Social Security professionals. *Soc Secur Bull* 65(4): 7–15.

Cohen, M.A., J. Miller, and M. Weinrobe. 2001. Patterns of informal and formal caregiving among elders with private long term care insurance. *Gerontologist* 41(2): 180–87.

Cohn, R. 1999. Direct contracting: Is it for you? *PT Magazine* 7(5): 22–24.

Crimmins, E.M., and M.D. Hayward. 2004. Workplace characteristics and work disability onset for men and women. *Sozial und Praventivmedizin* 49(2): 122–31.

D'Andrea, D.C., and J.D. Meyer. 2004. Workers' compensation reform. *Clin Occup Environ Med* 4(2): 259–71.

Davis, E., and T. Leach. 2002. Long term care insurance matures as a benefit. *Empl Benefits J* 27(4): 3–5.

Dembe, A. E., J. E. Himmelstein, B. A. Stevens, and M. P. Beachler. 1997. Improving worker's compensation health care. *Health Affairs* 16(4): 253–57.

Dembe, A.E. 2001. Access to medical care for occupational disorders: Difficulties and disparities. *J Health Pol Soc Policy* 12(4): 19–33.

Durbin, D. 1997. Workplace injuries and the role of insurance: Claims costs, outcomes and incentives. *Clin Orthop* 336: 18–32.

Fisher, T.F. 2003. Perception differences between groups of employees identifying the factors that influence a return to work after a work-related musculoskeletal injury. *Work* 21(3): 211–20.

Gabel, J.R., G.A. Jensen, and S. Hawkins. 2003. Self-insurance in times of growing and retreating managed care. *Health Affairs* 22(2): 202–10.

Garfinkel, S.A. 1995. Self-insuring employee health benefits. *Med Care Res Rev* 52(4): 475–91.

Goodyear, J. 2001. What is an employee benefit plan?: ERISA preemption of "any willing provider" laws after Pegram. *Columbia Law Rev* 101(5): 1107–39.

Green-McKenzie, J., S. Rainer, A. Behrman, and E. Emmett. 2002. The effect of a health care management initiative on reducing workers' compensation costs. *J Occup Environ Med* 44(12): 1100–05.

Green-McKenzie, J. 2004. Workers' compensation costs: Still a challenge. *Clin Occup Environ Med* 4(2): 295–398.

Guidotti, T.L. 2006. The big bang? An eventful year in workers' compensation. *Ann Rev Publ Health* 27: 153–66.

Guo, H. R., S. Tanaka, W. E. Halperin, and L. L. Cameron. 1999. Back pain prevalence in US industry and estimates of lost workdays. *Am J Pub Health* 89(7): 1029–35.

Health Insurance Association of America. Guide to Health Insurance. HIAA. http://www.hiaa.org/cons/guidehi.html#law (accessed March 3, 2000).

Hellinger, F.J., and G.J. Young. 2005. Health plan liability and ERISA: The expanding scope of state legislation. *Am J Public Health* 95(2): 217–23.

Himmelstein, J., J. L. Buchanan, A.E. Dembe, and B. Stevens. 1999. Health services research in workers compensation medical care: Policy issues and research opportunities. *Health Serv Res* 34(1 pt. 2): 427–37.

Hirsch, B.T. 1997. Incentive effects of worker's compensation. *Clin Orthop* 336: 33–41.

Kerns, W.L. 1997. Cash benefits for short term sickness, 1970–1994. *Soc Sec Bull* 60(1): 49–53.

Kiselica, D., B. Sibson, and J. Green-McKenzie. Workers' compensation: A historical review and description of a legal and social insurance system. *Clin Occup Environ Med* 4(2): 237–47.

Klein, R.W. Insurance regulation in transition: Structural change and regulatory response in the insurance industry. NAIC. http://www.naic.org/1misc/aboutnaic/about/regutra3.htm (accessed March 3, 2000).

LaDou, J. 2005. Occupational medicine: The case for reform. *Am J Prev Med* 28(4): 396–402.

Leigh, J.P., and S.A. McCurdy. 2006. Differences in workers' compensation disability and impairment ratings under old and new California law. *J Occup Environ Med* 48(4): 419–25.

Leigh, J.P., and J.A. Robbins. 2004. Occupational disease and workers' compensation: Coverage, costs and consequences. *Milbank Q* 82(4): 689–721.

Leigh, J.P., G. Waehrer, T.R. Miller, and S.A. McCurdy. 2006. Costs differences across demographic groups and types of occupational injuries and illnesses. *Am J Ind Med* 49(10): 545–853.

Lyles, A., J.P. Weiner, A.D. Shore, J. Christianson, L.I. Solberg, and P. Drury. 2002. Cost and quality trends in direct contracting arrangements. *Health Affairs* 21(1): 89–102.

Mariner, W.K. 1996. Liability for managed care decisions: The Employee Retirement Income and Security Act (ERISA) and the uneven playing field. *Am J Pub Health* 86(6): 863–69.

National Association of Insurance Commissioners. 1999. *A Shopper's Guide to Long-term Care Insurance.* Kansas City, MO: NAIC.

New York Life Insurance Company. 2006. Average Cost of Nursing Home Rises 6 Percent Year Over Year. http://www.newyorklife.com/cda/0,3254,15833,00.html (accessed April 11, 2007).

Patel, B., R. Buschbacher, and J. Crawford. 2003. National variability in permanent partial impairment ratings. *Am J Phys Med Rehabil* 82(4): 302–06.

Polzer, K., and P.A. Butler. 1997. Employee health plan restrictions under ERISA: Employee Retirement Income Security Act. *Health Affairs* 16(5): 93–102.

Prudential Insurance Company. 2006. 2006 Assisted Living Facility Monthly Rates. http://www.prudential.com/media/managed/2006_LTC_Cost_Data-Assisted_ Living_ Facility_Costs.pdf (accessed April 11, 2007).

Scharlach, A.E., N. Giunta, B. Robinson, and T.S. Dal Santo. 2003. Care management in long term care insurance: Meeting the needs of policyholders? *Care Manage J* 4(2): 73–81.

Tait, R.C., J.T. Chibnall, E.M. Andresen, and N.M. Hadler 2004. Management of occupational back injuries: Differences among African Americans and Caucasians. *Pain* 112(3): 389–96.

6
Managed Care and Beyond

CHAPTER OBJECTIVES

At the conclusion of this chapter, the reader will be able to:

1. Discuss the goals of managed care.
2. Define and describe the main principles employed by managed care organizations.
   a. limited access to the entire universe of providers
   b. payment mechanisms that reward efficiency
   c. enhanced quality-improvement monitoring
3. Describe the primary features of managed care products (plans).
   a. managed indemnity
   b. preferred provider organization
   c. health maintenance organization
   d. point-of-service plan
4. Define and discuss different provider-network models that contract with managed care organizations.
   a. staff model
   b. group model
   c. network model
   d. independent practice association
5. Discuss the advantages and disadvantages of managed care for physical therapists and occupational therapists.
6. Discuss successful strategies therapists have used to adapt to the age of managed care.
7. Summarize other payment trends in the health care insurance environment and how they relate to therapy practice (patient bill of rights, pay for performance, and consumer-directed health care).

KEY WORDS: Benchmarking, Bundled, Case Management, Credentialing, Gatekeeper, Leverage, Panel, Penetration, Pay for Performance, Consumer-directed Health Care, Health Savings Account (HSA)

Case Example

Ron, a physical therapist, and Steve, an occupational therapist, both work at a private clinic in the community. They follow a case load primarily of orthopedic patients. Although they are aware that most of their patient care is reimbursed by managed care organizations (MCOs) they do not pay close attention to the day-to-day management of billing and insurance issues. Two factors, however, increase their awareness of MCOs. The first is a denial of continued coverage for a patient that they both felt would benefit from more therapy. Second, they find out that their therapy clinic has lost a major contract with an MCO, as another therapy clinic undercut them when negotiating their annual contract. The loss of this contract will have major ramifications on staffing. Although Ron and Steve recognize that they cannot do anything about the loss of the MCO contract, they decide to do something about the denial of care for the patient that they are following. They make an effort to find out about the appeal process offered by the MCO and successfully work with the patient and the MCO to get continued therapy for the patient.

Case Example Focus Questions:

1. How could Steve and Ron have increased their awareness of managed care before it became an issue?
2. What are some proactive strategies the manager of the clinic might have taken to prevent the loss of the contract?

As you read this chapter, critically consider the impact of managed care and any discussed payment trends on therapy practice.

INTRODUCTION

Many forces (e.g., employer awareness of the cost of care, the disincentives that make fee-for-service inefficient) have come together to change the medical delivery system that was once based on solo providers receiving fee-for-service payments. Among the changes that have come about is a move toward an "integrated" delivery system that is often referred to as managed care. In the preceding chapter (Chapter 5), we introduced the basic purpose and characteristics of several types of health care insurance. In Chapters 7 and 8, we will discuss social insurance: the primary form of government-sponsored health insurance. This chapter addresses one of the most important developments regarding the organization and payment of health care services in recent decades: managed care. The principles of managed care affect both the private and government-sponsored health insurance systems. We will begin by defining managed care, historically examining how managed care became such an important player in the delivery of health care services. We will then discuss the basic principles of how managed care operates and how providers have responded to the changes it has brought. We will also discuss how managed care policies have affected physical and occupational therapist practice and how therapists have responded. The chapter concludes with a discussion about newer trends as a result of managed care, including consumer-directed health care.

Due to years of being sheltered from the rising costs of health care and the availability of the latest and greatest medical technology, many working Americans used the health care system without much restriction or awareness of costs (see Chapter 2). Likewise, hospitals and physicians did not feel constrained to contain costs or hold back on providing services. As concerns rose with regard to rising health care costs in the 1970s, the federal government and employers looked for new ways to reduce health care expenditures. One of their ideas was the use of provider prepayment in order to encourage cost-conscious, efficient, and effective care (Sultz and Young 1999). Though the concept of prepayment for services had been adopted by various employers in providing health insurance for their employees, it was not until the passage of the Health Maintenance Organization (HMO) Act in 1973 that managed care and the concept of prepayment were thrust into the forefront of health insurance policy. Employer concerns about the costs of health care expedited the growth of managed care plans beginning in the late 1980s. The growth of managed care was also propelled by the ERISA exemption that prevented states from regulating employer-sponsored, self-insured health insurance plans (Noble and Brennan 1999; see Chapter 5).

It is important to note the difference between managed care and HMOs. Whereas HMOs are organizations that serve beneficiaries for a fixed fee and provide both financing and the delivery of health care services, managed care is a broader concept referring to the principle that payment and the provision of service are interdependently linked. All HMOs represent some form of managed care; most insurance companies apply at least some managed care principles in different forms of their insurance products (see the section on managed care products later in the chapter).

DEFINING MANAGED CARE

David Mechanic (1994) commented that the term "managed care" is used so "promiscuously" that it has limited meaning. While many people use the term "managed care," they may all have different ideas about what it really means. Thus, the term may describe one type of system for some people and a totally different system to someone else. A minimal definition of managed care is "a system that integrates the financing and delivery of health services" (Barton 1999). Because of the widespread disparity in the definitions of "managed care," it has become an umbrella term to describe the many different organizational structures that try to accomplish the goal of linking the delivery and financing of health care services. This linkage between delivery and financing is very much different from the traditional, limited claims-processing and financing function of insurance companies.

Though managed care has many definitions, all managed care organizations (MCOs) have certain features in common (Kongstvedt 1999). Recall that in traditional indemnity insurance, the provider is paid a "reasonable and necessary" fee after delivering a service, without restriction on the number or type of services provided. The insurer acts as a processor of claims and makes no determination on the appropriateness of the care that was provided. Managed care health insurance plans expand the role of the insurer through three principles: (1) limited access to the universe of providers, (2) payment mechanisms that reward efficiency, and (3) enhance quality-control procedures. The insurer's role in managed care organizations is expanded from claims processing to determining, on some level, the appropriateness of the care and the access by the beneficiary to plan benefits.

How widely and strictly these principles are utilized varies between managed care products. In general, managed care plans that are more restrictive and uniform in their benefits packages (e.g., HMOs) are less expensive than other forms of managed care and traditional indemnity insurance. Other types of managed care organizations (e.g., PPO and POS plans) provide some, but not all, features of managed care. Open access to care is improved, but these plans are more expensive. Thus, a variety of insurance options at different prices are available to consumers in the marketplace. Before we discuss the specific types of managed care products, let us explore each of these managed care principles in more detail.

MANAGED CARE PRINCIPLES

The three major managed care principles are presented in Table 6–1 ■. A short description and application of each principle is included in the table. We will consider each principle separately.

Limited Access to the Universe of Providers

Managed care organizations typically establish a **panel** of health care providers (i.e., a group of physicians, therapists, hospitals, etc.) that are contracted with or employed by the managed care organization to deliver care to plan beneficiaries. The panel should

Table 6–1.   Managed Care Principles

Principle	*Description*	*Application*
Limited access to providers	Controlled number of providers	Open/closed panels
		Credentialing
	Controlled patient access	Gatekeeper
Payment rewards efficiency	Discounts	Discounted fee-for-service
	Bundling	Case-based payment
	Capitation	Per member per month
Quality improvement	Data collection	Utilization review
	Peer review	Clinical pathways
		Benchmarking
		Case management

be geographically distributed and include all necessary services in order to serve the population of patients covered by the plan. A panel is usually less than the universe of providers in the area. This is an important consideration because the highly competitive situation in marketplaces with heavy managed care **penetration** gives the MCO **leverage** to force providers to accept lower rates in order to maintain a patient base.

Provider panels may be either *open* or *closed*. An open panel allows any provider who agrees to the terms of the contract to join and be a part of the panel. A closed panel allows only a finite number of providers to participate in the panel, even if there are others who qualify and desire to be part of the panel. When HMOs organize their provider panels, the providers often go through a **credentialing** process that reviews their education, clinical experience, and professional behavior. Regardless of how a panel of providers is put together or how big the panel may be, the extent to which patients view the provider panel as sufficient is highly subjective and depends greatly on whether or not "their" provider is on the list. This situation has led to many consumer complaints about closed-panel managed care plans. Later in the chapter, we will discuss how providers organize themselves in response to the insurer's initiative to create panels (see the discussion of managed care provider structures).

Most MCOs also limit or refuse benefits to members if they receive care from noncontracted providers. In some managed care models, authorization is done through primary care physicians who act as **gatekeepers**. Patients who want to visit a specialist, such as a physical therapist or an occupational therapist, must first go to their primary care provider and obtain a referral. The purpose for using some form of authorization is to reduce the number of "unnecessary" visits to more expensive specialists and thus save money. A less strict pre-authorization policy may allow patients to visit any physician directly without getting a referral from the primary care physician, but requires them to get authorization for the more expensive procedures, such as hospital admissions. While all managed care products utilize a provider panel, authorization schemes vary.

Payment Mechanisms That Reward Efficiency

As stated at the beginning of the chapter, traditional indemnity insurance provides few incentives for patients or providers to be efficient users of health care. The financial risk of health care is borne by the insurer. Also, payment is made retrospectively, that is, after the intervention has occurred. In a managed care environment, providers are reimbursed for their services through a variety of mechanisms that either "bundle" individual services and procedures into one fee category or create new payment mechanisms altogether (e.g., discounted fee-for-service, case-based payment, capitation) (see Chapters 2 and 5). Some of these payment models utilize retrospective reimbursement (e.g., discounted fee-for-service), and other schemes utilize prospective payment systems (e.g., case-based payment, capitation). (For further discussion of retrospective and prospective payment systems in social insurance plans, see Chapter 7.) With these incentives, the provider assumes either some or all of the financial "risk" associated with patient care. Sharing of financial risk between the provider and the insurer is a very important concept in managed care:

No longer are providers not at risk of losing money for the decisions they make in providing care and allocating financial resources. Let us consider how this works.

In a discounted-fee schedule environment, providers accept a contract that is less than the full charge for certain services. In return for accepting this discounted fee, the provider is assured of a set of patients from those who subscribe to the contracted health plan and is paid per procedure, but at a lower rate than may be deemed "reasonable and necessary." Most of the financial risk in this system is still borne by the insurer, who must anticipate usage rates (e.g., number of therapy procedures) for plan benefits and collect enough premium dollars to pay providers. The insurer has relatively little control over the amount or types of services that are utilized, just the cost per procedure.

Under a **bundled** payment system, the insurer begins to further limit financial risk. This is done by paying one fee to the provider for a set of patient services. It may be as simple as an insurer collating several procedures on a fee schedule that are commonly performed together to create one new fee category (while typically discounting or eliminating certain fees). Or, as in the case of Medicare, the insurer may deny payment for certain procedures that are billed at the same time as another procedure. Bundling can also occur when payment is made for an entire visit, day, or episode of care, inclusive of all individual procedures and services. These payment mechanisms are all examples of case-based payment, which was introduced in Chapter 2. All of these payment mechanisms share financial risk between the insurer and provider. Unlike discounted fee-for-service, bundled and case-based payment systems control not only the cost per procedure, but also the number of procedures that can be billed. Instead of being paid more money for more individual procedures, providers receive fixed fees and are able to bill for fewer individual procedures.

Capitation completely separates payment from the incidence of treatment. Capitation prospectively pays the provider a predetermined sum for each covered member of the plan on a regular basis (usually monthly). The provider is paid even if the plan member does not access covered services during that month. Conversely, the provider is not paid extra for the cost of delivering services that exceed the capitation payment. Capitation payment systems transfer financial risk almost entirely to the provider. If the provider's expenses are greater than the capitation payment for the plan members for the month, then the provider loses money. However, if the provider can care for that population for less than the capitation reimbursement amount, then profits are realized. Thus, the incentive is to engage in coordinated preventive care and keep patients healthy while avoiding expensive or extensive health care services. These incentives are so powerful that, in some cases, the withholding of necessary services has been alleged against providers and MCOs that use capitated payment models.

Enhanced Quality Improvement Monitoring

Managed care plans integrate the financial and delivery mechanisms of health care. As we have discussed, they do this by controlling access to health care services and by creating payment mechanisms that encourage efficiency. But true integration of the financing and delivery of health care services requires policy related to *quality* as well as to access and cost. Since quality is clearly within the purview of providers, and not MCOs, this has been the most difficult policy principle for MCOs to implement.

To affect the quality of health care, MCOs perform utilization review, critical pathways, benchmarking, and case-management functions. Utilization review and critical pathways were discussed in Chapter 3 (see also Reynolds 1996). MCOs use these procedures to track the care of plan members. **Benchmarking** is an ongoing process of evaluating practice and outcomes against the evidence (i.e., industry standards, expert opinion, and scientific literature). The report cards discussed in Chapter 3 are an application of benchmarking. Case management is used to coordinate care that is provided to managed care plan members. In the conclusion of this chapter, we will have more to say about working with case managers.

In sum, managed care organizations use three principles: controlled access, cost incentives for efficiency, and quality-improvement mechanisms in order to integrate the financing and delivery of health care. A number of managed care products have been developed that incorporate the principles just discussed. The next section examines some of these managed care products.

MANAGED CARE PRODUCTS

Several types of managed care products exist that vary in their organizational structure and how they reimburse providers. Managed care plans range from less aggregated (discounted fee-for-service) to more aggregated (i.e., bundle payments either by episode of illness, per day or visit, or per member). *Aggregation* refers to the extent of integration between the financial and delivery components of the form of managed care. This section briefly discusses the following managed care products: managed indemnity, preferred provider organizations, health maintenance organizations, and point-of-service plans. The primary features of these products are described in Table 6–2 ■.

Managed Indemnity

Managed indemnity, the least aggregated form of managed care, is a fee-for-service reimbursement strategy that has a preauthorization component along with a utilization review. Thus, it is just one step removed from the fee-for-service systems of the past. The beneficiary in this system is required to obtain preauthorization for inpatient stays and other high-cost and relatively infrequent services. Failure to do so could result in no reimbursement. On a more positive note, beneficiaries in this system have maximum choice in selecting their health care provider, and there are few restrictions on the amount or types of services they can receive at the direction of their provider.

Preferred Provider Organizations

A preferred provider organization (PPO) is a contracted relationship between a panel of providers and the purchaser of health care services (i.e., the managed care

Table 6–2. Managed Care Products

Product	Characteristics
Managed indemnity	Open panel
	Discounted fee-for-service
	Preauthorization
	Utilization review
Preferred provider organization	Open or closed panel
	Discounted fee-for-service and case-based payment
	Preauthorization/utilization review
Health maintenance organization	Closed panel
	Discounted fee-for-service, case-based payment, or capitation
	Gatekeeper authorization
Point-of-service plan	Contains both HMO and PPO plans
	Rules based on which option patient chooses

organization). The contract is usually an agreed-upon discounted fee-for-service product for a set of specific services provided to beneficiaries. The PPO plan uses preapproval, utilization review, and discounted reimbursement to control costs. Health care providers benefit from an increased pool of patients, a low financial investment, and more autonomy than in other managed care products. Beneficiaries have a choice of providers within the panel. Limited or no reimbursement is available for providers who are not contracted panel members.

Health Maintenance Organizations

A health maintenance organization (HMO) is a highly aggregated form of managed care. HMOs typically utilize gatekeeper physicians, preapproval, and utilization review to control plan costs.

Beneficiaries can access plan benefits only upon referral from their primary care physician and only from panel (typically closed-panel) providers. There is no reimbursement for providers not on the HMO panel. Provider payment can take various forms, including discounted fee-for-service, case-based payment, and capitation.

Point of Service (POS)

A hybrid managed care plan is the point-of-service (POS) plan. POS plans contain both an HMO and a PPO form of managed care. In this plan, beneficiaries are able to choose their provider at the time services are needed. Benefits are typically paid at a higher percentage for persons choosing their primary care providers (HMO product) rather than other providers on the panel (PPO product). Thus, patients have more flexibility to choose the provider they think is most appropriate for their current condition.

Market Shares of Health Plan Types

The PPO health plan is the most common health plan that is offered to employees, followed by HMO plans, POS plans, and conventional plans (Claxton et al. 2006). Figure 6–1 ■ shows how PPO offerings have increased from 1988 to 2005, while

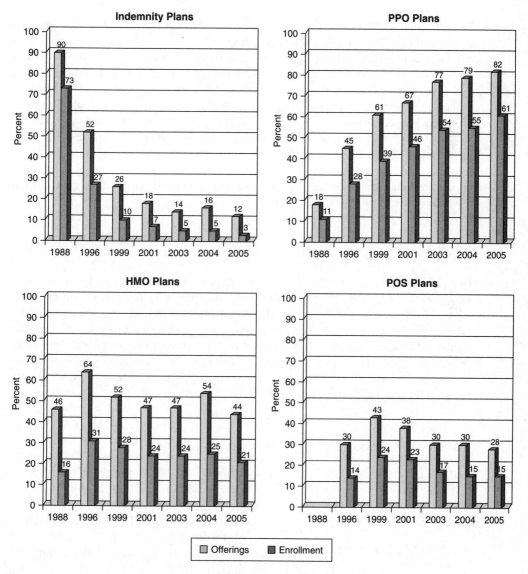

Figure 6–1.   Percentage of Plan Type Offerings and Enrollment
Source: Claxton et al. *Employer Health Benefits 2006 Annual Report.* The Kaiser Foundation and Health Research and Education Trust.
Note: No information on POS plans in 1988 was available.

conventional plans have decreased dramatically. Both HMO and POS plans have re-
mained relatively constant over this period. Enrollment in the various health plan
types also follows the same pattern (see Figure 6–1).

MANAGED CARE PROVIDER STRUCTURES

In order to establish managed care organizations, insurers or other entities must develop relationships and contracts with the provider community. These relationships
can take various forms that result in the provider panels discussed in the preceding
section. In broad terms, MCOs adopt four general types of model that describe how
provider contracts are established: a staff model, a group model, a network model,
and an independent practice association (IPA) model (see Table 6–3 ■). The more
integrated models are characterized by a tightly structured organization that allows
an MCO to have more control of the delivery and cost of health care service. These
models typically limit patient choices when it comes to how care is obtained. Those
models which have relatively less integration are less structured and offer more
choice to their patients. They also describe how providers choose to organize themselves in order to contract with MCOs.

Staff Model

In a staff model, individual providers are employed by an HMO and receive a base
salary for their services. Some HMOs may also pay incentives based on performance. The largest example of a staff model HMO is Kaiser of California, which
salaries its physicians and even owns many of its network hospitals. Other staff
model HMOs may not own but contract with hospitals while employing physician
providers. Beneficiaries in a staff model HMO receive coverage for a comprehensive set of conditions for a fixed price per month, but must be treated within the
HMO. This is a highly integrated form of managed care.

Table 6–3. Managed Care Provider Structures

Staff model	Providers are salaried employees of the MCO. MCO may own many of the institutional providers (e.g., hospitals).
Group model	MCO contracts with a multispecialty provider group for services.
Network model	MCO contracts with several provider groups for services.
Independent practice association (IPA)	Organization of independent or small group practices that contract with an MCO.

Group Model

Group model HMOs deliver health care services to their beneficiaries by contracting with provider group practices. The HMO contracts with just one multispecialty group to provide health care services. Some of these models have exclusive relationships with their provider group practice, referred to as a captive group, in which the provider group serves only patients from one HMO. In a nonexclusive relationship, also known as an independent group, the provider group practice may have contracts to provide service to multiple HMOs. The provider group may be paid by various mechanisms, including fee-for-service or capitation.

Network Model

The network model HMO is similar to the group model, but it contracts with multiple provider group practices, including both primary and specialty care groups. This model may offer greater geographical coverage than the group model. Compared with the staff and group models, the network model is significantly less integrated.

Independent Practice Associations

Independent practice associations (IPAs) are organizations that contract with individual providers or small provider group practices for the purpose of managed care contracting. The HMO then contracts with the IPA to provide health care services to the patients that belong to the HMO. Providers in this model are able to keep their individual or group practices. Thus, they see patients from multiple HMOs, as well as patients who do not participate in an HMO.

EFFECT OF MANAGED CARE ON PHYSICAL THERAPY AND OCCUPATIONAL THERAPY PRACTICE

Managed care has had an impact on all areas of health care, including physical and occupational therapy practice, and has become well integrated as a method of reimbursement for therapy practice. This section addresses the practical realities of

---

┌── Active Learning Exercise ──────────────

PTPN Corporation is a good example of a national independent practice association of physical therapists, occupational therapists, and speech–language pathologists. To learn more, go to http://www.ptpn.com/. From the site, identify what public policy issues PTPN is supporting and critically think about the company's reasons for supporting the issues.

therapy practice with managed care, including a discussion of typical benefits, concerns, and skills related to working with MCOs.

MCOs: Benefits and Concerns for Therapists

In the therapy literature, there is no clear consensus about whether managed care is beneficial or problematic (Poole 1996; Walker 2001; Wynn 1999). Table 6–4 ■ lists key benefits and concerns that have been voiced by therapists about MCOs.

Managed Care Benefits

Managed care results in patients needing to take more responsibility for their care, as visits are fewer than they were in the traditional fee-for-service-dominated market-

Table 6–4.   Benefits and Concerns About Managed Care

Benefit	Concern
Patients and caregivers take more responsibility for therapy secondary to fewer visits	Fewer patient visits with less therapy time
More outcomes research and use of evidenced-based practice	Less reimbursement
Stronger emphasis on preventive care	Less autonomy with therapy provision
Increased interprofessional team dependence and better communication	Patients with chronic conditions may not have adequate coverage
Better streamlined services with a business approach.	Patients with acute conditions are moved very quickly through the system
Improved care from preset treatment protocols, such as clinical pathways	Holistic (occupation) approach to patient care is incompatible with business emphasis
Improved care from educating other health professionals about the latest evidence-based treatments and from better defined therapy	Consumer may have less choice of health care providers
More consultation and supervisory roles	Consumers may have less choice of therapists
Increased problem-based learning in therapy education	Bureaucratic requirements may result in delayed treatment
Greater emphasis in therapy education on the health care environment and business principles	Ethical issues related to providing therapy within reimbursement guidelines

Source: Brayman 1996; Wynn 1999; Coffey et al. 1992; Spragins 1995; Vanleit 1996; Varela-Burstein et al. 1997; and Walker 2001.

place. With managed care, there is more application of outcome measures and research with evidenced-based practice, a stronger emphasis on preventive care, and increased health care team interdependence with better communication (Brayman 1996; Wynn 1999). A business streamlined approach is taken to the provision of therapy, as illustrated by the application of evidenced-based assessments, functional achievable goals, critical pathways, and more efficient documentation (Coffey et al. 1992; Walker 2001). Developing outcome measures and research has been very beneficial for therapists. Although therapists struggle with time constraints and the best methodology for doing clinical research, they recognize the importance of scientific research to validate the therapy fields (Foto 1996; Miller 1999; Wynn 1999). In some MCOs, physicians are educated about the most current treatments, which may ultimately improve therapy outcomes (Spragins 1998). Managed care has encouraged therapists to better clarify what they do. Working in the managed care environment has shifted some therapy roles from direct hands-on care to consultative roles with other health care providers and caregivers, and supervisory roles with assistants and aides.

A perceived impact of managed care on professional education is the increased usage of problem-based learning (Wynn 1999). There is also an emphasis on understanding the current health care environment and increased interest in the business aspects of therapy (Walker 2001; Wynn 1999). Students need to be trained to work quickly and competently in the health care environment and need to have a clear understanding of the "role and value" of therapy services (Walker 2001). Professional education highlights patient education, clinical research, and evidenced-based practice.

Managed Care Concerns

In managed care, therapists express concerns about having fewer visits with patients and less treatment time, lower reimbursement, and greater administrative demands, such as more involvement in treatment authorization and increased documentation (Walker 2001). Therapists also express concerns about feeling pressured to meet productivity demands (Vanleit 1996; Varela-Burstein, Voight, and Pantel 1997; Wynn 1999; Walker, 2001). Therapists voice dismay at their loss of autonomy in directing patient care to case managers and insurers making treatment referrals and reimbursement decisions (Walker 2001). Therapists are also concerned about having adequate coverage for patients with chronic conditions, because the managed care environment seems more supportive of the treatment of acute conditions (Wynn 1999). Yet acute care patients are moving through the system very quickly and getting sicker (Walker 2001). In addition, in a business-minded system, it is difficult to provide true holistic health care (Lohman and Brown 1997). Further concerns are that consumers have less choice of health care professionals, including therapy practitioners. This may result in patients being referred to generalist therapists who contract with a plan, rather than specialist therapists (e.g., a certified hand therapist). Moreover, because of the bureaucracy of MCOs, there often is a lapse of time from referral to treatment, which may adversely affect therapy results (Fisher 1997;

Miller 1999). Slower referrals are especially an issue with hand therapy patients because of the possible impact on therapy results (Walker 2001). Finally, therapists articulate apprehension related to ethical issues and the provision of managed care. A key issue is autonomy in providing adequate therapy within the confines of the managed care referral and approval guidelines (Lohman and Brown 1997; Sandstrom 2007). Other ethical concerns discussed are inappropriately billing occupational therapy services as physical therapy, wrongly using therapy aides for therapy treatment, and getting increased referrals for financial reasons. In addition, therapists feel pressured to meet productivity demands, and they worry over inappropriate application of group therapy for financial gain (Walker 2001).

ADAPTING TO THE CHANGES BROUGHT ABOUT BY MANAGED CARE

The changes shaped by managed care have revolutionized the delivery of therapy services in the United States. Therapists are adapting to the business approach to health care and many have a positive outlook about managed care (Walker 2001). Education about managed care and a good understanding of one's own organization help with this adaptation. We conclude this section with a discussion of successful strategies that have been adopted by occupational therapists and physical therapists to handle the changes brought about by managed care.

Importance of Good Communication

Good communication skills are crucial in today's health care environment. Several of the strategies we will discuss are summarized in Table 6–5 ■. It is important to develop rapport with key people in the managed care system, such as case managers, utilization review coordinators, and primary care gatekeepers. Regular communication helps increase other health care providers' awareness of what therapy can accomplish. Communication and demonstrating the effectiveness of treatment enhance

Table 6–5.   Good Communication Skills for Working in a Managed Care Environment

1. Develop and strengthen rapport with key players (e.g., case managers, utilization review coordinators, gatekeepers).
2. Learn the language of business to communicate better with the key players (Walker 2001).
3. Communicate the outcomes of your treatment to key players, use evidence-based assessments, and develop evidence-based research supporting your practice.
4. Be aware of the mission and goals of the MCO that you are working with.
5. Educate the MCO about the benefits and value of therapy.
6. Understand the needs and values of all of your customers.
7. Advocate for your patients and for your profession.

respect for therapy. Furthermore, effective communication will keep therapists aware of the MCO's goals, such as achieving quality care in a cost-effective, timely manner. Doing in-house **case management** by collecting and communicating outcome data to the MCO about the patient's length of stay, functional status at discharge compared with the same at entry, costs of providing care, and satisfaction with treatment enhances the working relationship with those in an MCO (Foto 1996). Since some case managers have nonmedical backgrounds, and even those from medical backgrounds may not have an in-depth understanding of therapy, good communication can make a big difference in the patient's ability to access and benefit from therapy services. Finally, good communication with all members of the interprofessional team ultimately helps improve patient care.

Therapists need to carefully analyze their customers and what they value. In the managed care environment, the key customers are MCOs, primary care physicians, patients' employers, and patients. Each may have a different perspective on what is expected from the therapist. MCOs usually value the most economical, streamlined, quality care (Foto 1997). Therefore, a therapy clinic that offers diversified care will have an edge in getting contracts over one that specializes in one type of care. Additionally, belonging to a therapy network can help with marketing to an MCO (Lansey 1996). Producing outcomes that are functional and sustainable will also enhance marketing efforts (Foto 1996). Practitioners from therapy clinics should also market to get coverage from several MCOs, so that if they lose a contract, they will still have adequate coverage.

Finally, patients are the main customers therapists regularly see. Patients value caring health care, clear and courteous communication, and an overall satisfactory experience from therapy (Foto 1997). One way to demonstrate care and improve patient satisfaction is to advocate for the patient. Advocacy is done by preauthorizing an adequate treatment amount and by communicating information about the treatment plan. Advocacy also means being assertive about the patient's rights for appropriate treatment if there are problems with the MCO. All MCOs offer appeal processes, which can be accessed if there is a perception of unfair treatment coverage or some other problem. If the appeals process is accessed, it is important to have clear, objective documentation. In addition, providing effective treatment through careful planning in the time-restricted managed care world is an important marketing tool for both the patient and the managed care provider (Miller 1999).

Case Managers and Managed Care

The key professionals in the managed care environment are the case managers, who coordinate, in a holistic manner, all aspects of a patient's care. Case management, as defined by the Commission for Case Management Certification, is a "collaborative process that accesses, plans, implements, coordinates, monitors, and evaluates the options and services required to meet an individual's health needs, using communication and available resources to promote quality, cost-effective outcomes (2006, p. 5)." Although nurses dominate the case management field, some occupational and physical therapists have assumed case management roles, as case management is not a profession, but rather an approach to managing care (Bracht-esende 2004). In the professional literature in both the case management field and the physical and occupational therapy field, there are articles addressing the role of therapists in case management (Baldwin and Fischer 2005; Fosnought 1996; American Occupational Therapy Association 1991; Fischer 1996; Lohman 1998, 1999), and some educational programs are presenting content about case management (Baldwin and Fischer 2005).

Therapists have much to offer case management, thanks to their background in rehabilitation practice (Fosnought 1996). Therapists who rehabilitate people who have work injuries also have a good skill set to be case managers, as they understand medical management and the vocational aspects of rehabilitation (Potocnik 2006). Geriatric case management can be a natural fit for therapists who are interested in helping older adults age successfully at home (Pett 2004; Wilder 2005). Working as case managers in a medical model may be difficult, because therapists often do not have the same depth of medical management knowledge as nurses (Lohman 1998), although they do bring a strong background in rehabilitation knowledge and skills. Lohman (1999) reflects that occupational therapists can assume case management roles in all settings, including medical settings, by learning the medical aspects of care from a functional perspective. One can also break into case management by demonstrating the ability to do the job and by making sure that the formal institutional policies include therapists as case managers (Lohman 1998, 1999), as some institutions may have policies allowing only nurses to provide case management.

Whether or not therapists assume case management roles, they will work with case managers. Therefore, it is beneficial to learn how to best work with case managers. One suggestion, as discussed earlier, is to think like a case manager when monitoring internal cases. Therapists who consider the perspective of the case manager will look at discharge planning from the initiation of therapy. It also helps to maintain good communication with the case manager from the initiation of treatment. Having regular communication and contact keeps communication open.

Active Learning Exercise

Objective: Find out about the case manager's role in managing patients. Network with a case manager, and ask for the case manager's perspective on how he or she reviews charts of patients who receive rehabilitation. Ask the case manager what he or she likes to see in documentation from therapists.

If possible, spend the day with this person and reflect about the experience.

Answer the Following Questions:

- Comment on how the case manager's perspective correlates or differs with your perception of patient care.
- Reflect about what you learned from him or her.

Another suggestion is to demonstrate the value of therapy by providing effective treatment that results in patient satisfaction and cost savings, and to share evidence of what works in practice (Fosnought 1996; Foto 1997). Additionally, therapists can educate case managers from other disciplines about the rehabilitation aspects of patient care (Lohman 1998).

HEALTH CARE ENVIRONMENT TRENDS RELATED TO MANAGED CARE

In this final section of the chapter, we will review three trends which have developed out of the managed care environment of the last 20 years: a patient "bill of rights," pay for performance, and consumer-directed health insurance. The patient "bill of rights" is a public policy which addresses issues about alleged managed care abuses that have adversely affected either access to or the quality of health care. Pay for performance is a newer movement and another approach to controlling health care costs by using evidence-based practice to pay a premium for higher quality health care. Consumer-directed health insurance, a recent development based on public policy, puts increased control and responsibility for health care spending back with the consumer. It is considered to be a departure from the managed care approach towards insurance and may eventually dominate the marketplace (Rosenthal and Milstein 2004). Therapists need to pay close attention to all these trends and how they might influence therapy practice.

Patient Bill of Rights

A number of ethical concerns about the effect of managed-care reimbursement structures have been raised, including potentially holding back needed services under a capitated payment model. In 1995, Spragins reported that physicians receive financial incentives, such as capitation or financial bonuses, to avoid referring patients to specialists. Unchecked, these incentives and others sometimes create the moral hazard of favorable selection—marketing a low-cost, but profitable, managed care plan to healthy people while avoiding persons who are less healthy (see Chapter 5). Additionally, there are concerns about access to emergency rooms, specialty care, therapy services, the appeals process, and the disclosure of financial incentives. These ethical concerns have raised a debate over the need for laws to protect patients that are enrolled in managed care plans. Proponents say that laws are necessary to protect vulnerable patients and consumers from inferior services and obstacles that patients face in seeking health care services (Rodwin 1996). Alternatively, opponents believe that laws are unnecessary, since there are no widespread problems and what problems that do exist the industry is correcting in response to public pressure (Hall 2005).

When societal issues are not solved in the private market, public policy can develop, as was the case with managed care. Since 1994, there have been several national attempts to pass bills to improve the delivery of managed care. To date, none of these bills have passed due to the political climate. Several bills, however, have passed on the state level. A number of states have enacted laws that include patients' rights provisions, such as patient-focused external review (*42 states*), direct access to specialists (*42 states*), and access to a prudent layperson for emergencies (*47 states*) (Hall 2004).

Pay for Performance

A movement in health care called Pay for Performance (P4P) suggests decreasing health care costs (Pawlson 2004) through better clinical accountability and positive outcomes based on the health care provider's performance with the patient (Fine 2006). P4P involves the use of evidence-based practice, better efficiency with patient care, and better usage of patient resources (AOTA 2005, July). P4P is currently being tested as a pilot program for therapy with Medicare Part B (AOTA 2007, January 26), and therapists should pay close attention to trends with Medicare, as other insurers, such as MCOs, do pick them up (Fine 2006; Pawlson 2004) (see also Chapter 7).

Consumer-Directed Health Plans

Used in conjunction with PPO models or other types of managed care plans, consumer-directed health plans allow individuals greater control over their health care utilization and, subsequently, over their health care spending. This greater control includes when, where, and how they access health care services and how much they spend on those services. One of the more recent consumer-directed health plan developments being offered by insurance companies and employers is known as a health savings account (HSA), which is usually coupled with a high-deductible health plan.

Created by the Medicare Modernization Act of 2003 (Pub. L. 108-173), health savings accounts (HSAs) consist of investment accounts that individuals own and subsequently use to pay for their current and future medical expenses. Used in conjunction with high-deductible health plans (HDHPs), these accounts help pay for first-dollar medical expenses not covered in HDHPs. Individuals can have an HSA only if they are covered by an HDHP, do not have any other health coverage, including Medicare, and cannot be claimed as a dependent on someone else's tax return (DOT 2007).

While the HSA is owned by the individual, contributions can be made by the employer, the individual, or both. HSA contributions made by the employer are not taxed, while individual contributions are tax deductible. Rules for contributions also include annual maximums that vary by year. For 2007, this maximum was $2,850 for individuals and $5,650 for families (DOT). Those individuals who are 55 years old or older can make "catch-up" contributions, as long as they are not enrolled in Medicare. Funds in HSA accounts earn interest, as well as additional income through various investment options, both of which can be used tax free to pay for qualified medical expenses. An advantage of HSAs over other tax-friendly accounts that pay for out-of-pocket expenses (e.g., flexible spending accounts) is that leftover funds can be carried over to a subsequent year.

High-deductible health plans are plans that have a minimal deductible (for 2007) of $1,100 for individual coverage and $2,200 for family coverage. Additionally, the annual out-of-pocket maximum for 2007 cannot exceed $5,500 or $11,000 for individuals and families, respectively (DOT 2007). Both of these limits change annually with inflation. It is also important to recognize that, within the various plans, there is quite a bite of variation in deductibles above the minimum required and out-of-pocket expenses below the maximum. No first-dollar benefit is allowed for services other than preventive services. That is, insurance will not pay for any percentage of the charges until the plan's deductible is met. This ban on first-dollar coverage also applies to prescription drugs. All prescription drugs are subject to the plan's deductible. Individuals choose to access the physician panel of their employer's plan and take advantage of negotiated rates or go elsewhere for their care.

Using HSAs as part of an HDHP may offer a number of advantages. HDHPs usually have much lower health insurance premiums than lower deductible plans. Monies in HSAs can be used at the discretion of the individuals to pay for current qualified medical expenses or can be saved for future health care–related needs. Individuals can decide when and how much money to put into the account, up to the maximum allowed limit. Once funds are in the account, they stay there until they are used to pay for qualified medical expenses. Additionally, HSAs are portable and stay with individuals, regardless of job status or geographic location. Finally, there is the potential tax savings associated with HSAs, including tax-deductible contributions, tax-free investment earnings, and tax-free withdrawals for qualified medical expenses. Another consumer option that is not as popular as the HSA is referred to as a health reimbursement account. These accounts are also used in conjunction with HDHPs. The main difference is that while HSAs are owned by the employee, HSRs are owned by the employer.

The use of HDHPs and HSAs is appealing to employers because the two types of plan represent a positive mechanism for controlling the growth of their health care expenditures. Figure 6–2 ■ shows that, since 2003, of those employers who offer health care benefits, there has been a steady increase in the percentage who offer an HDHP. In addition to the 20 percent of firms offering an HSA-qualified HDHP, 27 percent of employers who do not currently offer an HSA-qualified HDHP report that they are "somewhat likely" to "very likely" to do so the next year (Claxton et al. 2006). Supporters of these plans suggest that they help consumers become more aware of health care costs than they were with other types of insurances. Such plans may also help decrease the number of uninsured people, because of lower costs (Woo, Ranji, Salganicoff, and Claxton 2006).

However, as with any new initiative in the insurance industry, there are questions about how it will really work in a long-term implementation. A survey sponsored by the Employee Benefit Research Institute and the Commonwealth Fund (EBRI 2006, February; MacDonald 2006, February), found that people were more satisfied with comprehensive insurance plans than consumer-directed insurance plans. In addition, people were more likely to pass over or postpone needed health

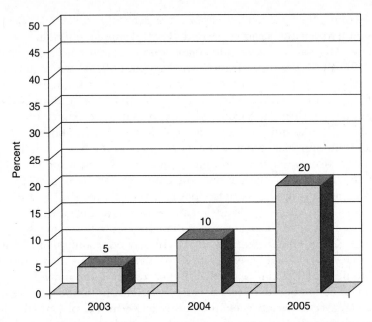

Figure 6–2. Percentage of Employers Offering Health Care Benefits Who Offer an HDHP
Source: Claxton et al. *Employer Health Benefits 2006 Annual Report.* The Kaiser Foundation and Health Research and Education Trust.

care because of costs. This last finding was most prevalent among those employees with incomes under $50,000. The survey did show that people with consumer-directed health care plans were making cost-conscious decisions, but that it was difficult to obtain adequate information to help with the decision-making process. Reiterated were concerns about the current uninsured population which may not have the financial resources to afford such plans (Champlin 2006; Woo et al. 2006, June). Another topic that was repeated was the moral hazard of favorable selection. If more healthy people choose these consumer-directed health plans, costs will go up for the less healthy people enrolled in traditional insurance plans. Lastly, most health care spending comes from a small segment of the population that has

---

⎯ Active Learning Exercise ⎯

Therapists need to keep abreast of trends regarding consumer-directed health plans. Go to the Employee Benefit Research Institute at http://www.ebri.org/pdf/notespdf/EBRI_Notes_02-20061.pdf and to the Kaiser Family Foundation at http://www.kaisernetwork.org to read more about these trends. Critically reason how the potential larger future dominance of such plans in the health care environment would affect therapy practice, and state what we need to do proactively to prepare for this possible.

tremendous health care needs. It is questionable whether these plans would really reduce the health care expenditures of these individuals (Woo et al. 2006). The verdict is still out on the long-run impact that these types of health plans, which will likely expand in the marketplace, will have on consumers as well as health care practitioners, such as therapists. More research will need to be completed on the impact of these plans on consumers and health care providers alike before a consensus can be reached (Woo et al. 2006).

CONCLUSION

In this chapter, we defined and described the philosophy and organization of managed care. Managed care has changed the traditional role of the insurer from actuarial analyst and claims processor to one that includes access/cost control and quality management. These functions are performed by limiting the size of the provider pool, implementing payment schemes that reward efficiency, and measuring provider performance and, in some cases, patient health status. Providers have responded to the emergence of managed care by organizing themselves into groups of practitioners and institutions that can provide the geographic coverage necessary for population-based contracts. Managed care has changed the practice of physical therapy and occupational therapy, and therapists must learn how to navigate the system effectively. Case management has emerged as a career option for therapists to explore, as well as to understand as an important player in the implementation of managed care. Finally, new trends, such as consumer-directed health care, may eventually have a stronger influence on the provision of therapy than will other models of managed care.

CHAPTER REVIEW QUESTIONS

1. Define managed care.
2. Identify and describe the three principles used by managed care organizations to influence the delivery of health care.
3. Compare and contrast the four types of managed care products (plans).
4. Compare and contrast the four types of managed care provider structures.
5. Discuss the advantages and disadvantages of managed care as it affects physical therapy and occupational therapy.
6. How are the following necessary for successful adaptation to working in managed care systems?
   a. communication skills
   b. case management
7. Discuss the impact of the health care environmental trends related to managed care (the patient "bill of rights," pay for performance, and consumer-directed health plans) on the provision of therapy.

CHAPTER DISCUSSION QUESTIONS

1. You have been working as a manager in a department that has contracted for the past two years with Happy MCO. Although its rates are on the low side, you have been able to meet your budget. This year, when you renegotiate the contract with Happy HMO, it will request even lower rates. You know that with the lower rate, your department will not be able to meet its budget. What will you do?

2. You are starting a clinic in an area that is highly penetrated by MCOs. Other therapy clinics currently have all the contracts. Provide a minimum of three suggestions as to how you might negotiate a contract that is financially feasible for your clinic.

3. You are following a patient who had a cerebral vascular accident (CVA) one month ago. The MCO discharged the patient and will not authorize any additional therapy time. What can you do?

4. Research the appeal process for therapy patients from a local MCO.

5. Meet with a manager of a therapy department, and discuss how he or she works effectively with managed care organizations.

6. Identify an employer who offers a consumer-directed health care plan. Meet with a representative from the organization, and discuss the pros and cons of offering that approach.

REFERENCES

American Occupational Therapy Association. 2007, January, 26. Medicare quality measures for occupational therapy coming soon. http://www.aota.org/nonmembers/area1/links/link22.asp (accessed February 26, 2007).

American Occupational Therapy Association. 2005, July. Federal Legislative Issues Update, July 2005. http://www.arota.org/pdfs/July2005legupdate.pdf (accessed February 26, 2007).

American Occupational Therapy Association. 1991. Statement: The occupational therapist as case manager. *Ameri J Occup Ther* 45: 1065–66.

Baldwin, T.M., and T. Fischer. 2005, July–August. Case management: Entry level practice for occupational therapists? *Case-Manager* 15(4): 47–51.

Barton, P.L. 1999. *Understanding the U.S. Health Services Systems*. Chicago: Health Administration Press.

Brachtesende, A. 2004, October, 18. Andrea asks: Alexandra "Allie Hafez", OTR/l, CDMS<CCM, QRC. *OT Practice* 9(19) 36.

Brayman, S.J. 1996. Managing the occupational environment of managed care. *Amer J Occup Ther* 50: 442–46.

Champlin, L. 2006, March 08. Consumer-directed health plans: Friends or foes? AAFP News Now. http://www.aafp.org/online/en/home/publications/news/news-now/professional-issues/20060308cdhp.html (accessed November 13, 2007).

Claxton, G., I. Gil, B. Finder, B. DiJulio, S. Hawkins, J. Pickreign, H. Whitmore, and Gabel. 2006. *Employer Health Benefits 2006 Annual Report*. Henry J. Kaiser Family Foundation, Menlo Park, California, and Health Research and Educational Trust, Chicago,

Illinois. http://www.kff.org/insurance/7527/upload/7527.pdf (accessed September 2007).

Coffey R. J., J.S. Richards, C.S. Remmert, S.S. LeRoy, R.R. Schoville, and P.J. Baldwin. 1992. Introduction to critical paths. *Quality Management in Health Care* 1: 45–53.

Commission for Case Management Certification. 2006. Definition of Case Management. CCM Certification Guide. http://www.ccmcertification.org/pages/14frame_set.html (accessed February 19, 2007).

Department of the Treasury. 2007. All About HSAs. U.S. Treasury Department, Washington: DC. http://www.treas.gov/offices/public-affairs/hsa/ (accessed September 2007).

Employee Benefit Research Institute. 2006, February. Executive summary: Survey of consumer-driven health plans raises key issues. EBRI. http://www.ebri.org/pdf/notespdf/EBRI_Notes_02-20061.pdf (accessed November 13, 2007).

Fine, A. 2006, Spring. Editor's perspective. *Managed Care Quarterly* 14(2): 1–2.

Fisher, T. 1996. Roles and functions of a case manager. *J Amer Occup Ther Assoc* 50: 452–54.

Fosnought, M. 1996. PT as case managers: An evolving role. *PT: Magazine of Physical Therapy* 4: 46–53.

Foto, M. 1996. Excelling in a managed care environment. *OT Practice,* January: 20–22.

———. 1997. Preparing occupational therapists for the year 2000: The impact of managed-care on education and training. *Amer J Occup Ther* 51: 88–90.

Freudenheim, M. 2001. "A changing world is forcing changes on managed care." *New York Times,* July 2, A1, A13.

Ginzberg, E., and M. Ostow. 1997. Managed care: A look back and a look ahead. *N Engl J Med* (14): 1018–20.

Hall, M.A. 2005. The death of managed care: A regulatory autopsy. *Journal of Health Politics, Policy, and Law* 30 (3): 427–52.

Hall, M.A. 2004. Managed care patient protection or provider protection? A qualitative assessment. *Am J Med* 117: 932–37.

Kassirer, J.P. 1997. Is managed care here to stay? *N Engl J Med* 336 (14): 1013–14.

Kauffman, S.H. 1996. "Management of Rapid Change." In *The Occupational Therapy Manager,* ed. Margo Johnson. Bethesda MD: American Occupational Therapy Association.

Kongstvedt, P.R. 1999. "Managed Health Care." In *Health Care Administration: Planning, Implementing, and Managing Organizational Delivery Systems,* ed. L. F. Wolper, 522–44, 3rd ed. Gaithersburg MD: Aspen.

Lansey, D. 1996. Reimbursement: Keeping track of managed care. *PT: Magazine of Physical Therapy* 4(12): 22–23.

Lohman, H. 1998. Occupational therapists as case managers. *Occupational Therapy in Health Care* 11: 65–76.

———. 1999. What will it take for more occupational therapists to become case managers? Implications for education, practice, and policy. *Ameri J Occup Ther* 53: 111–13.

Lohman, H., and K. Brown. 1997. Ethical issues related to managed care: An in depth discussion of an occupational therapy case study. *Occupational Therapy in Health Care* 10(4): 1–12.

MacDonald, J.A. 2006, February. Survey of consumer-driven health plans raises key issues. EBRI News, 27(2): 2–12. http://www.ebri.org/pdf/notespdf/EBRI_Notes_02-20061.pdf (accessed November 13, 2007).

Mechanic, D. 1994. Managed care: Rhetoric and realities. *Inquiry* 31(2): 124–28.

Miller, R.E. 1999. Hands in the new millennium: Therapist commentary. *J Hand Ther* 12: 182–83.

———— and H. S. Luft. 1994. Managed care plan performance since 1980. *JAMA* 271(19): 1512–19.

Nugent, J. 1996. Reimbursement: Planning for managed-care. *PT Magazine* 4: 32–34.

Pawlson, L.G. 2004, November. Pay for performance: Two critical steps needed to achieve a successful program. *American Journal of Managed Care.* http://www.ajmc.com/Article. cfm?Menu=1&ID=2771 (accessed February 25, 2007).

Peloquin, S.M. 1996. The issue is—now that we have managed care, shall we inspire it? *Amer J Occup Ther* 50: 455–60.

Pett, M.E. 2004. Geriatric care management: A viable practice area for the advanced occupational therapy practitioner. *Gerontology Special Interest Section Quarterly* 27(4): 2–4.

Poole, D.L. 1996. Editorial: Keeping managed care in balance. *Health and Social Work* 21: 163–65.

Potocnik, W.T. 2006, March. Navigating field and stream: Occupational therapists as work injury case managers. Part I: Theory and Practice. *Work Programs Special Interest Section Quarterly*, 20(1) 1–4.

Reynolds, J.P. 1996, February. LOS: SOS? *PT Magazine*: 38–47.

Rosenthal, M., and A. Milstein. 2004, August. *Health Services Research.* 39(4): 1055–70. http://www.pubmedcentral.nih.gov/articlerender.fcgi?artid=1361053 (accessed January 17, 2007).

Rowdin, M.A. 1996. Consumer protection and managed care: The need for organized consumers. *Health Affairs* 15(3): 110–23.

Sandstrom, R. The meanings of autonomy for physical therapy. *Phys Ther* 87(1): 98–105.

Spragins, E.E. Beware your HMO. *Newsweek,* October 23, 1995. 54–55.

Stahl, C. 1995. Who's doing the managing in managed-care? *Advance for occupational therapists,* 14–15.

Sultz, H.A., and K.M. Young. 1999. *Health Care USA: Understanding its Organization and Delivery.* Gaithersburg MD: Aspen.

Vanleit, B. 1996. Managed mental health care: Reflections in a time of turmoil. *Amer J Occup Ther* 50: 428–34.

Varela-Burstein, E. A., E. A. Voight, and E. S. Pantel. 1997. The impact of managed care on the practice of occupational therapy by hand therapists. *Occupational Therapy in Health Care* 10(4): 33–52.

Walker, K.F. 2001. Adjustments to managed health care: Pushing against it, going with it, and making the best of it. *Am J Occup Ther* 55(2): 129–37.

Wilder, L. 2005, May 18. Looking at the bigger picture. *Physiother-Frontline* 1(10): 11.

Woo, A., U. Ranji, A. Salganicoff, and G. Claxton. 2006, June. Consumer-directed health arrangements: Background brief. Kaiser Education http://www.kaiseredu.org/ topics_im.asp?id=500&imID=1&parentID=61 (accessed January 17, 2008).

Wynn, K. E. 1999. The pearls and perils of managed care. *PT: Magazine of Physical Therapy* 1: 34–44.

7
Medicare

CHAPTER OBJECTIVES

At the conclusion of this chapter, the reader will be able to:

1. Explain the history of the Medicare program.
2. Describe the organization and scope of the Medicare program.
3. Relate the eligibility criteria to the benefits in the Medicare Part A program.
   a. Hospital inpatient program
   b. Skilled nursing facility
   c. Hospice
   d. Home health care
4. Discuss the mechanisms of provider reimbursement under Medicare Part A.
   a. Cost-based reimbursement
   b. Prospective payment
      1. Hospitals: Diagnosis-Related Groups
      2. Skilled nursing facilities: Resource Utilization Groups
      3. Inpatient rehabilitation facilities: Case Mix Groups
      4. Home health agencies: Home Health Resource Groups
5. Relate the eligibility criteria to the benefits in the Medicare Part B program.
   a. Outpatient hospital programs
   b. Comprehensive Outpatient Rehabilitation Facilities (CORFs)
   c. Physical Therapist in Private Practice or Occupational Therapist in Private Practice
6. Discuss the structure of fee schedules as a method of provider reimbursement in the Medicare Part B program.
7. Relate the eligibility criteria and benefits in the Medicare Part C program.
8. Describe the quality-control procedures employed in the Medicare program.
   a. Recognize fraud and abuse in Medicare.
9. Define the structure and interaction of private health insurance plans with Medicare.
10. Relate the proposals for reform of the Medicare program.

KEY WORDS: Benefit Period, Case Mix Adjustment, Certification, Consolidated Billing, Cost-based Reimbursement, Cost Shifting, Defined Benefit Plan, Defined Contribution Plan, Entitlement, Fee Schedule, Intermediary, Medically Necessary, Medicare Assignment, Medigap, Peer Review Organization, Prospective Payment, Social Insurance, Vested

Case Example

Mrs. Smith is a 76-year-old widow who has health insurance coverage through Parts A and B of traditional Medicare. She worked for 15 years as a bookkeeper and made regular payroll contributions into the Hospital Insurance trust fund. She is vested in the Medicare program. When she became eligible for Medicare at age 65, she purchased the Part B program to help pay for her physician visits. More recently, she decided to participate in the Part D Medicare plan to help pay for her outpatient prescription drug costs.

Mrs. Miller has been experiencing pain and limited mobility in her left hip for many years. It has reached the point where she has elected to receive a total hip replacement to relieve the pain and disablement. She understands that Medicare will help pay for her hospital and post-hospital care. Mrs. Miller has her surgery in the local community hospital and stays for four days. She receives good nursing care, as well as visits from the occupational therapist and physical therapist. Her stay will cost her $992, and the government will pay the hospital a flat-rate payment for her surgery. Mrs. Miller then is transferred to a skilled nursing facility (SNF) to get stronger before she can return home. At the SNF, she is evaluated by the team, which uses the Minimum Data Set (see later), and her needs are identified. She stays 20 days and receives therapy each day. The facility is paid a flat rate by the government for each day of her care, based on the initial assessment and the amount of therapy time Mrs. Miller received. Mrs. Miller then goes home and receives a visit from a physical therapist and occupational therapist to help her adjust to her home environment and continue her recovery. This care lasts for one month, and the home health agency is paid a flat fee for the episode, based on her needs identified in a comprehensive initial evaluation. Mrs. Miller does not pay anything out of pocket for her SNF or home health care.

Two months after her total hip replacement surgery, Mrs. Miller is still experiencing some hip pain and weakness. Her surgeon sends her to a physical therapist for an evaluation. The standard fee schedule amount for this examination is $72.17. Mrs. Miller pays her physical therapist out of pocket for the examination, with the fee applied to her annual $100 deductible. Her course of therapy lasts one month, her pain is relieved, and her strength is improved. The cost of the therapy was $800. After her $100 deductible is paid, Mrs. Miller is responsible for 20 percent or $140, of the remaining fee schedule cost.

Case Example Focus Question:

1. Describe the types of benefits and out-of-pocket costs that are experienced by a Medicare beneficiary.

INTRODUCTION

Medicare is the most influential insurance program affecting the U.S. health care system. This is for two reasons. First, Medicare is the largest single payer of health care services in the United States. Second, it is organized and managed by the federal government, which has enormous statutory and regulatory authority over many activities performed by health care providers, including occupational therapists and physical therapists. It is important, then, for therapists and all health care providers to understand this program. Changes in the program affect the daily delivery of health care in the United States.

We will open this chapter by briefly reviewing the history of how Medicare came to be such a large and influential program. Then we will introduce how Medicare is organized and administered. Next, we will explore the major components, or "parts," of Medicare that provide services to many Americans. The reader should pay close attention to the methods by which providers, including therapists, are paid for services. These payment systems have powerful effects on the organization of the health care delivery system, especially how Medicare defines and regulates therapy services. Then we will review the organization of quality-control programs in Medicare, with special consideration given to fraud and abuse detection. Finally, we will examine efforts to reform Medicare, including proposals to increase private insurance participation in the delivery of Medicare services.

HISTORY OF MEDICARE

The origin of Medicare needs to be considered in the context of the movement to provide universal national health insurance to all Americans (Ball 1995; Friedman 1995). Prior to 1965, Americans who needed institutional health care services had two broad choices: pay privately or receive services in public health care facilities (Blaisdell 1992). This two-tiered system had developed in the first half of the century as medical care began to rely increasingly on technology (Blaisdell 1994). Medical care was no longer delivered primarily in the patient's home by a private physician. Hospitals became institutions where a person could receive the latest in medical technology applied to the treatment of his or her disease or illness. At the same time, social movements began to call for improved access to medical care for people with limited financial resources. Beginning in the late 19th century and into the 20th century, many European countries began to institute universal health insurance for their citizens. American efforts at universal coverage can be traced back to 1912 and are still ongoing (Friedman 1995).

Medicare has been identified as an interim step in the development of universal health insurance for all Americans. By the early 1960s, one in two elderly Americans lacked health care insurance to pay for hospital care (Davis and Burner 1995). Elderly Americans were known to have an increased need for hospital services, and they had fewer resources to pay for such care. Legislative attempts to enact an insurance program for older Americans commenced in 1957. Then, after the landslide election of Lyndon Johnson as President in 1964, proponents of public health insurance for older

Americans had firm control of the Congress and the executive branch. Medicare was vigorously opposed by organized medicine, which had defeated all previous attempts at establishing federal health insurance. In July 1965, however, Medicare was passed by Congress, and shortly thereafter it was signed into law by President Johnson.

Hospital insurance for elderly Americans was enacted as part of a package of benefits. This package is sometimes referred to as a "three-level cake" (Friedman 1995). Hospital insurance (HI), or Part A Medicare, provided coverage for inpatient hospital stays and short-term residential care for rehabilitation in other facilities. Supplementary Medical Insurance (SMI), or Part B Medicare, was intended to provide coverage for professional services (e.g., physicians, occupational therapists, physical therapists). Medicaid, the third tier of the cake, was enacted as an extension of the 1960 Kerr–Mills legislation that provided funds to states to care for the poor. We will discuss Medicaid in Chapter 8.

Until 2003, most major changes in the Medicare program were reforms to the payment systems. (These reforms will be discussed later in the chapter.) In 2003 (and to some extent in 1997), Congress enacted changes that increased the private insurance company role in designing competitive Medicare products. Part C, Medicare managed care, was enacted in 1997. The Part D outpatient prescription drug benefit (2003), the most significant benefit upgrade since 1965, uses private insurance contractors to develop and market competing prescription drug coverage products.

Medicare and Medicaid have been effective in increasing access to health care services for people who are older, people with a disability, people with low incomes (Medicaid), and people with end-stage renal disease (Medicare). These are populations that, in many cases, do not have access to private health insurance. The enactment of comprehensive national health insurance (the goal of the designers of Medicare), however, has not yet occurred. Rothman (1993) identified four reasons for this situation. First, private health insurers have been aggressive and successful in meeting most needs of middle-class Americans. Second, many components of the health care delivery system remain suspicious and opposed to more government involvement in health care. Third, the principle of charitable health care as a means of providing services for people who lack care remains alive in America. Finally, the existing programs (i.e., Medicare and Medicaid), appear to be adequate in meeting the needs of vulnerable Americans.

Another reason is the high cost of Medicare. Almost since its inception, concerns have arisen about the cost of the Medicare program (Russell and Burke 1978). In its first year, Medicare cost less than $2 billion. It was funded by a 0.35 percent payroll tax on the first $6,600 of a worker's earnings (Davis and Burner 1995). Today, Medicare pays out $406 billion in reimbursement for health care services (Medicare Trustees Report 2007). The government collects a 2.9 percent payroll tax on all earnings to fund Medicare Part A and uses general revenues and out-of-pocket costs from beneficiaries to fund the other parts of the program. As the "baby boom" population ages, more people are eligible for Medicare and the beneficiary–worker ratio increases, so there are concerns about the long-term financial viability of the program.

Since 1965, the Medicare program has changed the health care system in many ways. Friedman (1995) identifies these changes: an oversupply of hospitals, the birth of the for-profit hospital industry, the development of payment inequities and

cost shifting between private and public payers, the need to generate and use data to understand a very large health care system, and the formation of quality oversight bodies. Blaisdell (1994) notes that public hospitals have shrunk in size since Medicare's inception because private providers have gained access to public funds to care for persons who are indigent. Medicare was also an influential force in ending discrimination against the ability of minority Americans to access hospitals (Reynolds 1997).

As can be seen, Medicare is a very important and influential program. In the next section, we will review the Medicare program by examining how it is organized and looking at the size of its various components. We will follow this discussion with an explanation of its Parts A and B benefit packages.

SCOPE AND ORGANIZATION OF MEDICARE

Table 7–1 ■ describes the overall characteristics of the Medicare program. Medicare provides health insurance to about one in seven Americans. Medicare comprises two programs: original Medicare and Medicare Advantage. Original Medicare, the

Table 7–1. Characteristics of the Medicare Program

A. Enrollment: 44.8 million (2008)
  1. Aged: 37.6 million
  2. Disabled: 7.3 million
  3. Part A only: 3.6 million
  4. Part B only: 0.4 million
  5. Parts A and B: 40.9 million
B. Expenditures: $375 billion (2006)
  1. Part A: $184 billion
  2. Part B: $160 billion
  3. Part D: $32 billion
C. Persons served (2006):
  1. Hospital: 8.6 million
  2. Skilled Nursing Facility: 1.95 million
  3. Home Health: 3 million
  4. Hospice: 939 thousand
D. Number of Providers Receiving Medicare Payments (2007)
  1. Hospitals: 6,197
  2. Skilled Nursing Facilities: 15,057
  3. Home Health Agencies: 8,618
  4. OP Physical Therapy: 3,009
  5. Comprehensive OP Rehabilitation Facility: 589
E. Program Administrative Costs: 1.8 percent

Source: Centers for Medicare and Medicaid Services. 2007. Data Compendium http://www. cms. hhs.gov/DataCompendium/17_2007_Data_Compendium.asp#TopOfPage (accessed June 5, 2008).

most popular program, consists of Part A and, for most persons, Part B Medicare. Part A Medicare, the hospital insurance benefit, provides for hospital stays, short stays at a skilled nursing facility or an inpatient rehabilitation facility, and home health care or hospice care for eligible beneficiaries. Part B Medicare, or Supplementary Medical Insurance, provides coverage for outpatient hospital care, office visits to therapists and physicians, and durable medical equipment needs. The Medicare Advantage program was enacted by Congress in 2003 as a redesign of the 1997 Medicare Part C program. Unlike original Medicare, Medicare Advantage programs utilize private insurers to organize a benefit package that is comparable to original Medicare within a managed care framework. A fourth program, Medicare Part D, is the prescription drug benefit, which either is a privately sponsored stand-alone program or is included in a Medicare Advantage plan.

Medicare is the largest payer of health care services in the United States. In 2006, the Medicare program spent $375 billion on health care. In 2008, there are an estimated 44.8 million beneficiaries. It is the dominant form of insurance for persons over age 65 and persons with long-term disabilities. Slightly more than half of program expenditures are for Part A from the Hospital Insurance Trust Fund. Medicare operates in all states and territories and affects all providers. It operates at a less than 2 percent administrative cost.

Medicare is a good example of a federal **entitlement** program. In an entitlement program, eligible persons have a guarantee to services identified in the law. Once in place, entitlement benefits are difficult to change (see the discussion of public versus private policy in Chapter 1). Medicare (and Medicaid) is also an example of **social insurance**. Social insurance means that economic resources are transferred from one group to another group to meet a defined social need—in this case, health care. Taxes are paid by working Americans to provide health care benefits to nonworking Americans: the elderly and the permanently disabled. Unlike the situation with private health care insurance, those who pay the premiums (in this case, taxes) are usually not eligible for program benefits.

Medicare policy, (e.g., eligibility and program benefits), is established by congressional legislation. Changes in the policy structure of Medicare require changes in the statute and cannot be made administratively. Failure to provide benefits to eligible beneficiaries can be enforced in the courts. As an entitlement program, Medicare differs from Medicaid in one important aspect: Everyone who meets the eligibility requirements, regardless of income, can participate in Medicare. In contrast, Medicaid is a means-tested program that limits benefits to people who often have not made regular contributions to the program (e.g., low-income persons, children). The popularity of Medicare as the "third rail" of American politics can be tied to its structure as a "pay as you go" program with guaranteed benefits to those who have made regular contributions to the program. Unlike Medicaid, Medicare is not associated with welfare.

Medicare procedures (e.g., eligibility, reimbursement) are developed and implemented by the Centers for Medicare and Medicaid Services (CMS). This agency is part of the Department of Health and Human Services. Claims processing and review are performed by private organizations, usually insurance companies, for a defined region of the country. These claims-review organizations are called inter-mediaries. **Intermediaries** process and review claims for Medicare.

We are now ready to explore the Medicare program in detail. First, we will explore the eligibility criteria for Medicare. Then we will examine the benefit packages for Parts A, B, and D and for Medicare Advantage. In the sections that follow, we will use the case example of Mrs. Miller, a 76-year-old Medicare beneficiary, to illustrate how the program works.

MEDICARE ELIGIBILITY

Program eligibility is determined primarily by meeting the criteria of Medicare Part A. Persons participating in both Part A and Part B are also eligible to choose a Medicare Advantage plan in place of their Part A and B traditional benefits. The Part D prescription drug benefit is available to original Medicare or Medicare Advantage beneficiaries through the purchase of a stand-alone plan or through a Medicare Advantage plan that includes a prescription drug benefit.

Part A Eligibility

Eligibility for Medicare Part A benefits is based on a record of payroll or premium contributions, age, marital status, or the presence of permanent disability. Most individuals qualify on the basis of age (currently, age 65) and a record of payroll contributions into the program for 40 quarters (10 years). After paying into the program for 10 years, an individual is **vested** and is eligible for receiving benefits after reaching the minimum eligibility age. Spouses of vested Medicare beneficiaries are also eligible for Medicare at age 65. No monthly premium is required of vested beneficiaries or their spouses for participation in the Part A program.

Persons who are not vested in the program can receive Medicare benefits after reaching age 65 and agreeing to pay a monthly premium. Individuals younger than age 65 are eligible for Medicare benefits if they have been declared permanently disabled by the Social Security Administration for 24 months (see Chapter 4) or if they have end-stage renal disease.

Part B Eligibility

Persons who are eligible for premium-free Medicare Part A benefits (vested persons over age 65, spouses of vested beneficiaries, persons with permanent disabilities, and persons younger than age 65 with end-stage renal disease) are automatically eligible for Part B Medicare.

Part B Medicare is an optional benefit package. Many people enroll in Medicare Part B when they become eligible for Medicare Part A (see Table 7–1 ■). A person who declines Medicare Part B is eligible to enroll at a later date during

Table 7–2. 2008 Medicare Part B Monthly Premiums

If annual income is:

Individual Tax Return	Joint Tax Return	Monthly Premium
<$82,000	<164,000	$96.40
$82,001–$102,000	$164,001–$204,000	$122.20
$102,001–$153,000	$204,001–$306,000	$160.90
$153,001–$205,000	$306,001–$410,000	$199.70
>$205,000	>$410,000	$138.40

Source: Medicare Part B Monthly Premiums in 2008. http://questions.medicare.gov/cgi-bin/
medicare.cfg/php/enduser/std_adp.php?p_faqid=1980&p_sid=6e1rLWVi&p_lva=1979#
(accessed January 16, 2008).

special enrollment periods at a higher cost. About 25 percent of Medicare Part B
program costs are paid by enrollees. Monthly Medicare Part B premiums vary by annual income (see Table 7–2 ■) and are usually deducted automatically from Social
Security checks. There is a $135 annual Part B deductible and a 20 percent co-insur-
ance rate on Part B benefits beginning each January 1.

ORIGINAL MEDICARE

PART A: HOSPITAL INSURANCE

Benefits

Table 7–3 ■ outlines the three basic benefits included in Medicare Part A: inpatient
hospital care, short-term skilled nursing facility care, and home health/hospice
care. These benefits include room and board (at a hospital or skilled nursing facility) and **medically necessary** professional services provided by the institution. Medically necessary services, including physical therapy and occupational therapy, must
meet program requirements (see the Medicare and Therapy Services section) and
be authorized by a provider with physician status (e.g., a medical or osteopathic
physician). Although vested beneficiaries do not pay a monthly premium, the most
commonly used Part A benefits are not free. Beneficiary out-of-pocket costs include
a deductible (for hospital care) and a daily co-insurance fee (after 60 days of hospital care or 20 days of skilled nursing facility care).

Benefit Period

The Part A deductible and co-insurance are calculated with reference to a **benefit
period**. Unlike most forms of private health insurance, Medicare does not determine

Table 7–3.   2008 Medicare Part A Benefits/Beneficiary Costs

A. Monthly Premiums: $0 for vested individuals
                    $233 for persons with 30–39 quarters of payroll
                        contributions
                    $423 for persons with <30 quarters of payroll contributions
B. Hospital Inpatient Coverage
    1. Deductible: $1,024
    2. Ninety days of "medically necessary" care per benefit period.
        a. Co-insurance
            1. First 60 days: $0
            2. Day 61–90: $256 per day
    3. Sixty lifetime reserve days
        a. Co-insurance: $512 per day
C. Skilled Nursing Facility Coverage
    1. Deductible: $0
    2. One hundred days of post-hospital care
        a. Co-insurance
            1. First 20 days: $0
            2. Day 21 to 100: $128 per day
D. Home Health Care/Hospice
    1. No deductible or co-payment

Source: Medicare Premium Amounts for 2008. http://questions.medicare.gov/cgi-bin/ medicare.cfg/php/enduser/std_adp.php?p_faqid=1979 (accessed January 16, 2008).

out-of-pocket expenses for Part A benefits on the basis of an annual period. In-stead, a single episode of eligibility for Part A benefits (and the associated de-ductible) is defined as the time from admission to a hospital until the patient has been out of the hospital or skilled nursing facility for at least 60 days. All Part A benefits received during this period (including the case of a readmission) are cov-ered by one deductible and co-insurance fee. Conversely, a beneficiary who needs two episodes of Part A benefits in the same calendar year that are more than 60 days apart owes two deductibles and the appropriate co-insurance fee for each episode of care. This scenario would typically not occur in the private health insurance market.

In our hypothetical example, consider the implications of the benefit period on the potential cost of care to be paid by Mrs. Miller. She enters the hospital for a total hip replacement, paying the initial $1,024 in charges as her deductible. Sce-narios A and B in Case I illustrate the effect of the benefit period in calculating Medicare Part A benefits. Both scenarios describe another hospital admission for a complication related to her total hip replacement. In scenario A, Mrs. Miller owes nothing for the care, because it occurred within 60 days of her discharge from the skilled nursing facility (i.e., the two episodes of care were within the same benefit period). In scenario B, Mrs. Miller is required to pay another deductible expense for the care, because it occurred after the first benefit period expired. Even though her two episodes of care occurred within the same calendar year, Mrs. Miller needs to pay an additional $1,024 deductible for this hospital stay.

Case Example: Medicare Part A Benefit Period

Mrs. Miller is admitted to the hospital for a total hip replacement. She spends 4 days in the hospital and another 20 days in a skilled nursing facility, receiving nursing care, physical therapy, and occupational therapy services.

Out-of-Pocket Cost to Mrs. Miller

Deductible: *$1,024*
Co-Insurance: *$0*
Total: *$1,024*

A. *Ten days after returning home, Mrs. Miller develops hip pain due to a dislocation and re-enters the hospital for a five-day inpatient stay. She returns home after being discharged from the hospital.*

Out-of-Pocket Cost to Mrs. Miller

Deductible: *$0*
Co-Insurance: *$0*
Total: *$0*

OR

B. *Three months after returning home, Mrs. Miller develops hip pain due to a dislocation and re-enters the hospital for a five-day inpatient stay. She returns home after being discharged from the hospital.*

Out-of-Pocket Cost to Mrs. Miller

Deductible: *$1,024*
Co-Insurance: *$0*
Total: *$1,024*

Skilled Nursing Facility Benefit

The skilled nursing facility (SNF) benefit under Medicare Part A provides short-term (up to 100 days) nursing and skilled rehabilitation services in a Medicare-certified unit per benefit period that is related to the recovery from an acute hospital stay. Medicare does not pay for long-term institutionalization, nor can beneficiaries access the SNF directly without a hospital stay. Medicare-certified skilled nursing facility units are located both in freestanding nursing homes and in hospitals. Hospital units are commonly referred to as subacute, swing bed, transitional care, or restorative care units (see Chapter 10). Although they are physically within an acute care hospital, these units are licensed as skilled nursing facility beds, and Medicare patients receiving unit services are covered by the SNF benefit. Prior to admission to an SNF unit, a patient must have had at least a three-day stay in a hospital during the preceding 30 days and be certified for admission to the SNF by a physician.

Each Medicare beneficiary who receives services in an SNF is assessed and reassessed with a standardized examination set called the *Resident Assessment Instrument,* or RAI (Center for Medicare and Medicaid Services 2007). The RAI consists of three parts: the Minimum Data Set (MDS), Resident Assessment Protocols (RAPS), and Utilization Guidelines. The MDS provides a comprehensive description of the status and problems being experienced by the nursing home resident. Problems that are identified or changes in patient function trigger a RAPS. The Utilization Guidelines provide information about the implementation of the RAI, which represents a significant improvement in the coordination and planning of care for Medicare beneficiaries in skilled nursing facilities and has been applied internationally. Occupational and physical therapists working in such a facility will be involved with the RAI on a daily basis. In the next section, we introduce the main features of the RAI.

Minimum Data Set (MDS)   The MDS is a "core set of screening, clinical and functional status elements, including common definitions and coding categories, which forms the foundation of the comprehensive assessment for all residents of long-term care facilities certified to participate in Medicare or Medicaid." (Center for Medicare and Medicaid Services 2007). Currently, the MDS is implemented in a second version (v. 2.0); a third version is nearing implementation. The MDS is used in all Medicare- or Medicaid-certified SNFs. The MDS is required for any resident staying in a facility for more than 14 days. MDS assessment is coordinated by a registered nurse, with input from a variety of professionals, including physical and occupational therapists. A list of the major sections of the MDS can be found in Table 7–4 ■. In order to conduct the assessment, the resident must be observed, communicated with, and examined by staff over several days.

The schedule of MDS assessment depends on the anticipated length of stay and the reason for the beneficiary's stay. As part of their Part A benefit, persons in the facility for a short-term stay related to a hospital admission (e.g. rehabilitation for a total hip replacement) are assessed at days 5, 14, 30, 60, and 90 of the stay. The

---

Active Learning Exercise

Go to http://www.cms.hhs.gov/NursingHomeQualityInits. Navigate to the link to MDS 2.0 for Nursing Homes. Scroll down to the MDS All Forms Download link. Click on it to be able to review the MDS form. Familiarize yourself with this assessment. You will be providing information into the assessment when seeing clients and patients in a skilled nursing facility.

Table 7–4.   Major Sections of v. 2.0 Minimum Data Set

A. Identification and background information
B. Cognitive patterns
C. Communication/hearing patterns
D. Vision patterns
E. Mood and behavior patterns
F. Psychosocial well-being
G. Physical functioning and structural problems
H. Continence in last 14 days
I.   Disease diagnoses
J.   Health conditions
K. Oral/nutritional status
L. Oral/dental status
M. Skin condition
N. Activity pursuit patterns
O. Medications
P.   Special treatments and procedures
Q. Discharge potential and overall status

Source: Center for Medicare and Medicaid Services. Minimum Data Set v. 2.0. http://www.cms.hhs.gov/NursingHomeQualityInits/downloads/MDS20MDSAllForms.pdf (accessed May 17, 2007).

information obtained is used to set reimbursement rates for their stay (see Resource Utilization Group payment). For persons anticipating a longer SNF stay (see Chapter 8 on Medicaid), the MDS is administered at admission, quarterly, annually, and when a significant change in patient status occurs.

RAPS are a structured process whereby the care team identifies, analyzes, addresses, and follows up on patient problems. Most commonly implemented when patients are long-term residents of an SNF, RAPS will be explained in Chapter 8, on Medicaid.

Home Health Care Benefit

Patients qualify for the home health care benefit on the basis of a need for home confinement or skilled nursing and/or rehabilitation services, including physical therapy and occupational therapy. Home health care therapy is provided in the patient's residence, which need not be an institutional setting. Physician certification of home confinement is necessary. In general, patients may not leave the home, except for necessary medical treatments (e.g., a visit to a physician) or occasional community outings (e.g., attending a church service). Home health care services are ordered by a physician, who is required to recertify the continued need for skilled care every 62 days.

Patients may qualify for Medicare reimbursement of home health care as a Part A benefit or a Part B benefit. Those who are enrolled in both Part A and Part B Medicare are entitled to 100 visits of home health care if they meet the general

Table 7–5. Outcome Assessment and Information Set (OASIS) Major Sections

A. Demographics and patient history
B. Living arrangements
C. Supportive assistance
D. Sensory status
E. Integumentary status
F. Respiratory status
G. Elimination status
H. Neuro/emotional/behavioral status
I. ADL/IADLs
J. Medications
K. Equipment management
L. Need for therapy

Source: Center for Medicare and Medicaid Services. Outcome Assessment and Information Set. Start of Care Version. http://www.cms.hhs.gov/HomeHealthQualityInits/12_ HHQIOASISDataSet.asp#TopOfPage (accessed May 17, 2007).

eligibility criteria and have had a 3-day hospital stay within the prior 14 days. If they exceed the 100-visit limit, they are able to continue necessary home health care through Part B Medicare financing.

Everyone receiving home health care services is evaluated with a tool called the Outcome and Assessment Information Set, or OASIS (Center for Medicare and Medicaid Services 2007). OASIS assesses and describes the care needs of persons receiving home health care and serves as the primary data set used to determine home health prospective payment. OASIS can be completed by a physical therapist or an occupational therapist, and initial assessment must be completed within five days of referral for care. There are several forms of the OASIS survey: start of care and resumption of care, follow-up, transfer to an inpatient facility, and discharge. OASIS collects information in a checklist format about patient demographics, history, diagnosis, living arrangements, social support, attributes (e.g., sensation and integument), performance of activities of daily living, medications, equipment, and need for therapy (see Table 7–5 ■). OASIS is to be completed within five days of the start of a home health care episode, between day 55 and day 60 of a continuing episode, and within two days of the completion of a home health care episode. Data are reported to the Center for Medicare and Medicaid Services through state contacts on a monthly basis.

Active Learning Exercise

Go to http://www.cms.hhs.gov/HomeHealthQualityInits and navigate to the OASIS Data Set page. Scroll down and click on the Start of Care version of OASIS. Familiarize yourself with this assessment. For a therapy-only client, you will need to complete it when you provide therapy services for these Medicare beneficiaries in their homes.

**Table 7–6. Patient Diagnoses That Satisfy the 60 Percent Rule for Inpatient
Rehabilitation Facilities**

- Stroke
- Spinal cord injury
- Congenital deformity
- Amputation
- Major multiple trauma
- Fracture of the femur
- Brain injury
- Polyarthritis, including rheumatoid arthritis
- Neurological disorders, including multiple sclerosis, motor neuron disease, and
  polyneuropathy, muscular dystrophy and Parkinson's disease
- Burns

Source: Carter C.M., O. Hayden, B.O.Wynn. "Case Mix Certification Rule for Inpatient
Rehabilitation Facilities." Rand Corp. 2003. http://www.rand.org/pubs/drafts/2005/
DRU2981.pdf (accessed May 22, 2007).

Inpatient Rehabilitation Facility Benefit

The inpatient rehabilitation facility (IRF) benefit provides for intensive and coordinated therapy services in a rehabilitation hospital setting. Patients must require at least three hours of therapy each day to qualify for this benefit. The requirement is termed the "three-hour rule." Also, the facility must meet the "60 percent rule" to participate in this benefit: At least 60 percent of the facility's patients must be from certain diagnosis categories (Carter, Hayden, and Wynn 2003). The intent of the rule is to prevent overutilization of therapy for cases that do not require it. A list of the diagnoses can be found in Table 7–6 ■. A review of this list will provide the reader with a good sense of the problems found in patients in this setting.

Each Medicare beneficiary is evaluated with the use of a standard assessment tool called the Inpatient Rehabilitation Facility—Patient Assessment Instrument (IRF—PAI) (Center for Medicare and Medcaid Services 2001) (see Table 7–7 ■). The instrument should be completed within three days of admission and seven days of discharge from inpatient rehabilitation. All sections of the instrument are required to be completed, except the Medical Needs and Quality Indicator sections. The central evaluation piece of the IRF—PAI is the Functional Independence Mea-

---

Active Learning Exercise

Go to http://www.cms.hhs.gov/cmsforms/downloads/cms10036.pdf to view the Inpatient Rehabilitation Facility—Patient Assessment Instrument. If you work in an inpatient rehabilitation facility, this assessment will be used for every Medicare Part A beneficiary.

Table 7–7.   Inpatient Rehabilitation Facility—Patient Assessment Instrument Major Sections

- Background and demographic information
- Medical information
- Medical needs
- Functional modifiers
- Functional Independence Measure score
- Discharge information
- Quality indicators

Source: Center for Medicare and Medicaid Services. Inpatient Rehabilitation Facility-Patient Assessment Instrument. http://www.cms.hhs.gov/InpatientRehabFacPPS/downloads/CMS-100036.pdf (accessed May 22, 2007).

sure (the FIM^{TM}). This tool was widely used by inpatient rehabilitation facilities prior to the development of the IRF—PAI and was introduced in Chapter 3 as a quality measure.

Hospice Benefit

Hospice services are provided to Medicare beneficiaries who select this treatment option and have been diagnosed with a terminal illness. Core hospice services identified by Medicare for coverage are nursing, social services, medicine, and counseling. Physical therapy and occupational therapy are among the optional hospice benefits.

PART B: SUPPLEMENTARY MEDICAL INSURANCE (SMI)

Benefits

Medicare Part B pays for most of the costs of health-related professional services, outpatient care, home health care, durable medical equipment, prosthetics, and orthotics. Each beneficiary is responsible for a $135 annual Part B deductible before receiving program benefits and also is responsible for a 20 percent co-insurance rate (see Medicare Part B reimbursement). Medicare Part B will pay for therapy services provided in outpatient departments, homes, residential facilities, and, in certain circumstances, other inpatient environments (e.g., skilled nursing facilities).

Provider Types

Medicare Part B regulations define different types of therapy providers. All Medicare Part B provider types are reimbursed via a fee schedule (see Part B reimbursement).

Therapy services must meet program requirements (see Medicare and Therapy section), but some slightly different rules apply at each of these settings.

Outpatient Hospital Programs   Hospital outpatient programs (e.g., radiology, rehabilitation, laboratory services) provide a wide range of medically necessary, skilled services to community-dwelling Medicare beneficiaries.

Comprehensive Outpatient Rehabilitation Facility   A comprehensive outpatient rehabilitation facility (CORF) is a multidisciplinary provider that allows a beneficiary to receive multiple rehabilitation services at one location (CMS 2004).

A CORF consists of at least the following services: physician care, physical therapy, and social services. In addition, occupational therapy, speech/language therapy, respiratory therapy, nursing, prosthetics, and orthotics services can be offered through a CORF.

Physical Therapists and Occupational Therapists in Private Practice   Physical therapists in private practice (PTPP) and occupational therapists in private practice (OTPP) are two other recognized Medicare Part B provider types (Center for Medicare and Medicaid Services 2007). In Part B, physical and occupational therapists in solo practices, unincorporated partnerships, unincorporated group practices, and physician/non- physician group practices can be recognized as therapists in private practice. Physical therapists employed in institutional (Part A) environments are not eligible for this classification. These therapists apply for Medicare reimbursement through their regional intermediary. They must maintain an independent office with sufficient equipment to practice in order to qualify as a Medicare provider under Part B.

MEDICARE AND THERAPY SERVICES

The need for rehabilitation is a major criterion that qualifies an individual for a Medicare-funded stay in a skilled nursing facility, for services at home through a home health agency, or for therapy as an outpatient in a clinic environment. The intent of the benefit is for the patient to continue the process of recovery after an acute illness and hospital stay. The Medicare program defines certain requirements for outpatient therapy services that qualify as meeting a Medicare benefit (Center for Medicare and Medicaid Services 2007):

- Therapy services were required by the condition of the beneficiary.
- The beneficiary must be under the care of a physician or a nonphysician practitioner.
- A plan of care exists that was designed by the therapist or physician/nonphysician practitioner and is periodically reviewed and approved by the physician or nonphysician practitioner.
- Services must be provided on an outpatient basis (outpatient benefit only).

- All of the above requirements are certified by the physician or nonphysician practitioner as having been met.

Let's explore each of these requirements in detail.

Therapy Services The Medicare program defines therapy services as physical therapy, occupational therapy, and speech-language pathology. Other professions (including recreational therapy, athletic training, kinesiotherapy, and massage therapy) are not eligible to participate in the therapy benefit. Therapy services must be provided by licensed providers (not students or aides). Physical therapists, occupational therapists, speech language pathologists, physical therapist assistants, and occupational therapy assistants can participate in the Medicare program under the therapy benefit. If care is provided by the assistant, then "general supervision" must be provided by the therapist, except for the physical therapist in private practice, where "direct supervision" is required. Physicians and, if allowed by state law, nonphysician providers, may also participate under the therapy benefit "incident to" services provided in their practice, as long as they meet the other program requirements (e.g., documentation).

Therapy Services Are Required by the Condition of the Patient Implicit in the purpose of the therapy benefit is the assumption that the care is "reasonable and necessary" on the basis of the needs and condition of the beneficiary. The determination of reasonable and necessary care is based on the plan of care (see shortly) and a definition of "skilled" physical therapy and occupational therapy. Table 7–8 ■ summarizes the components of the Medicare definition of skilled therapy services. Table 7–9 ■ provides some examples of skilled therapy services. The definition of skilled therapy

Table 7–8. Medicare Definition of Skilled Therapy Services

1. The services must be of a level of complexity and sophistication, or the condition of the patient must be of a nature, that requires an occupational or physical therapist.
   a. Or the supervision of a therapist (i.e., the services of a physical therapist assistant or occupational therapy assistant).
      1. Services must be provided with proper supervision.
   b. The diagnosis or prognosis of the beneficiary is not enough to demonstrate the need for skilled therapy services.
2. The services must be provided with the expectation that the condition of the patient will improve in a reasonable and generally predictable period of time, the services must be necessary for the establishment of a safe and effective maintenance program, or, in the case of a progressive degenerative disease, periodic visits are permitted to make equipment changes or provide services to maximize function.

Source: Center for Medicare and Medicaid Services. "Sec. 220.01 Conditions of Coverage for Outpatient Physical Therapy, Occupational Therapy and Speech-Language Pathology Services" www.cms.hhs.gov/manuals/Downloads/bp102c15.pdf (accessed May 17, 2007).

Table 7–9. Selected Examples of Medicare Definitions of Skilled Rehabilitation Services

A. Physical Therapy
    1. Evaluation and reevaluations
    2. Designing a plan of care
    3. Regular assessment of the patient's condition
    4. Patient and family instruction
    5. Selection of adaptive equipment

Source: Center for Medicare and Medicaid Services. "Sections. 220 and 230 Conditions of Coverage for Outpatient Physical Therapy, Occupational Therapy and Speech-Language Pathology Services." www.cms.hhs.gov/manuals/Downloads/bp102c15.pdf (accessed May 17, 2007).

services is important because most private insurance companies also will utilize this definition in determining the appropriateness of therapy services for reimbursement.

Care that does not meet the definition of skilled therapy services is nonskilled therapy care and is not reimbursed by the Medicare program. Maintenance therapy is one example of nonskilled care. For example, general exercise and routine assistance with activities of daily living and ambulation are not covered by the Medicare benefit. However, a therapist who develops a maintenance therapy program is providing a skilled service. In addition, therapy services are skilled when they are provided to a beneficiary with a progressively degenerative condition who needs periodic services (e.g., equipment updates) to improve function.

The condition of the patient is an important determinant of the need for therapy services. For example, diagnosis, age, comorbidities, social status, acuity/stability of the condition, risk to the patient if unskilled care is provided (e.g., for a recent fracture), and prognosis are all determinants of the need for therapy services. It is important that the status of these issues be included in the patient record.

Beneficiary Must Be Under the Care of a Physician or a Nonphysician Practitioner
The Medicare program will reimburse for therapy services only if they are provided with a referral and certification (see next subsection) of a physician or a nonphysician provider. This requirement persists irrespective of state law, which may permit a form of direct access to therapy services. A physician is defined as an allopathic physician (M.D.), an osteopathic physician (D.O.), a podiatrist, or an optometrist (low-vision services only). Dentists and chiropractors are not able to refer or certify Medicare beneficiaries for therapy services. A nonphysician practitioner is a physician assistant, a nurse practitioner, or a clinical nurse specialist. Typically, these providers practice under a practice agreement with a medical physician.

A Plan of Care Exists That Was Designed by the Therapist or the Physician or Non-Physician Practitioner
A written, active plan of care must be developed and maintained for each Medicare beneficiary. Most commonly, these plans are developed by the therapist upon referral of the physician or nonphysician practitioner.

Each plan of care must be signed by the person who developed it and must include the person's professional designation (e.g., PT or OTR). At a minimum, each plan must contain the following elements:

- Patient diagnosis
- Long-term treatment goals
- Type, amount, frequency, and duration of therapy services

The type of therapy includes the procedures to be used. The amount of therapy is the number of procedures or visits per day. The frequency of therapy is the number of visits or encounters per week. The duration of therapy is the number of weeks or sessions over time. Therapists can make minor changes in the plan of care independently (e.g., decreasing the frequency or duration of therapy). Major changes in the plan of care require certification. A change in long-term goals is an example of a major change.

Certification Occupational therapy and physical therapy services under the Medicare program must be periodically reviewed and approved by a physician or a nonphysician practitioner as meeting program requirements. Therapy services need to be certified at no less than 90-day intervals. Certifications should occur on or before the 90-day period expires. If certifications are not present on a timely basis, this is a justification for denial of payment, unless extenuating circumstances preventing such certification can be explained with the billing. A physician may request recertification at less than 90-day intervals, or a recertification should occur if there is a significant change in the patient's status.

Services Must Be Provided on an Outpatient Basis This requirement applies only to the Part B benefit. Beneficiaries receiving therapy services under Part A—in the hospital, skilled nursing facility, or home health agency—are not subject to these rules. The Medicare outpatient therapy benefit defines four groups of persons as eligible for therapy services:

- Providers to outpatients in the patients' homes
- Providers to outpatients who come to the outpatient clinic
- Providers to inpatients of other institutions
- Suppliers to outpatients in the patients' homes or in outpatient clinics.

Therapy services at home and in an outpatient clinic are covered by the Part B therapy benefit. A supplier is a therapist employed by a physician/nonphysician group practice.

Therapy Documentation The Centers for Medicare and Medicaid Services have identified several reports, with specific expectations for each report, that need to be submitted with a Part B Medicare claim. Documentation rules are important policies to understand, since noncompliance will delay or prevent reimbursement for

┌─ **Active Larning Exercise** ─────────────────────────────────┐

Go to http://www.apta.org. Type in the word "optimal" in the search box to
learn more about OPTIMAL.

└──┘

care. There are three types of therapy documentation: evaluation/reevaluation,
progress reports, and treatment notes.

Evaluation Reevaluation Therapist evaluation/reevaluation of the Medicare patient should demonstrate the need for therapy services and outline the plan of care.
The criteria for the need for therapy services and the plan of care have already
been discussed. Three comprehensive patient examination tools will provide, but
are not required for, a comprehensive documentation format needed for physical
therapists and occupational therapists:

- Patient Inquiry by Focus on Therapeutic Outcomes (FOTO)
- Activity Measure—Post-Acute Care (AM—PACS)
- OPTIMAL by Cederon by the American Physical Therapy Association

Reevaluations are typically done by therapists when the goals change (this may require new certification) or when the patient is nearing discharge from therapy.

Progress Reports/Treatment Notes Progress reports are required with each recertification in order to continue therapy services. These reports justify the continuing need for therapy care and should also demonstrate improvement in the
patient's condition. Physical therapist assistants and occupational therapy assistants
may contribute to the progress report for the patient.

Treatment notes are the daily or per-visit record of the patient's condition, the
intervention, and the patient's responsiveness to therapy. Each treatment note
needs to be dated and must include the interventions the patient received, the treatment time in minutes for any timed procedure codes, and the total treatment time.

"Incident To" Therapy Procedures

Therapy services are also a Medicare benefit when provided by a physician or a nonphysician practitioner who, within the scope of his or her state practice act, provides
care that meets all of the preceding program requirements (see also the "in-office
ancillary exception" for physician self- referral). Providers who are prohibited from
participating in the therapy benefit (e.g., athletic trainers, massage therapists, or ki-
nesiotherapists) are also prohibited from providing services incident to the physician or nonphysician practitioner care. In addition, a therapy assistant may not
provide services that are incidental to therapy in a physician's or nonphysician practitioner's office.

PART A: PAYMENT STRUCTURES

From the time Medicare was established up to 1983, Part A providers were paid based on the costs they could reasonably justify when caring for Medicare beneficiaries. The intent was to reimburse providers a fee for each service received by a beneficiary, based on "reasonable and necessary" charges in the provider's region. This method of payment, common to private insurance plans at the time, was known as **cost-based reimbursement**. Under the cost-based reimbursement mechanism, Part A providers were paid a preliminary amount for providing care during the year, and final reimbursement amounts were determined at the end of the year, after reconciliation between a cost report and the periodic interim payment. Every provider was required to produce a detailed cost report to Medicare on the direct and indirect costs of caring for beneficiaries for the year. At the end of the year, providers and the government reconciled the difference between the interim payment and final costs for the year. This retrospective system of payment offered few incentives for providers to be efficient when delivering services. As long as costs could be documented and were allowed by Medicare, providers had every incentive to provide as much care as possible and expect government payment.

Beginning with hospitals in 1983 and, since 2000, continuing with skilled nursing facilities, home health agencies, and rehabilitation hospitals, Medicare has phased out cost-based reimbursement as a Part A payment mechanism in favor of various forms of prospective payment. Cost reports are still required as an accounting report, but payment is determined on the basis of sets of predetermined criteria. Prospective payment identifies payment amounts up front, based on sets of patient characteristics, service needs, and facility characteristics determined at the time of admission to, during, or upon discharge from a Part A service. These mechanisms are all examples of case-based payment systems. Instead of being paid for each individual service (e.g., nursing, physical therapy) and procedure (e.g., ADL training) on the basis of individual facility costs, providers are paid an all-inclusive rate for a day or multiple days (an episode) of care. This case-rate payment is a lump sum for all Medicare services, with few exceptions. As we will see, prospective payment is determined with the use of a sophisticated process of classifying patients or procedures and through the calculation of average, adjusted, national costs of the services. Provider behavior incentives in prospective payment systems are the opposite of those in cost-based reimbursement systems. Acceptance of a case rate incentivizes the provider to keep the cost of care (number or intensity of services) lower than the fixed case rate amount. In effect, providers are placed on a predetermined budget with which to deliver care. We discussed the incentives of these systems in Chapter 2.

Hospital Prospective Payment

In 1983, the federal government initiated prospective payment for inpatient hospital stays by classifying patients into groups that could predict resource utilization.

This system of patient classification is called **case mix adjustment**. Several patient characteristics are used to determine which group a patient should be assigned to: diagnosis, surgery, patient age, patient sex, and discharge destination. Using these criteria, the Center for Medicare and Medicaid Services has established 579 Diagnosis-Related Groups, or DRGs, in order to classify patients at discharge from the hospital into payment groups (Center for Medicare and Medicaid Services 2006). The top 10 DRGs for hospitals in 2005 are listed in Table 7–10 ■. Reimbursement amounts for each group are established on the basis of cost report and billing information collected by CMS. DRG payments are intended to be inclusive of all direct and indirect hospital costs. Hospitals can receive other payments for patients who justifiably exceed day or cost limits and if the hospital treats a "disproportionate share" of low-income Medicare beneficiaries. The DRG methodology has been adopted internationally (Chaix-Couturier et al. 2000; Forgione and D'Annunzio 1999).

Payment to a hospital for a Part A stay is determined by multiplying a national standardized rate (approximately $4,800) by a DRG relative weight that accounts for the severity of the condition and the cost of care. For example, the surgical DRG 210 (Hip and Femur Procedures for a Person Older than Age 17) is listed with a relative weight of 1.9022. The actual payment is further modified by adjusting the labor portion of the standardized rate for local conditions and for any "add-on" payments for treating a large number of poor Medicare beneficiaries or if the facility is a teaching hospital. The average Part A hospital payment is $8,540. This payment varies significantly by location. For example, a large metropolitan hospital's average payment is $9,368, while the average rural hospital payment is $6,228. Much of this discrepancy can be attributed to labor cost differences, case severity, and add-on payment differences.

When hospital prospective payments were introduced in the 1980s, their effect on the health care system was dramatic. The DRG cost-control mechanism resulted in a sharp reduction in inpatient hospital utilization (Whetsell 1999; Takemura and Beck 1999; Menke et al. 1999). Patients spent fewer days in the hospital

Table 7–10.   Top 10 Diagnosis Related Groups in the United States (2005)

1. Heart Failure and Shock
2. Simple Pneumonia and Pleurisy
3. Major Joint and Limb Reattachment Procedures
4. Chronic Obstructive Pulmonary Disease
5. Psychoses
6. Esophagitis, Gastritis, and Digestive Diseases
7. Septicemia
8. Rehabilitation
9. Specific Cerebrovascular Disorders, except TIA
10. Gastrointestinal Hemmorrhage

Sources: Medicare Rankings for All Short Stay Hospitals by Discharges. Fiscal Year 2005 vs 2004. http://www.cms.gov/MedicareFeeForSvcPartsAB/Downloads/SSDischarges0405.pdf (accessed on May 18, 2007).

and received fewer services than in the previous cost-based reimbursement environment. The effect of the DRG system on occupational therapists and physical therapists, however, was positive. Patients needed rehabilitation services to move out of inpatient hospitals. In addition, the need for rehabilitation qualified patients for a recuperative stay in a skilled nursing facility, an inpatient rehabilitation facility, or at home. Cost-based reimbursement was maintained in skilled nursing facilities, inpatient rehabilitation facilities, outpatient hospital rehabilitation, and home health care. As a result, the demand for rehabilitation expanded in all of these settings in order to meet the needs of an increasing number of patients who were being discharged from hospitals to these levels of care at ever earlier periods. Care that was originally provided in hospitals was transferred to skilled nursing facilities and home health agencies. The demand for therapists increased.

The reorganization of care from inpatient hospital care to subacute or SNF care has caused CMS and Congress to act to limit the ability of providers to profit unfairly from an early patient discharge from a hospital to an SNF or to home health care. In 1997, Congress established a "transfer rule" that reduces the DRG payment to an acute care hospital for patients who are discharged more than one day earlier than the average for the 10 DRGS with the highest rate of acute hospital transfers to post-acute care (Gilman et al. 2000).

Part A Prospective Payment for Post-Hospital Services

As was discussed earlier, Medicare Part A includes a hospitalization benefit as well as benefits for recovery after a hospitalization in a skilled nursing facility, at home with home health services, in an inpatient rehabilitation facility, or in a hospice. The Balanced Budget Act of 1997 authorized the implementation of a national prospective payment system for Medicare Part A post-hospital services that replaced the facility-specific, cost-based reimbursement system that existed prior to 1997. The prospective payment system was phased in over six years.

Each of the payment systems calculates a case rate payment for care on the basis of the results of a standardized assessment and categorization into like patient groups. As in the hospital Diagnosis Related Groups system, payments are adjusted for local cost of living and case outliers. This case rate payment is all-inclusive; that is, each service (e.g., physical therapy) is not billed individually, but rather is included in one payment amount to the facility. Each payment does differ by the unit of service (e.g., day or episode). In this section, we will explore the three patient categorization systems and provide an example of how a case rate payment is developed.

Skilled Nursing Facility Prospective Payment Skilled nursing facility (SNF) prospective payment is based on the classification of persons residing in nursing homes into Resource Utilization Groups (RUGS) (Centers for Medicare and Medicaid Services 2007). The determination of the RUGS class for a person is based on the results of the MDS assessment, the medical diagnosis, documented therapist contact time, nursing restorative interventions, and certain behavioral observations.

MDS assessment is regularly completed by SNF staff for a 5-day, 14-day, 30-day, 60-day and 90-day report on patient status.

The intent is to identify the service needs of persons in skilled nursing facilities and to pay an all-inclusive per diem payment to providers for this care. There are 53 RUGS in one of eight categories: rehabilitation plus extensive services, rehabilitation, extensive services, special care, clinically complex, impaired cognition, behavior problems, and reduced physical function. The last 18 RUGs (making up the impaired cognition, behavior problems, and reduced physical function categories) typically do not qualify a person for skilled nursing facility payment. These patients have needs that require custodial (residential services with little expectation for improvement), not skilled, care.

The rehabilitation categories are of most interest to occupational and physical therapists working in skilled nursing facilities. Table 7–11 ■ describes the Rehabilitation subcategories of the RUGS-III classification system. Patients are classified into a group on the basis of an ADL Index Score, the number of therapy disciplines involved in the patients' care, and the amount of time spent in therapy each week. The Rehabilitation Plus Extensive Services group consists of nine RUGS categories that have differing levels of therapy intensity and functional ability, as well as at least one extensive nursing care procedure. The other rehabilitation categories are classified on the basis of therapy intensity and functional ability alone. Prospective payment for skilled nursing facility care is based on the calculation of a per diem amount that is in turn based on a federal standard base rate that is adjusted by (1) a conversion factor related to the Resource Utilization Group classification and (2) a cost-of-living factor for local wage conditions. (An example is provided later.) These payments are updated each year for inflation.

Home Health Agency Prospective Payment   Home health agency prospective payment was implemented in 2000 (Centers for Medicare and Medicaid Services 2007). In this system, home health agencies are paid on the basis of a 60-day episode of care. This payment is intended to cover all home health services (including physical therapy and occupational therapy) received by the beneficiary during that period. Durable medical equipment is excluded from this payment mechanism and is paid on the basis of a fee schedule (see Part B reimbursement). Using historical claims and cost report data, CMS determines a "standardized prospective payment rate." In 2007, the rate was $2,339 per episode of care (Center for Medicare and Medicaid Services). Similar to the SNF prospective payment formula, the prospective payment rate is adjusted for individual patient needs and regional differences in the cost of care.

The effect of individual patient needs on provider reimbursement is based on the determination of a home health resource group (HHRG) classification. Data for this classification are generated from the OASIS that is completed at admission and from a record of the number of therapy hours received by the beneficiary. These data determine three domains used to classify the patient into one of 80 HHRGs: clinical severity factors, functional severity factors, and services utilization factors (see Table 7–12 ■). Points are awarded for patient status in each of these

Table 7–11.   Resource Utilization Groups: Rehabilitation Subcategories

Rehabilitation Plus Extensive Services

Receiving one of the following extensive services:
Parenteral/IV medication
IV Medication
Suctioning
Tracheostomy care
Ventilator or respirator AND

Ultra-High Rehab and ADL Score 16–18	RUGS Group RUX
Ultra-High Rehab and ADL Score 7–15	RUGS Group RUL
Very High Rehab and ADL Score 16–18	RUGS Group RVX
Very High Rehab and ADL Score 7–15	RUGS Group RVL
High Rehab and ADL Score 13–18	RUGS Group RHX
High Rehab and ADL Score 7–12	RUGS Group RHL
Rehab Medium and ADL Score 15–18	RUGS Group RMX
Rehab Medium and ADL Score 7–14	RUGS Group RML
Rehab Low and ADL Score 7–18	RUGS Group RLX

Ultra-High

At least 720 minutes of therapy per week
At least two disciplines involved, one at
  least five days per week

ADL Index Score 16–18	RUGS Group RUC
ADL Index Score 9–15	RUGS Group RUB
ADL Index Score 4–8	RUGS Group RUA

Very High

At least 500 minutes of therapy per week
At least one discipline with patient five
  days per week

ADL Index Score 16–18	RUGS Group RVC
ADL Index Score 9–15	RUGS Group RVB
ADL Index Score 4–8	RUGS Group RVA

High

At least 325 minutes of therapy per week
One discipline five days per week

ADL Index Score 13–18	RUGS Group RHC
ADL Index Score 8–12	RUGS Group RHB
ADL Index Score 4–7	RUGS Group RHA

(continued)

Table 7–11. **Resource Utilization Groups: Rehabilitation Subcategories**
(*Continued*)

Medium

At least 150 minutes of therapy per week	
Five days of therapy across three disciplines	
ADL Index Score 15–18	RUGS Group RMC
ADL Index Score 8–14	RUGS Group RMB
ADL Index Score 4–7	RUGS Group RMA

Low

45 minutes of therapy per week over at least three days	
Nursing rehabilitation six days per week, two activities	
ADL Index Score 14–18	RUGS Group RLB
ADL Index Score 4–13	RUGS Group RLA

Source: Center for Medicare and Medicaid Services. Medicare Program: Prospective Payment System and Consolidated Billing for Skilled Nursing Facilities; Final Rule 42 CFR Parts 409, 411, 424 and 489. 2006. http://www.cms.hhs.gov/snfpps/downloads/cms-1282-f-display.pdf (accessed May 22, 2007).

Table 7–12. **Home Health Prospective Payment: HHRG Case Mix Classification**
Criteria

Clinical Severity	Functional Status	Service Utilization
Primary home care diagnosis	Dressing	No discharge last 14 days
IV/infusion/parenteral/ enteral therapies	Bathing	IP rehab/SNF discharge past 14 days
Vision	Toileting	10 or more therapy visits
Pain	Transfers	
Wound/lesion	Locomotion	
Multiple pressure sores		
Most problematic pressure ulcer stage		
Stasis ulcer status		
Dyspnea		
Urinary incontinence		
Bowel incontinence		
Bowel ostomy		
Behavioral problems		

Source: Health Care Financing Administration, 42 CFR Parts 409, 410, 411, 413, 424 and 484. Medicare Program; Prospective Payment System for Home Health Care Agencies; Final Rule. Table VII. *Federal Register* 65(128): 41194.

criteria, and the total in each domain scores the domain as minimum, low, moderate, high, or maximum. The combination of three domains with five different scores creates 80 Home Health Resource Groups (HHRGs). As with RUGS, each HHRG is assigned a case mix weight factor that reflects the intensity of services received or health problems experienced by the beneficiary. This case mix factor is used in combination with a local wage condition factor to determine the prospective payment rate.

After the implementation of home health prospective payment, there remain fewer home health agencies across the country, but nearly all Medicare beneficiaries are receiving necessary services (Office of the Inspector General 2000). There has been no increase in hospital admissions or emergency room visits as a result of this new payment system (Office of the Inspector General 2000).

Inpatient Rehabilitation Facility Prospective Payment

The third Part A prospective payment system is for inpatient rehabilitation facilities. The structure of the system is similar to that used by hospitals and home health agencies. Each patient is evaluated with the use of the Inpatient Rehabilitation Facility—Patient Assessment Instrument (IRF—PAI). Information from the IRF—PAI is used to classify patients into Case Mix Groups (CMGs) that are used for payment purposes (Centers for Medicare and Medicaid Services 2007). Each CMG is assigned a weight that is multiplied by a national standard payment conversion factor. In 2007, this payment conversion factor was $12,981. As with hospitals and home health agencies, this is a per episode payment, and as in the examples of hospitals, skilled nursing facilities, and home health agencies, the final payment to the facility is adjusted for local wage conditions and certain outlier characteristics.

Case Example of a Part A Prospective Payment System Calculation

Each of the Part A prospective payment systems utilizes a common method to derive a payment to a provider for beneficiary services. The payment systems share the following characteristics:

- Use of a standardized patient assessment instrument
- Classification of patients into homogeneous groups based on the results of the assessment (case mix adjustment)
- Adjusting a standardized payment amount by a case mix adjustment weight factor and certain other factors (e.g., local wage conditions)
- Consolidated or all-service inclusive billing

The results of most of these systems is a per episode payment to the facility. The skilled nursing facility payment is per day, not per episode. The SNF RUGS system

Table 7–13. SNF Prospective Payment: Federal Per Diem Rate Calculations for RUX

Unadjusted Federal Per Diem Rate (Urban) $335.62

Nursing case mix: $142.05	Therapy case mix: $106.99
Therapy non-case mix: $14.09	Non-case mix: $72.49

RUX Conversion

Nursing case mix (1.9): $269.88
Therapy case mix (2.25): $240.73
Non-case mix: $72.49
Total per diem rate: $583.10

Wage Conditions Adjustment

Total labor-related component: $442.22
Adjusted for Omaha: $417.89 (× 0.9450)
Adjusted for San Francisco: $670.67 (× 1.5166)
Total non-labor-related component: $140.80
Total per diem rate in Omaha: $558.69
Total per diem rate in San Francisco: $811.47

Source: Center for Medicare and Medicaid Services. Medicare Program. Prospective Payment System and Consolidated Billing for Skilled Nursing Facilities Update Notice. *Federal Register.* CMS-1530-N. http://www.cms.hhs.gov/snfpps/downloads/cms-1530-n.pdf (accessed May 22, 2007).

provides a common and useful example to see the application of these systems. Table 7–13 ■ illustrates an example from the SNF PPS.

In this example, the RUX Resource Utilization Group has been selected. The RUX group is in the Rehabilitation Plus Extensive Services category and would be used for a beneficiary requiring one of the extensive services and the most intensive therapy services in a skilled nursing facility. The baseline for the per diem rate is an unadjusted federal rate, either for an urban facility or a rural facility. In this example, an urban facility has been selected. Four components of the base rate are identified: nursing case mix, therapy case mix, therapy non-case mix, and non-case mix. The case mix costs vary by RUGs group. No therapy case mix or non-case mix cost is included in RUGs that do not include a rehabilitation service. The unadjusted per diem federal rate is $335.62. As can be seen in the example, the unadjusted rates are then updated in a two-step process. First, the RUGs' conversion rate is applied to the case mix value. In this example, the RUX conversion factor is 1.9 for a nursing case mix and 2.25 for a therapy case mix. This changes the per diem rate to $583.10, reflecting the greater service needs of these beneficiaries. The second step is to adjust the rate for the local-cost-of-living condition, specifically labor costs. To do so, the labor portion of the per diem rate is multiplied by a conversion factor. In this example, the Omaha conversion factor is .9450 and the San Francisco conversion factor is 1.5166. As can be seen, this results in a final per diem rate that is lower in Omaha than in San Francisco, reflecting differences in the cost of living between these two communities.

MEDICARE PART B: PAYMENT STRUCTURE

Earlier in this chapter, we reviewed the criteria for the Part B Medicare therapy benefit. Physical therapists and occupational therapists who bill for these services use the Physicians Fee Schedule. This is the same billing system used by physicians in outpatient practice, except that a financial limitation called a "therapy cap" (see shortly) has been placed on the benefit.

Fee Schedule

The Medicare Part B payment methodology for physical and occupational therapy services is the **fee schedule**. A Medicare fee schedule is a list of procedures with associated payments based on the estimated costs of delivering them. This list of procedures is coded in Current Procedural Terminology, or CPT (American Medical Association 2002). Physical therapists and occupational therapists use codes in the 97000 series, or "Physical Medicine and Rehabilitation" section, of the CPT. Some of the therapy codes are procedure-only codes and some are timed codes. For example, evaluation codes are one-unit procedure-only codes, irrespective of time spent on the evaluation. Many procedures (e.g., therapeutic exercise) are timed codes, which are based on a 15-minute procedure length called a unit of therapy. CMS has further defined treatment units (see Table 7–14 ■).

Fee schedule payments for each code are determined with the use of a cost-determination method called the Resource-Based Relative Value Scale, or RBRVS.

Table 7–14.   Counting Minutes for Timed Codes in 15-Minute Units

< 8 minutes	0 Units
>= 8 minutes through 22 minutes	1 Unit
>= 23 minutes through 37 minutes	2 Units
>= 38 minutes through 52 minutes	3 Units
>= 53 minutes through 67 minutes	4 Units
>= 68 minutes through 82 minutes	5 Units
>= 83 minutes through 97 minutes	6 Units
>= 98 minutes through 112 minutes	7 Units
>= 113 minutes through 127 minutes	8 Units

Source: Center for Medicare and Medicaid Services. Medicare Claims Processing Manual. "Chapter 5: Part B Outpatient Rehabilitation and CORF/OPT Services." http://www.cms.hhs.gov/manuals/downloads/clm104c05.pdf (accessed May 22, 2007).

The fee schedule payment for each procedure can be calculated by the following formula (Center for Medicare and Medicaid Services 2006):

[Resource Value Unit for Work × BN Adjuster × Geographic Practice Cost Index] + [Resource Value Unit for Practice Expense × Geographic Practice Cost Index] + [Resource Value Unit for Malpractice × Geographic Practice Cost Index] × National Conversion Factor = Fee Schedule Payment

Each year, CMS calculates a "value unit" for each procedure. This unit represents the technical ability, knowledge, and skill required to perform the procedure. In 2007, a "budget neutrality" factor was added to the work relative value unit to limit any program cost increase. Similarly, value units are determined for the overhead costs that are necessary to perform the procedure (practice expense and malpractice). Each of these three components of the RBRVS is adjusted for differences in local costs of providing the procedure to beneficiaries. The sum of the adjusted factors is multiplied by a standard national payment amount to determine the fee schedule payment.

Consider the example in Table 7–15 ■. We will use the Physical Therapy Evaluation CPT code to illustrate how a fee-schedule payment amount is determined. The

Table 7–15. Medicare Part B Reimbursement: Fee Schedule

Physical Therapy Evaluation: CPT 97001

2007 National Conversion Factor: $37.8985
Work-related RVU: 1.20
  Geographic practice cost index adjustment
    Omaha (× 0.959) = 1.151
    San Francisco (× 1.06) = 1.272
Practice expense RVU: 0.67
  Geographic practice cost index adjustment
    Omaha (× 0.876) = 0.587
    San Francisco (× 1.546) = 1.036
Malpractice expense RVU: 0.05
  Geographic practice cost index adjustment
    Omaha (× 0.47) = 0.024
    San Francisco (× 0.64) = 0.032
Total relative value units (RVU) = 1.92
  Adjusted total for Omaha = 1.762
  Adjusted total for San Francisco = 2.34
Fee schedule payment for 97001
  Standard amount (1.92 × 37.8985) = $72.77
  In Omaha (1.762 × 37.8985) = $66.78
  In San Francisco (2.34 × 37.8985) = $88.68

Source: Medicare Program. Revisions to Payment Policies Under the Physician Fee Schedule for Calendar Year 2007; Final Rule. *Federal Register.* http://www.cms.hhs.gov/quarterlyproviderupdates/downloads/cms1321fc.pdf (accessed May 22, 2007).

occupational therapy evaluation CPT Code (97003) has similar resource value units. Each relative value unit (RVU) has a factor applied to it that accounts for the work-related and practice-overhead costs associated with the procedure. Each RVU is further adjusted by a local cost index (the GPCI). As can be seen, this adjustment increases the RVU factor in San Francisco compared with Omaha. The sum total of the adjusted RVUs is multiplied by the national conversion factor to determine the fee schedule amount for this CPT code. The fee-schedule payment in San Francisco is about one-third more than a physical therapist in Omaha would expect.

Provider Participation

Medicare Part B providers, including physical therapists and occupational therapists in private practice, can elect to accept or not to accept the fee schedule amount as payment in full. This is called accepting or declining **Medicare assignment**. A provider who accepts the Medicare assignment agrees to the fee schedule amount as payment in full for the procedure, less the deductible and 20 percent co-insurance that is the responsibility of the beneficiary. A provider who does not accept Medicare assignment can still obtain Part B reimbursement, but agrees to accept a 5 percent reduction in payment from the Medicare fee schedule reimbursement. This provider can charge the beneficiary the full charge for the procedure, up to 15 percent over the fee schedule amount. The difference between the fee schedule amount and the provider charge, along with the deductible and co-insurance, is the responsibility of the beneficiary.

Financial Limitations on Medicare Part B Therapy Services

For many years, there has been a financial limit on the responsibility of Medicare to pay for therapy services provided by physical therapists or occupational therapists in private practice. Nonphysician practitioners providing therapy are also included under the cap (APTA 2007). In 2007, the limit was set at $1,780 per beneficiary per year. The $1,780 limit applies separately to occupational therapy, but is a combined limit for speech/language pathology and physical therapy. Beneficiaries receiving services in outpatient clinics, at home, and in skilled nursing facilities are affected. Beneficiaries receiving services in outpatient hospital environments are not subject to the therapy cap.

For some beneficiaries, this "therapy cap" has been burdensome, so Congress has acted since to place a moratorium on the therapy caps for most of the period

---

Active Learning Exercise

For current information on the terapy cap, visit http://www.apta.org and type in the word "therapy cap" in the search feature.

since 2000. More recently, Congress has acted by providing an "exceptions process" for medically necessary therapy that exceeds the cap. A KX coding modifier is being used to note services exceeding the cap.

MEDICARE ADVANTAGE PLANS

The Balanced Budget Act of 1997 created a new part of the Medicare program: Part C reorganized and expanded the Medicare-managed care programs and choices for beneficiaries. Currently, most beneficiaries can choose either to continue with traditional Medicare (Parts A and B) or to receive their Medicare benefits through a range of managed care options (Part C). In 2003, Congress reformed Medicare again by enactment of the Medicare Prescription Drug, Improvement, and Modernization Act of 2003 (Sculley and Roskey 2004). This act represented a shift in policy towards increasing competition by encouraging private companies and unions to contract with the government, and providers to provide Medicare benefits, as opposed to the traditional policy of the government contracting directly with providers (Gold 2005). The Part C plans were included in what are termed **Medicare Advantage** plans.

There are four types of Medicare Advantage plans (Center for Medicare and Medicaid Services 2007):

- Medicare health maintenance organizations (HMOs)
- Medicare preferred provider organizations (PPOs)
- Private fee-for-service plans
- Medicare Special Needs Plans

Medicare health maintenance organizations are similar in structure to the HMOs discussed in Chapter 6. Medicare HMOs are paid a capitated member rate based on the county of residence of the beneficiary. They are associated with lower hospitalization rates, fewer inpatient days (Zeng et al. 2006), and being less expensive (Safran, Wilson, Rogers, Montgomery, and Chang 2002). For the more seriously ill beneficiaries, however, the out-of-pocket costs can be higher (Biles, Hersch-Nicholas, and Guterman-Stuart 2006). Medicare PPOs are new to the program and are also patterned after PPOs in the private insurance market. The Centers for Medicare and Medicaid Services have established 26 market regions for PPO development (Benko, 2004). During the demonstration project, most PPOs were found in metropolitan areas, had a prescription drug benefit, and had mid-range monthly premiums and out-of-pocket costs, compared with HMOs, traditional Medicare, and Medigap plans (Pope, Greenwald, Kautter, Olmsted, and Mobley 2006). Private fee-for-service plans are offered by private insurance companies, but, as opposed to the HMO option, the provider is paid on a per service basis (Center for Medicare and Medicaid Services 2004). These plans can raise out-of-pocket costs, and providers may bill the beneficiary up to 15 percent more than the fee schedule amount (see Provider Participation section). Medicare Special Needs Plans are new and provide a managed care option for persons who have certain chronic diseases or disabling conditions, live in institutional environments (e.g., a nursing home), or are Medicare–Medicaid dual eligible (see Chapter8) (Piper 2006).

About 8.5 million Medicare beneficiaries receive their benefits through a Medicare Advantage Plan (Centers for Medicare and Medicaid Services 2007). About three in four enrollees have some form of a health maintenance organization that includes a prescription drug benefit (see Medicare Part D). Favorable selection (i.e., selecting healthier beneficiaries), market instability, and lack of rural access have been identified as problems in Medicare-managed care plans (Morgan, Vernig, DeVito, and Persily 1997; Khan, Tsai, and Kung 2002; Biles, Dallek, and Nicholas 2004; McBride, Terry, and Mueller 2006). Higher government payments to insurance companies have been enacted to improve plan availability, but at an increased cost to the program (Biles, Nicholas, and Cooper 2004).

MEDICARE PART D

Medicare Part D was added to the Medicare program in 2003 with the enactment of the Medicare Modernization Act (Center for Medicare and Medicaid Services 2007). Medicare Part D establishes an outpatient prescription drug benefit for beneficiaries. The Medicare Part D program is a continuation of the policy to increase private health plan activity in the Medicare program. Rather than being a government-sponsored standard benefit, the Medicare Part D benefit uses competing private pharmacy benefit plans. There are two mechanisms for participating in Medicare Part D: a stand-alone prescription drug plan and a plan integrated into a Medicare Advantage plan.

To participate in Medicare Part D, a beneficiary pays a monthly premium and other co-payments. The amount of these out-of-pocket costs varies by the type of plan. Payment of these fees provides the beneficiary with access to outpatient prescription drugs at a reduced cost. The types of drugs are limited by the formulary developed by the plan and, in certain cases, prior approval of the health plan. A formulary is a list of drugs that are covered by the plan. The government requires at least two drugs per class to be included in the formulary. In addition, the Part D benefit has a coverage gap for annual costs between $2,400 and $3,850. This means that if a person's drug costs are between these two amounts, there is no insurance coverage. The standard plan covers most costs under $2,400 or over $3,850 per year. Low-income beneficiaries are eligible for assistance with out-of-pocket costs.

PRIVATE HEALTH INSURANCE AND MEDICARE

As we have seen, the traditional Medicare program provides many insurance benefits for beneficiaries, but also has significant deductibles and co-payments. In addition, the benefit package does not cover foreign medical care services or some preventive health care services. As a result, some private insurance companies offer a Medicare supplemental, or **Medigap**, policy that beneficiaries can purchase to cover these other expenses (Center for Medicare and Medicaid Services 2007). Medigap plans cannot be used to pay for out-of-pocket Medicare Advantage plan costs.

Ten Medicare supplemental plans are defined under Medicare law. An insurance company will decide which type of plan it will offer and in what states. All Medigap plans cover Part A hospital co-insurance costs and 365 extra days of care after Medicare ends, as well as Part B co-insurance costs and the cost of the first three pints of blood each year. Other plans include skilled nursing facility costs, foreign medical insurance, and certain preventive services not covered by Medicare.

QUALITY AND MEDICARE

The Medicare program ensures quality health care services through four primary processes: report cards, provider certification, utilization review, and oversight by peer review organizations (PROs). Report cards were discussed in Chapter 3 and are publicly available for several post-acute providers. Providers must submit an application to CMS in order to participate in the Medicare program. **Certification** ensures that providers are licensed and meet other minimum requirements for participation. For hospitals, accreditation by the Joint Commission on Accreditation of Healthcare Organizations (JCAHO) is evidence of certification. CMS independently surveys a small percentage of JCAHO-accredited hospitals each year. Besides certifying providers, CMS certifies managed care organizations.

Utilization review is a process of internal audit and review of the care received by beneficiaries, primarily in hospitals. Health care professionals audit patient records, discuss the plan of care with the health care team, and make recommendations regarding the appropriateness of the level of care. Utilization review committees regularly review the quality and appropriateness of care.

Utilization review is also performed by external organizations, including intermediaries, carriers, and **peer review organizations** (PROs). Intermediaries and carriers routinely monitor Medicare claims and investigate possible fraud (see next section). PROs independently contract with CMS to perform two primary functions. First, PROs conduct beneficiary protection and education functions (e.g., utilization review, investigation of providers, beneficiary complaint hot lines). Second, PROs conduct special quality-improvement projects focusing on specific areas of concern.

FRAUD AND ABUSE

Medicare fraud and abuse constitute a multibillion-dollar problem. Much of this fraud and abuse can be attributed to illegal beneficiary activity and unethical and illegal provider behavior. The False Claims Act of 1986 and the Health Insurance Portability and Accountability Act of 1996 strengthened the ability of the government to find and prosecute fraud and abuse. The most common forms of Medicare

Table 7–16.   Common Types of Medicare Fraud

- Billing for services not furnished.
- Altering claim forms to receive a higher payment.
- Duplicate billing to the beneficiary, a private insurer, or Medicare.
- Falsely representing the nature of the services provided.
- Soliciting, offering, or receiving a kickback.
- Billing a person who has Medicare for services provided to someone who does not have Medicare.
- Using another person's Medicare card for services.

Source: Centers for Medicare and Medicaid Services. Definitions and Examples of Fraud. 20.3.1 In *Medicare General Information, Eligibility and Entitlement.* Chapter 1: General Overview. http://www.cms.hhs.gov/manuals/downloads/ge101c01.pdf (accessed May 23, 2007).

fraud are listed in Table 7–16 ■. In addition to these types of fraud, provider waivers of beneficiary payment of the Medicare deductible or co-insurance are another form of Medicare fraud.

Fiscal intermediaries, carriers, and "program safeguard contractors" perform routine and special audits of many types of provider activities, including practice patterns. Utilization review by these organizations has three levels. Level I reviews the utilization pattern against an "edit" (i.e., a defined number of visits or days of treatment, used to initially screen claims for appropriateness). A Level II review is a focused review by a health professional (e.g., an occupational therapist or physical therapist), who reviews the documentation to determine whether the care meets Medicare guidelines for appropriateness (e.g., did the care deliver a skilled or a nonskilled service? was the physician certified to deliver such care?). A Level II review may result in a denial of payment on a Medicare claim or referral to a Level III review. A Level III review is an onsite review of patient-care documentation and Medicare billing records. In response to the increased efforts of the government to reduce Medicare fraud and abuse, compliance programs are being established by providers in order to avoid allegations of fraud. These programs emphasize timely and accurate documentation and the avoidance of improper business relationships between Medicare providers and contractors.

Fraud is defined as "making false statements or representations of material facts in order to obtain some benefit or payment for which no entitlement would otherwise exist" (Medicare General Information, Eligibility and Entitlement p. 9). Abuse is considered to be "practices that either, directly or indirectly, result in unnecessary costs to the Medicare program" (Medicare General Information, Eligibility and Entitlement p. 10). The difference between fraud and abuse is often the intent of the person committing the crime. Examples of Medicare abuse can be found in Table 7–17 ■.

It is important for therapists to understand the definitions and common causes of Medicare fraud and abuse. A conviction of Medicare fraud can result in

Table 7–17. Common Types of Medicare Abuse

- Overcharging for service and supplies
- Providing medically unnecessary services that do not meet professional standards
- Billing Medicare on a higher fee schedule than that for non-Medicare patients
- Submitting bills to Medicare that are the responsibility of another insurer

Source: Centers for Medicare and Medicaid Services. Definitions and Examples of Abuse. 20.3.2 in *Medicare General Information, Eligibility and Entitlement.* Chapter 1: General Overview. http://www.cms.hhs.gov/manuals/downloads/ge101c01.pdf (accessed May 23, 2007).

Active Learning Exercise

The Office of the Inspector General of the Department of Health and Human Services is responsible for combating fraud and abuse in the Medicare and Medicaid programs. Go to http://www.oig.hhs.gov and learn more about the activities of this office. Examine the List of Excluded Individuals and Entities to see the public listing of persons or organizations who are suspended from participation in Medicare or Medicaid.

---

expulsion from participation in the program, financial penalties, and/or prison time. A finding of Medicare abuse risks a fraud investigation and also will result in denial of payment for the claim.

Physician Self-Referral Restrictions

Section 1877 of the Social Security Act prevents physicians from making referrals to certain health care providers or organizations that they or their families own or for which they receive a financial compensation. The intent of this law is to prevent unnecessary utilization of Medicare benefits. Therapists are one type of provider that is restricted by this law. The restriction is subject to an "in-office ancillary exception," which allows a physician or another person in the physician's office who is under direct supervision to provide therapy procedures. The procedures must be applied in an identified building and must use the physician's or group's billing number in the claim that is filed (APTA 2004).

MEDICARE REFORM

Reform of Medicare has been ongoing since the program's inception. The first 15 years of the program were marked by an expansion of eligibility (e.g., persons with disabilities or end-stage renal disease) and program benefits (the program has funded numerous medical innovations, e.g., joint replacements). Since 1983, the

Medicare program has implemented multiple cost-restraint initiatives (e.g., prospective payment systems). In its 35-year existence, Medicare has become the largest funder of the health care system. Bruce Vladeck (1999), a former Medicare administrator, described the relationship between the growth of the Medicare program and the U.S. medical care system in the last quarter-century as the development of a "Medicare-industrial complex." For many communities, hospitals and health care are as valuable for their economic effect as for their effect on health. The strength of Medicare, then, has a direct effect on the viability of the economic and medical care systems.

Wilensky and Newhouse (1999) outline several major challenges for Medicare in the future. First, the current system of controlled pricing is inefficient, is difficult to administer, and adds significant indirect costs to the system. Second, the benefits package has not been comprehensively updated since the program's inception and is out of date. This has created a large market for Medigap plans that are often too expensive for the poor and other vulnerable populations. Persons without Medigap coverage face significant out-of-pocket expenses and, as a result, probably do not have access to necessary services. Third, the aging of the baby-boom generation will put additional strain on the program to deliver benefits while the number of Americans paying into the system in relation to those receiving benefits declines.

To face these challenges, Congress has so far employed primarily provider payment restrictions. These restrictions are politically acceptable because they affect few beneficiaries, but they are bureaucratic, do not address beneficiary utilization rates, and reinforce interest-group politics. Other proposals for reform include means-testing the program, similarly, in principle, to the way Medicaid is means-tested, and raising the age of eligibility. The new Part B premiums are an example of this reform. Raising the eligibility age is politically unpopular and transfers the cost of health care for persons currently covered by the program (at age 65) to the private sector, which is becoming increasingly reluctant to bear the costs of health care.

Medicare reform is likely to continue into the coming decades, as Congress and the president struggle with the rising demand for health care by elderly and disabled Americans and as the numbers of workers who pay into the program decline. Physical therapy and occupational therapy will be affected by whatever changes are enacted in the future.

CONCLUSION

Medicare is the largest single source of funding for medical care in the United States. Established in 1965 as a federal entitlement program, namely, Title XVIII of the Social Security Act, Medicare has four parts: hospital insurance, supplementary medical insurance, managed care plans, and an outpatient prescription drug benefit. Medicare Part A covers inpatient hospital stays and services, home health care and hospice care, and short-term skilled nursing facility care. Medicare Part B covers outpatient services, including physical therapy and occupational therapy. Medicare Part C provides a range of managed care options for beneficiaries. Medicare Part D provides an outpatient prescription drug benefit, either as part of a managed care plan or as a stand-alone benefit. Medicare has been effective in improving the quality of life for persons over age 65 and for persons with permanent disability or end-stage renal disease. It has revolutionized reimbursement systems for providers by defining provider types and implementing cost-based reimbursement models, prospective payment systems, and the fee schedule. As the population ages, Medicare will continue to grow in importance as a major influence on the health care system.

CHAPTER REVIEW QUESTIONS

1. Describe the social and political reasons for the development of Medicare.
2. Define the four parts of Medicare.
3. Who is eligible for Medicare Part A?
4. Define and describe the services of Medicare Part A.
5. What is cost-based reimbursement? Prospective payment?
6. Identify the patient classification systems used for
    a. inpatient hospital care
    b. skilled nursing facility care
    c. home health care
    d. inpatient rehabilitation hospital care
7. What three factors determine a prospective payment rate?
8. Who is eligible for Medicare Part B?
9. Define and describe the services of Medicare Part B.
10. Define the types of therapy providers in Medicare Part B.
11. Identify the criteria and describe how Medicare defines therapy services.
12. What is a fee schedule and how are fee schedule payments determined?
13. Who is eligible for Medicare Part C plans and what are the benefits offered?
14. Describe how the Medicare program ensures the quality of its health plans.
15. Define the most common forms of Medicare fraud and abuse.
16. Review the challenges that will confront the Medicare program in the next decade.

CHAPTER DISCUSSION QUESTIONS

1. Medicare's founders have stated that the Medicare program is one step on the road toward national health insurance. From your understanding of the program, what would be the advantages and disadvantages of using the Medicare model as a template for national health insurance?

2. Discuss how the Medicare definition of the therapy benefit promotes and inhibits the development of occupational therapy and physical therapy as autonomous professions.
3. Consider the examples of Medicare fraud and abuse. Discuss how you can practice so as to avoid committing Medicare fraud.

REFERENCES

American Medical Association. 2002. *Current Procedural Terminology: CPT.* Chicago: American Medical Association.

American Physical Therapy Association (APTA). 2004. *Highlights of the Stark II Phase II Regulations.* http://www.apta.org/AM/Template.cfm?Section=Fraud_and_Abuse&Template=/CM/ContentDisplay.cfm&CONTENTID=22176 (accessed May 24, 2007).

American Physical Therapy Association (APTA). 2007. *Medicare Therapy Cap Resource Center.* http://www.apta.org/AM/Template.cfm?Section=Therapy_Cap&Template=/TaggedPage/TaggedPageDisplay.cfm&TPLID=188&ContentID=18639 (accesed May 23, 2007).

Ball, R.M. 1995. What Medicare's architects had in mind. *Health Affairs* 14(4): 62–72.

Benko, L.B. 2004. CMS creates 26 PPO regions. *Mod Healthc* 34(50): 8–9, 16.

Biles, B., G. Dallek, and L.H. Nicholas. 2004. Medicare advantage: Déjà vu all over again? *Health Aff Suppl Web Exclusives*: W4-586-97.

Biles, B., L.H. Nicholas, and B.S. Cooper. 2004. The cost of privatization: Extra payments to Medicare Advantage plans. Issue Brief. *Commonw- Fund* 750: 1–12.

Biles, B., L. Hersch-Nicholas, and S. Guterman-Stuart. 2006. Medicare beneficiary out-of-pocket costs: Are Medicare Advantage plans a better deal? Issue Brief. *Commonw-Fund* 19: 1–6.

Blaisdell, F.W. 1992. The pre-Medicare role of city/county hospitals in education and health care. *J Trauma* 32(2): 217–28.

———. 1994. Development of the city/county (public) hospital. *Arch Surg* 129(7): 760–64.

Carter, C.M., O. Hayden, and B.O. Wynn. 2003. Case Mix Certification Rule for Inpatient Rehabilitation Facilities. Rand Corp. http://www.rand.org/pubs/drafts/2005/DRU2981.pdf (accessed May 22, 2007).

Center for Medicare and Medicaid Services. 2001. IRF—PAI Training Manual. http://www.cms.hhs.gov/InpatientRehabFacPPS/downloads/irfpai-manualint.pdf (accessed May 22, 2007).

Center for Medicare and Medicaid Services. 2004. *Medicare Benefit Policy Manual.* "Comprehensive Outpatient Rehabilitation Facility (CORF) Coverage." http://www.cms.hhs.gov/manuals/Downloads/bp102c12.pdf (accessed May 18, 2007).

Center for Medicare and Medicaid Services. 2004. Your guide to private fee for service plans. Pub. No. CMS-10144. http://www.medicare.gov/Publications/Pubs/pdf/10144.pdf (accessed May 11, 2007).

Center for Medicare and Medicaid Services. 2006. Data Compendium. http://www.cms.hhs.gov/DataCompendium/18_2006_Data_Compendium.asp#TopOfPage (accessed March 21, 2007).

Center for Medicare and Medicaid Services. 2006. Medicare Program; Hospital Inpatient Prospective Payment Systems and Fiscal Year 2007 Rates; Notice. *Federal Register* 71(196): 59886–60043.

Centers for Medicare and Medicaid Services. 2007. Definitions and Examples of Fraud. Definitions and Examples of Abuse. 20.3.1 in *Medicare General Information, Eligibility and Entitlement.* http://www.cms.hhs.gov/manuals/downloads/ge101c01.pdf (accessed May 23, 2007).

Center for Medicare and Medicaid Services. 2007. Home Health PPS. http://www.cms.hhs.gov/HomeHealthPPS/ (accessed May 17, 2007).

Centers for Medicare and Medicaid Services. 2007. Inpatient Rehabilitation Facilities PPS. http://www.cms.hhs.gov/InpatientRehabFacPPS/ (accessed May 22, 2007).

Centers for Medicare and Medicaid Services. 2007. "Your 2007 Medicare Premiums" in *Medicare and You 2007*, 103. http://www.medicare.gov/publications/pubs/pdf/10050.pdf (accessed May 17, 2007).

Centers for Medicare and Medicaid Services. 2007. MDS 2.0 for Nursing Homes. http://www.cms.hhs.gov/NursingHomeQualityInits/20_NHQIMDS20.asp#TopOfPage (accessed May 15, 2007).

Center for Medicare and Medicaid Services. 2007. Coverage of Outpatient Rehabilitation Services (Physical Therapy, Occupational Therapy, Speech/Language Pathology) Under Medical Insurance. 120–173. http://www.cms.hhs.gov/manuals/Downloads/102c15.pdf (access May 17, 2007).

Center for Medicare and Medicaid Services. 2007. Medicare Advantage Plans. http://www.medicare.gov/Choices/Advantage.asp (accessed May 10, 2007).

Center for Medicare and Medicaid Services. 2007. Medicare Prescription Drug Coverage. http://www.medicare.gov/pdphome.asp (accessed May 23, 2007).

Center for Medicare and Medicaid Services. 2007. Choosing a Medigap policy: A guide to health insurance for people with Medicare. http://www.cms.hhs.gov/Publications/Pubs/pdf/02110.pdf (accessed May 23, 2007).

Center for Medicare and Medicaid Services. 2007. Skilled Nursing Facilities PPS. http://www.cms.hhs.gov/SNFPPS/ (accessed May 17, 2007).

Center for Medicare and Medicaid Services. Medicare Program. Prospective Payment System and Consolidated Billing for Skilled Nursing Facilities: Update: Notice. *Federal Register.* CMS-1530-N. http://www.cms.hhs.gov/snfpps/downloads/cms-1530-n.pdf (accessed May 22, 2007).

Center for Medicare and Medicaid Services. "Part B Outpatient Rehabilitation and CORF/OPT Services" in *Medicare Claims Processing Manual.* http://www.cms.hhs.gov/manuals/downloads/clm104c05.pdf (accessed May 22, 2007).

Center for Medicare and Medicaid Services. 2007. Therapy Services. http://www.cms.hhs.gov/TherapyServices (accessed May 21, 2007).

Chaix-Couturier, C., I. Durand-Zaleski, D. Jolly, and P. Durieux. 2000. Effects of financial incentives on medical practice: Results from a systematic review of the literature and methodological issues. *Int J Qual Health Care* 12(2): 133–42.

Davis, M.H., and S.T. Burner. 1995. Three decades of Medicare: What the numbers tell us. *Health Affairs* 14(4): 231–43.

Forgione, D. A., and C.M. D'Annunzio. 1999. The use of DRGs in health care payment systems around the world. *J Health Care Fin* 26(2): 66–78.

Friedman, E. 1995. The compromise and the afterthought. Medicare and Medicaid after 30 years. *JAMA* 274(3): 278–82.

Gilman, B. H., J. Cromwell, K. Adamache, and S. Donoghue. 2000. *Study of the Effect of Implementing the Post-Acute Care Transfer Policy under the Inpatient Prospective Payment System.* Waltham, MA: Health Economics Research Institute.

Gold, M. 2005. Private plans in Medicare: Another look. Even if regional plans are not widespread, MMA is likely to dramatically expand the private-sector role in Medicare. *Health Affairs* 24(5): 1302–10.

Health Care Financing Administration. 1998. Medicare Home Health Benefit: The Balanced Budget Act of 1997: Financing Shift of Home Health Services from Medicare Part A to Part B. Transmittal No. A-98-49.

Khan, M.M., W.C. Tsai, P.T. Kung. 2002. Biased enrollment of Medicare beneficiaries in HMO plans: Implications for Medicare costs. *J Health Care Finance* 28(4): 43–57.

McBride, T.D., T.L. Terry, and K.J. Mueller. 2006. Medicare Part D: Early findings on enrollment and choices for rural beneficiaries. *Rural Policy Brief* 10(8): 1–9.

Medicare Program. 1998. Changes to the Inpatient Hospital Prospective Payment Systems and Fiscal Year 1998 Rates, Final Rule. 42 CFR Parts 410 et. al., *Federal Register* (63) 26318–26360.

Medicare Program. Revisions to Payment Policies Under the Physician Fee Schedule for Calendar Year 2007; Final Rule. *Federal Register.* http://www.cms.hhs.gov/quarterlyproviderupdates/downloads/cms1321fc.pdf (accessed May 22, 2007).

Medicare Trustees Report. 2007. http://www.ssa.gov/OACT/TR/TR07/ (accessed May 24, 2007).

Menke, T.J., C.M. Ashton, N.J. Petersen, and F.D. Wolinsky. 1998. Impact of an all-inclusive diagnosis-related group payment system on inpatient utilization. *Med Care* 36(8): 1126–37.

Morgan, R.A., B.A. Vernig, C.A. DeVito, and N.A. Persily. 1997. The Medicare–HMO revolving door: The healthy come in and the sick go out. *N Engl J Med* 337(3): 169–75.

Piper, K.B. 2006. Medicare advantage: Understanding special needs plans. *Manag Care* 15(7 Suppl 3): 25–27.

Pope, G.C., L. Greenwald, J. Kautter, E. Olmsted, and L. Mobley. 2006. Medicare preferred provider organization demonstration: Plan offerings and beneficiary enrollment. *Health Care Financ Rev* 27(3): 95–109.

Reynolds, P.P. 1997. The federal government's use of Title VI and Medicare to racially integrate hospitals in the United States, 1963 through 1967. *Am J Pub Health* 87(11): 1850–58.

Rothman, D.J. 1993. A century of failure: Health care reform in America. *J Health Polit Policy Law* 18(2): 271–86.

Russell, L.B., and C.S. Burke. 1978. The political economy of federal health programs in the United States: A historical review. *Int J Health Serv* 8(1): 55–77.

Safran, D.G., I.B. Wilson, W.H. Rogers, J.E. Montgomery, and H. Chang. 2002. Primary care quality in the Medicare program: Comparing the performance of Medicare health maintenance organizations and traditional fee-for-service Medicare. *Arch Intern Med* 162(7): 757–65.

Scully, T.A., and C.T. Roskey. 2004. New directions in Medicare managed care. *Healthc Financ Manage.* 58(5): 64–68.

Takemura, Y., and J.R. Beck. 1999. The effects of a fixed-fee reimbursement system introduced by the federal government on laboratory testing in the United States. *Rinsho-byori* 47(1): 1–10.

Vladeck, B. 1999. The political economy of Medicare. *Health Affairs* 18(1): 22–36.

Whetsell, G.W. 1999. The history and evolution of hospital payment systems: How did we get here? *Nurs Adm Q* 23(4): 1–15.

Wilensky, G., and J.P. Newhouse. 1999. Medicare: What's right? What's wrong? What's next? *Health Affairs* 18(1): 92–106.

Zeng, F., J.F. O'Leary, E.M. Sloss, M.S. Lopez, N. Dhanani, and G. Melnick. 2006. The effect of Medicare health maintenance organizations on hospitalization rates for ambulatory care-sensitive conditions. *Med Care* 44(10): 900–07.

8

Medicaid, SCHIP, Military/Veterans Medical Insurance, and Indian Health Service

CHAPTER OBJECTIVES

At the conclusion of this chapter, the reader will be able to:

1. Describe the statutory authorization, size, and purpose of the Medicaid program.
2. Identify and relate the criteria for eligibility for Medicaid benefits.
   a. Discuss the impact of welfare and immigration reform on eligibility for Medicaid benefits.
3. Describe the services covered by the Medicaid program.
4. Describe the organization of services in the Medicaid program.
   a. Medicaid managed care
   b. Medicaid waiver programs
5. Describe the statutory authorization, size, and purpose of the State Children's Health Insurance Program.
6. Relate the eligibility criteria and health insurance benefits for active military and veterans' health benefit programs.
7. Describe the purpose and organization of the Indian Health Service.

KEY WORDS: Categorical Eligibility, Dual Eligibility, Means-tested, Medically Needy Eligibility, Personal Care Services, Presumptive Eligibility, Safety-net Provider, Spend down, Spousal Impoverishment, State Option, Waiver Program

Case Example

Sophia is a physical therapist working in a U.S. Public Health Service hospital for the Indian Health Service. In her role, she provides treatment and consultation services for community members seeking services. She is often asked by physicians and physician's assistants to provide consultation on whether to refer a patient to a medical specialist. She works actively in the community to provide prevention and wellness services to address diabetes mellitus, which is endemic to this population. Very few of her patients have private health insurance. It is funding from the Indian Health Service and Medicaid that provides the resources for her to work in this community.

Case Example Focus Question:

1. Consider and explain how social insurance programs support health care services in underserved communities.

INTRODUCTION

The preceding three chapters introduced and described several large insurance mechanisms that finance much of the health care system in the United States. In Chapter 5, we discussed the purpose of insurance and introduced several ways that health insurance products are organized. In Chapter 6, we learned about managed care, the dominant form of private health care insurance today. In Chapter 7, we considered Medicare, an example of social insurance and the largest insurance program, in terms of dollars spent, in the world. In this chapter, we turn our attention to other governmental health care insurance programs: Medicaid, the State Children's Health Insurance Program (SCHIP), insurance for active military personnel and veterans, and health care programs for American Indians and Alaska natives.

These insurance programs target populations that have historically not been able to obtain private health care insurance or, as in the case of the military, for whom the government has a direct responsibility for the health care of plan members. Medicaid and SCHIP serve a large and vulnerable component of our society: the poor, persons with disabilities, women, and children. The structure of Medicaid and SCHIP displays the societal tension concerning the roles of government and the private sector in providing solutions to the dilemma of access to health care insurance for everyone in the country. Both programs are federal–state partnerships. Eligibility requirements are sophisticated and limited to certain groups. Benefit packages are generous, but are increasingly relying on managed care and private insurance contracting to deliver the services.

First, we will consider Medicaid, the largest health care insurance plan, in terms of persons served, in the United States. In 1997, the increasing number of uninsured children spawned an effort to improve health care for poor children in the United States—an effort that became the State Children's Health Insurance Plan. We will explore the Veterans' Health Plan and TRICARE, a major source of funding for active and retired military beneficiaries. Finally, we will introduce the Indian Health Service.

MEDICAID

What Is Medicaid?

Medicaid is a joint federal–state medical insurance program designed to meet the health care needs of people who meet certain low-income requirements, have high medical costs, or are in certain defined, disadvantaged populations (e.g., low-income pregnant women and children). Medicaid is a **means-tested** program. Unlike eligibility in Medicare, in Medicaid a beneficiary must qualify by demonstrating a level of need usually based on low income and personal assets or on excessive medical expenses. Medicaid insures more Americans, about 49 million persons, than any other health care insurance program in the country.

Medicaid was established in 1965 as Title XIX of the Social Security Act. Medicaid replaced the small medical insurance programs for indigent persons that were offered by several states with one large national program. Medicaid insurance has improved access to medical care for poor families (Newacheck, Pearl, Hughes, and Halfon, 1998). Medicaid was one of the cornerstones of President Lyndon Johnson's Great Society program.

All 50 states and the District of Columbia participate in the Medicaid program. Each state has its own Medicaid plan that sets eligibility criteria and benefits within federal guidelines. The federal government shares with the states the cost of providing a defined package of medical care benefits to Medicaid beneficiaries. The federal share of a state's program ranges from at least 50 percent up to 76 percent of the total program cost. Poor states pay less than wealthy states. For many states and territories, these shared payments for the Medicaid program are the largest grant they receive from the federal government, and the cost of the program is one of the largest annual expenditures of state funds.

The total cost of the Medicaid program in 2005 was $313 billion (Catlin, Cowan, Heffler, and Washington 2007) (see Table 8–1 ■). Of this amount, $179 billion (57 percent) was paid by the federal government and $124 billion (43 percent) was paid by state governments. A study by the Kaiser Family Foundation found that five percent of Medicaid enrollees account for about half of program expenditures (Kaiser Commission on Medicaid and the Uninsured 2006). These persons are primarily elderly or disabled beneficiaries residing in institutional environments. Medicaid is

Table 8–1.   Medicaid General Statistics

- Total Number of Enrollees (2006): 49.3 million
- Number of Children Enrolled: 23.9 million
- Number of Adults Enrolled: 11.4 million
- Number of Persons Who Are Blind or Disabled and are Enrolled: 8.8 million
- Number of Elderly Persons Enrolled: 5.2 million
- Number of SCHIP Eligible Who Are Enrolled: 4.4 million
- Medicaid Medical Assistance Payments (2005): $313 billion
- Total Federal Share: $172 billion (57.5%)

Sources: Medicaid Enrollment and Beneficiaries, Selected Fiscal Years. 2006. Center for Medicare and Medicaid Services. http://www.cms.hhs.gov/DataCompendium/18_2006_Data_Compendium.asp#TopOfPage (accessed June 19, 2007). Catlin, Cowan, Heffler, and Washington. 2007. National health spending in 2005: The slowdown continues. *Health Affairs* 26(1): 142–53.

Table 8–2.   Medicaid Expenditures

• Hospital Care: $106 billion	• Prescription Drugs: $38 billion
• Professional Services: $78 billion	• Program Administration: $21 billion
• Nursing Home Care: $54 billion	• Home Health Care: $16 billion

Source: Catlin et al. 2007.

the largest purchaser of long-term care in the United States (Centers for Medicare and Medicaid Services 2007). Children make up about 50 percent of the Medicaid beneficiary population (Centers for Medicare and Medicaid Services 2007). However, children are typically low-cost (average $1320 per child) users of Medicaid benefits. While Medicaid is often associated with welfare and public assistance programs, it is important to recognize that it is a vital program providing insurance coverage for persons with complex medical needs related to nursing home care ($54 billion in 2005; see Table 8–2 ■).

Who Is Eligible for Medicaid?

Eligibility for the Medicaid program is determined through a complicated process of meeting one or more sets of criteria: **categorical eligibility**, **medically needy eligibility**, and Medicare–Medicaid **dual eligibility**. As a means-tested government program, Medicaid has rules which stipulate that potential participants must demonstrate that they meet certain income or assets criteria in order to receive benefits. In general, single men and childless couples are not eligible for Medicaid. Participation in the Medicaid program has been significantly affected by welfare and immigration reforms enacted in the mid-1990s. We will have more to say about the effect of these governmental actions on Medicaid after we introduce the basic eligibility criteria.

Table 8–3 ■ summarizes the basic qualifications for Medicaid benefits. The first six items outline the criteria for becoming a categorically eligible beneficiary. All states must cover individuals who meet the criteria for at least one of these categories. This type of eligibility defines the criteria that qualify many poor women, infants, and children for Medicaid benefits. Many people with disabilities receive Supplementary Social Income payments (SSI) from the Social Security program that qualify them to also receive Medicaid. Wards of the state are covered by these criteria. Besides these basic eligibility requirements, the federal government will match state costs for more liberal program-eligibility qualifications. For example, many states increase the opportunity for Medicaid eligibility by raising the family income level to 185 percent of the federal poverty level for infants in poor families (annual income of $38,205 for a family of four, based on a federal poverty level of $20,650 for a family of four [U.S. Department of Health and Human Services 2007]).

Table 8–3. Medicaid Eligibility

Mandatory Categories

1. Low-income families with children
2. Recipients of Supplemental Security Income payments
3. Children under age six and pregnant women whose family income is at or below 133 percent of the federal poverty level
4. Caretakers of children under age 18
5. Individuals and couples living in a medical institution with an income up to 300 percent of the federal poverty level

Medically Needy

Required
1. Pregnant women through a 60-day postpartum period
2. Children under age 18
3. Certain newborns to age one
4. Certain persons who are blind

Optional
1. Children ages 19 to 21 who are full-time students
2. Caretaker relatives
3. Persons age 65 or older, persons who are blind or disabled

Special Groups

1. Medicare–Medicaid Dual Eligibles
   a. Qualified Medicare beneficiary
      1. Low income: Less than or equal to 100 percent of the federal poverty level
      2. Limited personal assets: Twice the limit for SSI eligibility
2. Qualified Working Disabled Individuals

Medicaid Waiver Program

1. Expanded eligibility for persons enrolled in Medicaid managed care, either voluntarily or, under some circumstances, mandatory

Source: Center for Medicare and Medicaid Services. Medicaid At-A-Glance. 2005. http://www.cms.hhs.gov/MedicaidGenInfo/ (accessed June 18, 2007).

The medically needy eligibility criteria are a **state option** that can be included or not included in each state's Medicaid program. As an example, the criteria used in Nebraska are listed in Table 8–4 ■. These criteria allow individuals with high medical care expenses to **spend down** their assets to a certain level, after which the Medicaid program will pay for the continuing costs of care. This qualification enables many elderly persons and persons with disabilities who have high medical costs and limited private insurance to access medical and long-term care insurance benefits.

Table 8–4.   Medically Needy Criteria for Medicaid Benefits—Nebraska (2005)

1. Able to maintain $4,000 in assets/$6,000 per couple
   a. Home is exempt until the patient leaves it for a nursing home
   b. $1,500 in life insurance/$3,000 per couple
   c. One car
   d. $3,000 in a burial expense account/$6,000 per couple
2. Meet monthly income guidelines: Must be less than $392 per month.
3. Spousal Impoverishment: If one married spouse enters a nursing home, joint resources less than $19,620 remain with the community-dwelling spouse. Resources from $19,620 up to $184,000 of the couple's assets are divided in half. Any resources above $184,000 should be spent for the care of the nursing home spouse. The spouse entering the nursing home uses his or her share of the split assets and assets above $184,000 to pay for nursing home expenses until the $4,000 threshold is reached.

Source: Nebraska Medicaid Eligibility Categories. http://www.hhs.state.ne.us/med/reform/eligibility.htm (accessed June 20, 2007).

In order to qualify, one must meet two sets of financial criteria based on resources and income. Personal assets (e.g., savings and investments) must be used to pay for medical care expenses until a financial threshold is reached. The person's monthly income must also be below another threshold value. Once both these criteria are met, the person qualifies as a medically needy Medicaid beneficiary. The spend-down provision requires the person in need of care to use up personal assets first, but in most instances protects some assets and the income of a surviving spouse. A community-dwelling spouse is not forced to use up all of a couple's assets to pay for nursing home care, thus preventing a situation termed **spousal impoverishment**. States are able to prevent the transfer of assets to children, recover some previously transferred assets, and recover expenses by applying a lien on the assets of an estate in probate if a couple attempts to hide resources that could be used to pay for nursing home care.

The third method of obtaining Medicaid coverage is by qualifying for dual eligibility, which allows a low-income Medicare beneficiary to qualify for Medicaid payment of Medicare deductibles and co-insurance (see Chapter 7). Examples of dual-eligible status are persons who are "qualified Medicare beneficiaries" or "specified low-income Medicare beneficiaries." Lamphere and Rosenbach (2000) have found that many dual-eligible beneficiaries do not take advantage of this benefit because they are unaware that they qualify and the eligibility process is quite complex.

In sum, Medicaid is another example of a social insurance program. In most cases, the persons paying for the benefits are not eligible to receive the benefits. The benefits are instead transferred to another social group to meet a defined social need. Medicaid is an excellent example of an egalitarian government program (see Chapter 1). Medicaid is also a very important program for the health care industry, since it provides payment for care to persons who are uninsured and have very limited income and resources.

Medicaid Managed Care

Medicaid costs have been growing rapidly in the last decade. As a result, reform of the program has been an annual issue for most state legislatures. A common answer to increased costs has been the introduction of managed care principles into Medicaid (see Chapter 6). Unlike Medicare, managed care is the dominant form of health care delivery in state Medicaid programs. About 60 percent of Medicaid beneficiaries are enrolled in a managed care plan (Centers for Medicare and Medicaid Services 2006). In 1991, 2.7 million beneficiaries were enrolled in a managed care plan. By 2004, the number had grown to 24 million, an increase of 900 percent (Centers for Medicare and Medicaid Services 2006). Only Alaska, New Hampshire, and Wyoming do not encourage or require managed care enrollment for their Medicaid population.

Medicaid managed care takes two forms: primary care case management and capitation (Regenstein and Anthony 1998). Primary care case management contracts with physicians who provide routine care and coordinate the referral and utilization of specialty care services. Capitation forms contracts with managed care organizations to provide all the services needed by the beneficiary at a predetermined monthly rate.

Medicaid managed care has reduced health disparities, improved access to primary care, and decreased the number of unnecessary hospitalizations. Cook (2007) found that participation in Medicaid managed care lowered disparities in having a source of primary care for African Americans and Hispanic Americans, compared with other racial or ethnic groups. Managed care has been associated with a decrease in hospital utilizations (Bindman, Chattopadhyay, Osmond, Huen, and Bacchetti 2005) and the use of emergency rooms (Garrett and Zuckerman 2005; Baker and Afendulis 2005). Felland, Lesser, Staiti, Katz, and Lichiello (2003) found that the "health care safety net" for communities has been improving.

Medicaid Services

State agreement to participate in Medicaid and acceptance of matching federal funds mandates the provision of a basic set of benefits in each state's Medicaid program. The Medicaid program offers a three-tier package of benefits. A basic benefit package is established for states that offer Medicaid benefits only to categorically eligible populations. An additional benefit package is established for states that offer

---

Active Learning Exercise

Why has managed care been successful in Medicaid, but less successful in Medicare? Read *Medicare and Medicaid: A Tale of Two Trajectories*, by Hurley and Retching, available online in the *American Journal of Managed Care* (2006) at http://www.ajmc.com/Article.cfm?Menu=1&ID=3074.

Table 8–5.   Medicaid Benefits

A. Categorically Eligible Populations
1. Inpatient and outpatient hospital services
2. Laboratory and radiology services
3. Certified pediatric and family nurse practitioners
4. Nursing facility services for age 21 or over
5. Early and periodic screening, diagnosis, and treatment (EPSDT) services for those under age 21
6. Family planning services and supplies
7. Physicians' services
8. Dental services
9. Home health care for persons eligible for nursing facility services
10. Pregnancy-related services (e.g., nurse-midwife services, 60-day postpartum care)

B. Medically Needy Populations
1. Prenatal care and delivery services for pregnant women
2. Postpartum care services for persons under age 18 and persons entitled to institutional services
3. Home health services

C. Examples of Optional Benefits
1. Occupational and physical therapy
2. Prosthetics and orthotics
3. Personal care services

Source: Center for Medicare and Medicaid Services. Medicaid At-A-Glance. 2005. http://www. cms.hhs.gov/MedicaidGenInfo/ (accessed June 18, 2007).

a medically needy program. Finally, states are able to include several optional benefits at their discretion. Table 8–5 ■ lists the benefit packages offered in Medicaid.

Like other health insurance programs, Medicaid provides insurance coverage for inpatient and outpatient hospital care and physician services. Unlike the situation with most private health insurance plans, states are required to provide coverage for skilled nursing facilities for everyone over age 21. Unlike Medicare, many state Medicaid programs provide a prescription drug benefit. Medically necessary physical therapy and occupational therapy are optional services in the Medicaid program. In reality, all states must cover necessary therapy services provided to children in the early and periodic screening, diagnosis, and treatment (EPSDT) program and to categorically eligible persons over age 21 who reside in skilled nursing facilities. These are federally mandated benefits. Some therapy services are commonly covered in the hospital benefit package, but the type and intensity of the therapy that is covered varies. States may or may not pay for outpatient or home health physical therapy or occupational therapy services.

The high cost of institutionalization has encouraged the development of alternatives to expensive skilled nursing facility care. **Personal care services** are an optional

Medicaid benefit that provides for payment of a nonrelative to assist with activities of daily living or, in some cases, instrumental activities of daily living in the patient's residence. This service can allow persons with disabilities to leave their homes and be employed or enjoy other community activities. The home- and community-based **waiver program** is a comprehensive state plan to provide a benefit package to persons with disabilities in community settings rather than skilled nursing facilities.

Physical therapy and occupational therapy services are an optional benefit in the Medicaid program. Table 8–6 ■ lists states that include therapy services in their Medicaid plan. Eight states do not include therapy services. Thirty-five states and the District of Columbia cover physical therapy and occupational therapy for both their categorical and medically needy eligible populations. The remainder of the states cover therapy services only for their categorically eligible population.

Medicaid is an important part of the financing of the U.S. health care system. It is the largest insurance program in terms of persons served in the United States. It provides access to health care insurance for many groups of Americans who would otherwise have impaired access due to a lack of employment-based private

Table 8–6.   Medicaid and Therapy Services (2005)

1. States that Cover Physical and Occupational Therapy for the Categorical and Medically Needy Groups.

Arkansas	Illinois	Montana	North Dakota	Vermont
Arizona	Kansas	Nebraska	Ohio	Virginia
California	Kentucky	Nevada	Pennsylvania	W.Virginia
Colorado	Maine	New Hampshire	South Carolina	Wisconsin
District of Columbia	Maryland	New Jersey	South Dakota (PT)	Wyoming
Florida	Massachusetts	New Mexico	Tennessee	
Georgia	Minnesota	New York	Texas (PT)	
Hawaii	Mississippi	North Carolina	Utah	

2. States that Cover Physical and Occupational Therapy for the Categorical Eligibility Group.

Alaska	Oregon
Idaho (PT)	Washington
Indiana	

3. States that Do Not Cover Occupational or Physical Therapy Services in the State Medicaid Plan.

Alabama	Michigan
Connecticut	Missouri
Delaware	Oklahoma
Louisiana	Rhode Island

Source: Center for Medicare and Medicaid Services. Medicaid At-A- Glance. 2005. http://www.cms.hhs.gov/MedicaidGenInfo/ (accessed June 18, 2007).

Active Learning Exercise

Medicaid services, including occupational therapy and physical therapy, vary from state to state. The Kaiser Family Foundation maintains a current listing of state Medicaid plans, including therapy services, at http://www.kff.org/medicaid/benefits.

---

insurance. Medicaid supports safety-net providers who serve individuals in these communities. It provides a package of medical care benefits and certain social benefits that are not covered in traditional health care insurance plans (e.g., personal care services, long-term skilled nursing facility care). Access to occupational therapy and physical therapy services is generally available, but is not consistent among states. Medicaid is also the best example of the utilization of managed care principles in a public health care insurance program.

STATE CHILDREN'S HEALTH INSURANCE PROGRAM (SCHIP)

The State Children's Health Insurance Program (SCHIP) is a federal–state program that provides health insurance to about 4 million children in the United States (Centers for Medicare and Medcaid, Services 2007). The program is organized as a stand-alone insurance program in 18 states, an expansion of existing state Medicaid program in 11 states, and a combination of both in 21 states. After the enactment of SCHIP in the late 1990s, the percentage of uninsured children living in homes with incomes below 200 percent of the federal poverty level decreased from 21 percent in 2000 to 14 percent in 2005 (Kaiser Commission on Medicaid and Uninsured 2007). SCHIP offers eligible children a health insurance benefit package that is similar to the health insurance package offered by their state to its employees or by the largest health maintenance organization in the state to its members. Recently, access to health insurance through SCHIP has been expanded to include the parents of uninsured children in some states.

The consensus on the SCHIP program is that it has been successful in decreasing rates of uninsured persons and in improving access to health care for low-income children and children with special needs (Kenney and Yee 2007; Seid, Varni, Cummings, and Schonlau 2006; Duderstadt, Hughes, Soobader, and Newacheck 2006; Kempe et al. 2005). Medicaid or SCHIP covers two out of five of the 13.5 million children with disabilities in the United States (Tu and Cunningham 2005). Shone, Dick, Klein, Zwanziger, and Szilagyi (2005) found a reduction in racial/ethnic disparities related to access, continuity, and quality of care due to SCHIP. Davidoff et al. (2005) found similar improvements for children with chronic conditions. Data indicate that SCHIP programs administered through an expansion of state Medicaid plans have been more effective in achieving these gains than have plans administered through a separate program (Kronebusch and Elbel 2004; Yu and Seid 2006).

VETERANS ADMINISTRATION AND MILITARY HEALTH INSURANCE PROGRAMS

The Veterans Administration (VA) operates the largest health care system in the world. In this section, we will explore the unique eligibility requirements and the benefit package offered to veterans who utilize this system. Veterans' health benefits date to the beginning of the country and the government's sense of responsibility for caring for those who have served in the military. Occupational therapists and physical therapists are important members of the VA health care team. Therapists provide services to the thousands of veterans who have experienced disability as a result of military service. Like Medicaid, the VA health system is an important component of the health care safety net for poor or disabled veterans (Hughes 2003).

Table 8–7 ■ lists the eligibility categories that qualify an individual for veterans' health benefits. Except for Priority Group 8, veterans who meet the criteria for at least one of these categories are eligible for benefits. Veterans with service-related or service-aggravated disabilities are given the highest enrollment priority. Impoverished veterans also receive priority enrollment in the VA system. Non-service-connected veterans are veterans who have not incurred or aggravated a disability while in military service. Non-service-connected veterans typically have to meet

Table 8–7. Veterans Administration Health Program Eligibility

A. Priority Group 1
 1. Veterans with at least a 50 percent service-related disability
B. Priority Group 2
 1. Veterans with a 30 to 40 percent service-related disability
C. Priority Group 3
 1. Veterans who are former prisoners of war or who have received a Purple Heart
 2. Veterans who were discharged for disability-related reasons
 3. Veterans with a 10 to 20 percent service-related disability
D. Priority Group 4
 1. Veterans who are receiving homebound benefits
 2. Veterans who are classified as "catastrophically disabled"
E. Priority Group 5
 1. Veterans receiving VA pension benefits or are Medicaid eligible
F. Priority Group 6
 1. Veterans who are not disabled, but who are receiving VA compensation
G. Priority Groups 7 and 8
 1. Non-service-connected veterans who do not meet the criteria for the other groups and agree to pay the required co-payment for services

Source: Department of Veterans Affairs. All Enrollment Priority Groups. http://www.va.gov/healtheligibility/eligibility/PriorityGroupsAll.asp (accessed June 21, 2007).

Table 8–8.   Veterans' Health Uniform Benefit Package

A. Inpatient and outpatient hospital care
B. Prescription drugs
C. Physician services
D. Mental health care
E. Home health and hospice
F. Rehabilitation therapies
G. Prosthetics and orthotics
H. Home improvements to improve structural access
    1. $4100 for service-connected disability and $1200 for non-service-connected disability.
I. Vocational rehabilitation and supported employment programs
J. Services for veterans who are blind.
K. Long-term care
L. Disability compensation
M. Automobile adaptations (one time, up to $11,000)
N. Annual clothing allowance

Source: Department of Veterans Affairs. Federal Benefits for Veterans and Dependents. http://www1.va.gov/opa/is1/9.asp (accessed June 21, 2007).

income/asset requirements or pay deductibles and copayments to receive veterans' health benefits.

Eligible veterans are entitled to a comprehensive package of health care benefits. Table 8-8 ■ lists the main components of this benefit package. Unlike private health insurance or Medicare/Medicaid, VA health insurance includes a rich benefit package for long-term care and support for persons with disabilities. Physical therapy and occupational therapy are mandated benefits in the VA health plan. In addition, prosthetics and orthotics are routinely covered. The inclusion of these benefits reflects the common connection between disability and veterans' health benefits.

The veterans' benefit package is not free to all eligible veterans. The VA health plan has established co-payments for prescription drugs, inpatient and outpatient hospital services, and nursing home care. Veterans with service-related disabilities do not pay these costs. Non-service-connected veterans are required to meet income and asset thresholds or demonstrate financial hardship to avoid making the required co-payments. The private insurance companies of insured veterans who receive care in VA health care facilities are routinely billed for the services.

The accessibility and acceptability (see Chapter 2) of VA health care is influenced by information about available benefits, the sense of entitlement by veterans, perceptions of VA benefits as welfare, and respect for the veteran by health professionals and staff (Damron-Rodriguez et al. 2004). A reversal of the racial disparities observed in the civilian health system has been reported in the VA health care system. Jha, Shilipak, Hosmer, Frances, and Browner found lower mortality rates for African Americans compared with white Americans for common conditions treated in VA facilities. They attributed this finding to better access to care and quality of treatment (2001). An emerging issue in veterans' health care is treating women veterans (Washington, Yano, Simon, and Sun 2006).

Active military personnel receive their health care through a system of military hospitals. Certain services or services for eligible dependents, however, are provided in the civilian health care system. The government insurance plan for active military personnel and their families is called TRICARE.

TRICARE consists of three insurance options for military personnel (Department of Defense 2006). TRICARE Prime uses military hospitals and clinics as the primary provider of care. It is provided at no cost to the member and with low co-payments. Access is limited to the military health care system. TRICARE Extra is a preferred provider organization that utilizes contracted civilian providers in the community. Members must use these providers and pay plan deductibles and co-payments. TRICARE Standard is the fee-for-service option. Members have an open choice of providers who will accept TRICARE, but members are responsible for claims management, paying all deductibles and co-payments, and may be responsible for claims above the allowable charge (similar to a Medicare beneficiary utilizing a nonparticipating Medicare provider).

The introduction of a managed care product into the military health plan has been demonstrated to be effective. Kravitz et al. (1998) found that managed care reduces emergency department costs, especially among repeat users with nonsevere illnesses. Zwanziger et al. (2000) concluded that a test of a military health maintenance organization product resulted in lower utilization of services, adequate patient access to services, good patient satisfaction, and little change in the cost to the government. Mangelsdorff, Finstuen, Larsen, and Weinberg's (2005) study found high patient satisfaction with the military's health care system.

INDIAN HEALTH SERVICE

The Indian Health Service (I.H.S.) was organized in 1955 as an agency of the federal government to provide health care to 1.5 million American Indians and Alaska Natives from the 557 recognized tribes living in 35 states (Indian Health Service 2007). Health care is provided for this population, which often lives in rural and isolated communities with poor access to a health care system. Health care is provided through one of two mechanisms: direct delivery and tribal self-determination. The I.H.S. operates 176 hospitals, health centers, health stations, and urban Indian health projects, all provided through the direct delivery of health care. In addition, the tribes operate 518 hospitals, health centers, residential treatment centers, health stations, and Alaska village clinics through tribal self-determination contracts with the federal government. Physical therapy and occupational therapy services have been offered through I.H.S. since the early 1960s. Therapists provide services either as civilians or as commissioned members of the Public Health Service.

Active Learning Exercise

To learn more about rehabilitation services in the Indian Health Service, go to
http://www.ihs.gov/NonMedicalPrograms/NC4/nc4-pt.asp.

CONCLUSION

In this chapter, we have explored health insurance plans other than Medicare
that are operated by the federal and state governments. Combined with
Medicare, these governmental plans fund nearly half of the United States health
care system. Eligibility for such programs reflects a public consensus that government should provide health insurance for the poor, children, persons with disabilities, active military personnel, veterans, American Indians, and Alaska
Natives. Because these classifications include so many people of so many different
backgrounds, the eligibility criteria, types of included benefits, and provider payment methods represent some of the largest and most influential health policy
decisions made by government. Recent innovations in these programs highlight
the importance of managed care as a defining mechanism for contemporary payment of health care in America.

Although Medicaid is an important source of health care insurance for low-income people with disabilities, the provision of physical therapy and occupational
therapy services is a state option. The lack of a consistent national Medicaid policy
for the disabled means that many of these individuals lack access to rehabilitation
services, especially in community-based environments. For military personnel and
veterans, rehabilitation services are a mandated benefit. This provision reflects a
belief that government has a responsibility to care for people who have served society in certain capacities.

CHAPTER REVIEW QUESTIONS

1. Review the history and origins of the Medicaid program.
2. Describe the partnership arrangement between the federal government and
   the states as it pertains to Medicaid.
3. Define the eligibility criteria for receiving Medicaid benefits.
   a. categorical eligibility
   b. medically needy
   c. Medicare–Medicaid dual eligible
4. What is included in the Medicaid benefits package?
   a. Define the position of occupational therapy and physical therapy in the
      Medicaid program.
5. Describe how managed care is utilized in state Medicaid programs.

6. Recall how welfare reform and immigration reform affected the Medicaid program in the 1990s.
7. Define the purpose of the State Children's Health Insurance Program (SCHIP), and describe its effectiveness in achieving that purpose.
8. Identify the eligibility criteria and benefits package for Veterans Affairs health insurance benefits.
9. What is TRICARE and how is it organized?
10. What are the two mechanisms of organizing health care delivery in the Indian Health Service?

CHAPTER DISCUSSION QUESTIONS

1. Physical therapy and occupational therapy are included as benefits in the Medicaid and Department of Veterans Affairs health insurance programs. Both of these insurance plans serve persons with disabilities. Compare and contrast the benefit packages. What are the reasons for these differences? Do you agree with them?
2. The eligibility criteria for the Medicaid program are good examples of the policy "balancing act" between the egalitarian and libertarian views of the role of government in health care. Examine closely the traditional criteria and the recent immigration criteria. Analyze and discuss these criteria from both the egalitarian and libertarian points of view.
3. Managed care is increasingly being used in public insurance programs. Managed care has been more easily implemented in the Medicaid, SCHIP, and TRICARE programs than in Medicare. What are the reasons for this situation? How does it reflect our political and social realities?

REFERENCES

Baker, L. C., and C. Afendulis. 2005. Medicaid managed care and health care for children. *Health Serv Res* 40(5 Pt 1): 1466–68.

Bindman, A. B., A. Chattopadhyay, D. H. Osmond, W. Huen, and P. Bacchetti . 2005. The impact of Medicaid managed care on hospitalizations for ambulatory care sensitive conditions. *Health Serv Res* 40(1): 19–38.

Catlin, A., C. Cowan, S. Heffler, and B. Washington. 2007 National health spending in 2005: The slowdown continues. *Health Affairs* 26(1): 142–53

Centers for Medicare and Medicaid Services. 2006. Medicaid Managed Care Overview. http://www.cms.hhs.gov/MedicaidManagCare/ (accessed June 20, 2007).

———. 2007. SCHIP Enrollment Reports. http://www.cms.hhs.gov/NationalSCHIP Policy/SCHIPER/itemdetail.asp?filterType=none&filterByDID=-99&sortByDID=2 &sortOrder=ascending&itemID=CMS1199248&intNumPerPage=10 (accessed June 20, 2007).

Cook, B. L. 2007. Effect of Medicaid managed care on racial disparities in health care access. *Health Serv Res* 42(1 Pt 1): 124–45.

Damron-Rodriguez, J., W. White-Kazimepour, D. Washington, V. M. Villa, S. Dhanani, and N.D. Harada. 2004. Accessibility and acceptability of the Department of Veterans Affairs health care: Diverse veterans' perspectives. *Mil Med* 169(3): 243–50.

Davidoff, A., G. Kenney, and L. Dubay. 2005. Effects of the State Children's Health Insurance Program expansions on children with chronic health conditions. *Pediatrics* 116(1): e34–42.

Department of Defense. Tricare Handbook. http://www.tricare.mil/tricarehandbook/ (accessed June 21, 2007).

Duderstadt, K. G., D.C. Hughes, M.J. Soobader, and P.W. Newacheck. 2006. The impact of public insurance expansions on children's access and use of care. *Pediatrics* 118(4):1676– 82.

Felland, L.E., C.S. Lesser, A.B. Staiti, A. Katz, and P. Lichiello. 2003. The resilience of the health care safety net, 1996– 2001. *Health Serv Res* 38(1 Pt 2): 489–502.

Garrett, B., and S. Zuckerman. 2005. National estimates of the effects of mandatory Medicaid managed care programs on health care access and use, 1997–1999. *Med Care* 43(7): 649–57.

Holahan, J., S. Zuckerman, A. Evans, and S. Rangarajan. 1998. Medicaid managed care in thirteen states. *Health Affairs* 17(3): 43–63.

Hu, H. T., and P. J. Cunningham. 2005. Public coverage provides vital safety net for children with special health care needs. Issue Brief. *Cent Stud Health Syst Change* 98: 1–7.

Hughes, J.S. 2003. Can the Veterans Affairs health system continue to care for the poor and vulnerable? *J Amb Care Manage* 26(4): 344–48.

Indian Health Service. 2007. About the Indian Health Service. http://www.ihs.gov/ AboutIHS/index.asp (accessed October 9, 2007).

Jha, A. K., M.G. Shilipak, W. Hosmer, C.D. Frances, and W. S. Browner. 2001. Racial differences in mortality among men hospitalized in the Veterans Affairs health care system. *JAMA* 285(3): 297–303.

Kaiser Commission on Medicaid and the Uninsured. 2006. Medicaid's high cost enrollees: How much do they drive program spending? http://www.kff.org/medicaid/ 7490.cfm (accessed June 20, 2007).

———. 2007. The State Children's Health Insurance Program: Lessons and outlook. http://www.kff.org/medicaid/7628.cfm (accessed June 20, 2007).

Kempe, A., B.L. Beaty, L.A. Crane, J. Stokstad, J. Barrow, S. Belman, and J.F. Steiner. 2005. Changes in access, utilization and quality of care after enrollment into a state child health insurance plan. *Pediatrics* 115(2): 364–71.

Kenney, G., and J. Yee. 2007. SCHIP at a crossroads: Experiences to date and challenges ahead. *Health Aff* 26(2): 356–389.

Kravitz, R. L., J. Zwanziger, S. Hosek, S. Polich, E. Sloss, and D. McCaffrey. 1998. Effect of a large managed care program on emergency department use: Results from the CHAMPUS reform initiative evaluation. *Ann Emerg Med* 31(6): 741–48.

Kronebusch, K., and B. Elbel. 2004. Enrolling children in public insurance: SCHIP, Medicaid, and state implementation. *J Health Polit Policy Law* 29(3): 451–89.

Lamphere, J. A., and M. L. Rosenbach. 2000. Promises unfulfilled: Implementation of expanded coverage for the elderly poor. *Health Serv Res* 35(1 Pt. 2): 207–17.

Mangelsdorff, A.D., K. Finstuen, S.D. Larsen, and E.J. Weinberg. 2005. Patient satisfaction in military medicine: Model refinement and assessment of Department of Defense effects. *Mil Med* 170(4): 309–14.

Newacheck, P., M. Pearl, D. C. Hughes, and N. Halfon. 1998. The role of Medicaid in ensuring children's access to care. *JAMA* 280(20): 1789–93.

Regenstein, M., and S. E. Anthony. 1998. Assessing the new federalism: Medicaid managed care for persons with disabilities. *http://www.newfederalism.urban.org/pdf/occal1.pdf* (accessed July 14, 2000).

Seid, M., J.W. Varni, L. Cummings, and M. Schonlau. 2006. The impact of realized access to care on health-related quality of life: A two year prospective cohort study of children in the California State Children's Health Insurance Program. *J Pediatr* 149(3): 354–61.

Shone, L.P., A.W. Dick, J.D. Klein, J. Zwanziger, and P.G. Szilagyi. 2005. Reduction in racial and ethnic disparities after enrollment in the State Children's Health Insurance Program. *Pediatrics* 115(6): e697–705.

U.S. Department of Health and Human Services. 2007. 2007 HHS Federal Poverty Guidelines. http://aspe.hhs.gov/poverty/07poverty.shtml (accessed January 17, 2008).

Washington, D., E.M. Yano, B. Simon, and S. Sun. 2006. To use or not to use: What influences why women veterans choose VA health care. *J Gen Intern Med* 21 (Suppl 3): S11–8

Weissman, J. S., R. Witzburg, P. Linv, and E. G. Campbell. 1999. Termination from Medicaid: How does it affect access, continuity of care, and willingness to purchase insurance? *J Health Care Poor Under* 10(1): 122–37.

Yu, H., and M. Seid. 2006. Uninsurance among children eligible for the State Childrens Health Insurance Program: Results from a national survey. *Manag Care Interface* 19(5): 31–39.

Zwanziger, J., R. L. Kravitz, S. D. Hosek, K. Hart, E. M. Sloss, D. Sullivan, J. D. Kallich, and D. P. Goldman. 2000. Providing managed care options for a large population: Evaluating the CHAMPUS reform initiative. *Mil Med* 165(5): 403–10.

9

The Acute Medical Care System

CHAPTER OBJECTIVES

At the conclusion of this chapter, the reader will be able to:

1. Explain the historical development of the hospital.
2. Describe the administrative structure of hospitals.
3. Define a hospital by size, ownership, and scope of services.
4. Compare and contrast primary, secondary, tertiary, and quaternary care.
5. Describe the development of integrated health care systems.
6. Discuss the development and results of physician–hospital integration in the acute medical care delivery system.

KEY WORDS: Hospitals, Integrated Health Care System, Matrix System, Patient-focused Care, Physician–Hospital Organization, Primary Care, Product-line Team, Quaternary Care, Secondary Care, Tertiary Care

Case Example

Jim M. Charge is the director of occupational therapy in Anytown Hospital. Jim is responsible for patient care and the supervision of four occupational therapists in his area. The administration of Anytown Hospital has decided to expand its rehabilitation services, which include physical therapy and speech–language pathology. The reason for this expansion is that the hospital wants to develop a unit to treat persons who have suffered either a stroke or a hip fracture. As a result of the change, Jim has been asked to lead the stroke team. This will require him to manage not only the occupational therapists in the hospital, but also physical therapists and speech–language pathologists who are working with the patients with stroke, in order to develop stronger "patient-focused care" in the hospital. This is an example of a matrix management system—a system in which people with similar skills are pooled together to accomplish certain tasks.

Case Example Focus Questions:

1. What are some reasons for, or benefits derived from, using a matrix management system?
2. How does making this change affect the hospital's organizational structure?

INTRODUCTION

In the preceding chapters, we have introduced and focused on health care policy and various forms of reimbursement for health services. With this chapter, we will begin to discuss the health care system. Upcoming chapters will discuss the post-acute care system (Chapter 10), the mental health care system, public health, educational environments, and alternative medical providers (Chapter 11). In Chapter 12, we will discuss advocacy, or how therapists can act to change the system.

When we think of the U.S. health care system, we commonly break it down into two broad categories: an acute care medical delivery system and a post-acute care delivery system (see Figure 9–1 ■). The acute care medical delivery system includes primary, secondary, tertiary, and quaternary care systems. The post-acute care system consists of a mix of subacute care, long-term care, outpatient services, home health care, and hospice care. This chapter focuses mainly on the acute care medical delivery system and, in particular, on one of the biggest players in this system: the hospital.

Hospitals are arguably one of the most recognized and least understood entities of the health care system. Hospitals are home to many activities related to health care, including patient care, medical education, and research functions. Additionally, hospitals are usually one of the major employers in a community and are major employers of occupational therapists, physical therapists, and therapist assistants. In this chapter, we examine hospitals and the acute care medical system more closely and explain their role in the health care system. We discuss the historical development of hospitals, their diverse functions and characteristics, their management structures, and their position within the primary, secondary, tertiary, and quaternary health care system. We conclude with a discussion of the various forces that both constrain and promote change in the hospital industry. An understanding of the hospital's role in the health care system and the external forces that influence it is critical to therapists because it is, in large part, within the health care environment that they must interact.

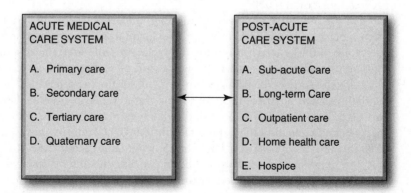

ACUTE MEDICAL CARE SYSTEM	POST-ACUTE CARE SYSTEM
A. Primary care	A. Sub-acute Care
B. Secondary care	B. Long-term Care
C. Tertiary care	C. Outpatient care
D. Quaternary care	D. Home health care
	E. Hospice

Figure 9–1.   The United States Health Care System

HOSPITALS

Historical Development

The hospitals that existed in early America were very different from the hospitals that we have today. The first hospitals were primarily charitable religious organizations whose missions were focused more on providing care to those they served than on curing their illnesses (Freymann 1974; Starr 1982). Early hospitals tended to care for and shelter the poor, elderly, orphaned, and homeless, in addition to protecting society from those who were contagious or dangerously insane (Sultz and Young 1999). Thus, these early hospitals were nothing more than infirmaries for the sick and the poor, and people with sufficient financial resources received care at home. Hospitals were commonly characterized as dirty and overcrowded environments with limited medical capabilities. The focus was on the caring not the curing of patients.

From the late 1800s to the early 1900s, hospitals began to evolve into the physician's workshop. Advances in biomedical science and technology made it more difficult and complex for physicians to have everything they needed in their "black bags" (Kovner 1995). While earlier hospitals had provided more care than cure, hospitals during this period were better able to provide a cure and a means of intervention. Because of improvements in science and technology, the hospital industry experienced a large growth in the number of hospitals, and by 1909 there were more than 4,300 hospitals, compared with just 178 in 1873 (Stevens 1971).

A second major era of growth took place between 1945 and 1980. Two major events contributed to this growth: Federal monies became available to build new hospitals under the Hill-Burton Act, and the rapid growth of hospital insurance, including Medicare and Medicaid, increased the diversity and number of services offered to a hospital's inpatients (Kovner 1995). Without clear and consistent oversight, however, these policies resulted in creating a hospital environment characterized by overbuilding and overcapacity, which resulted in a call for hospitals to become more accountable and efficient. During this era, the number of hospitals grew to more than 6,000.

In part because of this overbuilding and overcapacity, hospitals in the 1990s experienced consolidation through the formation of networks and through closure. One of the several reasons for these changes included the cost of building and maintaining a hospital, especially in a period of cost control. In some cases, hospitals have closed because of a declining demand for their services. Mergers or consolidations were pursued to establish integrated delivery systems. **Integrated health care systems** are discussed in more detail later in this chapter. Partially due to these mergers and consolidations, the total number of community hospitals for the years 1999 through 2005 has been stable at approximately 4,900 (KFF 2007).

An overview of this developmental process on therapy services was presented in Chapter 1. As physical therapy and occupational therapy services developed in the first half of the 20th century, much of this growth occurred within hospitals. Physical therapy and occupational therapy were commonly viewed as an extension of medical care, another service in the "physician's workshop." In the second half of the 20th century, private practice (primarily in outpatient environments) emerged as a workplace for therapists. With this development, an autonomous identification of occupational therapy and physical therapy as distinct fields increased. However, the emergence of integrated health systems represents new threats and opportunities for therapists to respond and shape the health care system of the 21st century. Hospitals and outpatient clinics will remain an important site of therapy services in this system. In the next several subsections, we briefly examine the managerial structure of hospitals and their unique characteristics.

Hospital Structure

Hospitals have a complex administrative structure that is reflective of their growth into established organizational institutions. Since physicians have the ability to control the type and amount of services patients consume, physicians have always had, and still have, an important role in the organization and management of hospitals. For years, physicians or leaders of religious organizations managed hospitals. However, the complexity of hospital management led to the creation of the field of health services management. A traditional hospital structure includes a board of directors, an administrative structure, and a medical staff structure (see Figure 9–2 ■). Physical therapy and occupational therapy services may be positioned under the health services administrator or the medical director.

A board of directors is selected that retains fiduciary responsibility to manage and govern the hospital. This includes the hiring of a management team. Physicians are commonly represented on the hospital's board of directors. Therapists and other health professions (e.g., nursing) are not typically represented at this level of governance. Historically, hospital administrators were responsible primarily for nonclinical matters, such as finance, personnel, community/public relations, and the hospital's "hotel" functions (laundry, housekeeping, etc.). However, in today's environment, strategic planning and negotiating ability are critical skills for the successful health care executive.

A hospital structure also includes a medical division, usually headed by a physician known as the chief of the medical staff who is the liaison to the hospital administration and who commonly serves on the board of directors. A medical division is commonly divided into departments by medical specialty (e.g., internal medicine, surgery). The medical division has important oversight over the credentialing of health care professionals (i.e., determining their right to admit patients, perform surgery, etc.) and provides consultation about the quality of care in the hospital.

Other clinical professions are represented in various ways. Organizationally, these professions may be placed under the hospital administration component of the structure or under the medical division. The largest unit is usually the nursing division, which is traditionally organized into subunits by types of patient treatment/pathology (e.g., orthopedics, pediatrics). Physical therapy, occupational

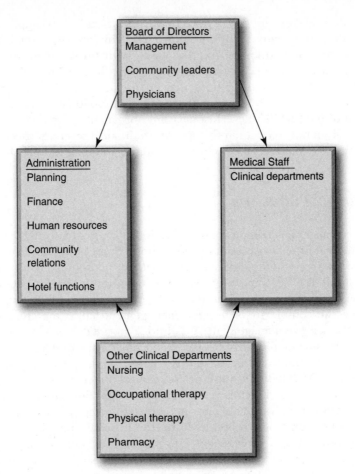

Figure 9–2.   Traditional Structure of Hospitals

therapy, and the other rehabilitation disciplines are customarily organized by discipline.

The development of **patient-focused care** caused a radical reorganization of this system. Patient-focused care organizes providers around perceived patient needs rather than professional disciplines or procedures. This type of organization avoids certain problems typical of traditional structures, such as poor communication and redundancy of services. Therapists may be organized into **product-line teams** organized around common patient conditions (e.g., stroke teams, joint-replacement teams). In this case, occupational therapists and physical therapists may be responsible to a team leader for their activities and performance. In some cases, a dual-management structure called a **matrix system** is established whereby a physical therapist may be responsible to a team leader for clinical matters and to a physical therapy manager for nonclinical matters (e.g., personnel issues) (Boissoneau 1983) (see Figure 9–3 ■).

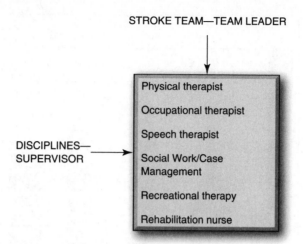

STROKE TEAM—TEAM LEADER

DISCIPLINES—
SUPERVISOR

Physical therapist

Occupational therapist

Speech therapist

Social Work/Case
Management

Recreational therapy

Rehabilitation nurse

Figure 9–3.   "Matrix" Hospital Organizational Structures

Hospital Characteristics

Hospitals differ along various dimensions, including size and scope, ownership, general versus specialty hospitals, acute care versus long-term care hospitals, teaching versus nonteaching hospitals, and independent hospitals versus those in multihospital systems or networks. This section explores these issues in greater detail.

Size

The number of inpatient beds that are set up and staffed is one indicator of the size of a hospital. Figure 9–4 ■ shows the distribution of hospitals by bed size and indicates that most hospitals are under 200 beds. The larger hospitals most likely represent large tertiary-care centers that care not only for a general population, but for a large indigent population and persons in need of advanced specialty services (e.g., trauma care).

Ownership

Hospital organizations generally have one of three types of ownership classification:

1. Hospitals operated by nonprofit organizations are referred to as not-for-profit hospitals.
2. Hospitals owned and operated by profit-making corporations are known as investor-owned or for-profit hospitals.
3. Hospitals owned and managed by either federal, state, or local government bodies are referred to as public hospitals.

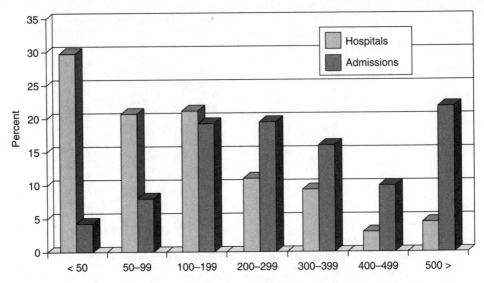

Figure 9–4.   Percentage of U.S. Hospitals by Admissions and Bed Size
Source: 2005 AHA Annual Survey Copyright 2006 by Health Forum LLC

Almost two-thirds of all community hospitals are not-for-profit organizations (Kaiser State Health Facts 2007) that are managed by community boards or religious organizations (see Figure 9–5 ■). For example, orders within the Roman Catholic Church operate some of the largest systems of medical care facilities in the United States. These hospitals are more commonly associated with local decision-making

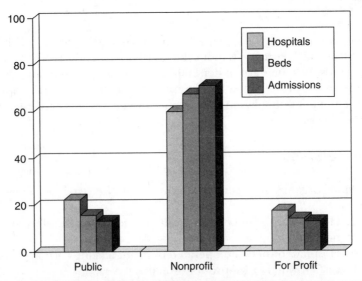

Figure 9–5.   Percentage of Hospitals, Beds, and Admissions, by Ownership
Source: 2005 AHA Annual Survey Copyright 2006 by Health Forum LLC

and the provision of charity care. In return for the latter service, the federal government has historically granted an exemption from state and federal taxation to hospitals operated by not-for-profit organizations.

Investor-owned or for-profit hospitals are dominated by national chains (e.g., Tenet Healthcare). Since the 1980s, private investment in hospitals and the development of hospital chains have grown significantly. The net revenue from for-profit hospitals is shared with outside investors, who are co-owners of the hospital. Investor participation in the hospital industry increases the amount of private capital available for medical care investment. It also has increased the emphasis on financial management in all hospitals. For-profit companies own approximately 17 percent of the hospitals in the United States (Kaiser State Health Facts 2007). Whatever its profit status, every hospital must generate some type of profit—the difference lies in how that profit is used. In a not-for-profit facility, profits are returned to the organization or community, whereas a for-profit organization distributes the profits to its shareholders.

The last type of ownership structure is the public hospital. The public hospital was the primary source of health care for the poor and indigent before the advent of Medicaid in 1965. Examples of public and government-controlled hospitals include city and county hospitals (e.g., John H. Stroger, Jr., Hospital of Cook County in Chicago), military hospitals, VA hospitals, and U.S. Public Health Service hospitals (e.g., Indian Health Service hospitals). Public hospitals provide an important safety net for the poor and for populations for which private organizations have chosen not to provide services.

In addition to these three distinct categories, a number of hybrid ownership structures exist. Some hospitals have multiple owners. For example, when a not-for-profit hospital is sold to a for-profit company, the not-for-profit organization may retain some ownership short of a majority. Additionally, some local government hospitals may be leased and managed by a for-profit organization while the government retains ownership of the hospital.

General vs. Specialty

A general hospital provides general medical services, such as ambulatory surgery, pediatric inpatient care, rehabilitation outpatient care, emergency services, open-heart surgery, angioplasty, obstetric services, and community health promotion. Alternatively, specialty hospitals provide services for either specific diseases or specifically defined populations. Examples of specialty hospitals include children's hospitals, long-term care centers, rehabilitation hospitals, mental health or psychiatric hospitals, and substance abuse centers.

Acute Care vs. Long-Term Care

Many general hospitals are acute care facilities as well. Acute care hospitals serve inpatients that have an average length of stay of no more than 30 days. Most of the patients admitted to these hospitals actually stay for less than 10 days. Patients in such

hospitals have acute short-term illnesses, compared with patients with chronic illness, who may require prolonged treatment.

Long-term care hospitals include such facilities as nursing homes, psychiatric
hospitals, and rehabilitation hospitals, as well as home health agencies. Increasingly, long-term acute care hospitals are emerging to care for persons with complex
medical problems outside of an acute care hospital. Long-term care hospitals provide care for those experiencing diminishing functional capabilities, which may
vary across age categories and chronic conditions. Care provided to these individuals may be continuous or intermittent, but will be carried on over a long time or
throughout the patient's life (Kane and Kane 1987).

Teaching Hospitals

Teaching hospitals are an important part of America's health care system. In addition to their offering sophisticated technology and cutting-edge research, they deliver a large percentage of health care services throughout the country (Iglehart
1993). They also deliver a disproportionate share of charity and indigent care. Although only a small percentage (approximately 6 percent) of all short-term nonfed-
eral acute care hospitals are classified as members of the Council of Teaching
Hospitals and Health Systems (COTH), they represent approximately one-fifth of
all the beds and admissions across the country (AHA 2006).

The Council of Teaching Hospitals, part of the Association for Academic Medical Centers (AAMC), specifies (1) that member hospitals must sponsor four approved medical residency programs and (2) that at least two of the four programs
must be in either medicine, surgery, pediatrics, family practice, OBGYN, or psychiatry. Teaching hospitals have the additional responsibility of educating our nation's
physician base and conducting medical research, as well as providing quality patient
care. Though other hospitals may participate in training physicians through various
residency programs, they have not demonstrated the commitment outlined in the
COTH definition.

Safety-net Hospitals

Many different types of provider organizations, including hospitals, come together
to make up the nation's safety net that provides care for vulnerable patient populations, including those without health care insurance or the ability to pay for health
care services. Every year, these hospitals provide uncompensated care that is worth
billions of dollars (Fishman 1997). Such hospitals typically are both academic medical centers and public hospitals. From a policy perspective, it is important to understand the role that these hospitals play in care for the poor and uninsured.
Safety-net hospitals receive funding from local, state, and federal government agencies. They also bill for Medicare, Medicaid, and private insurers. Thus, policies or
environmental changes that affect these sources of payment have a relatively

greater negative impact on safety-net hospitals than on their "non-safety-net" hospital counterparts.

For example, from the late 1990s through the early 2000s, a number of forces affected the hospital industry in general. During the late 1990s, health maintenance organizations gained power and used their leverage to negotiate deals with hospitals that lowered the hospital's reimbursement for services (Bazzoli et al.). Additionally, during this time hospitals felt the impact of the Balanced Budget Act of 1997 in terms of Medicare and Medicaid payments. Despite changes to the act in 1999 and 2000, hospitals still saw a decline in their payment growth, coupled with higher expenses resulting from higher operating costs (Strunk and Ginsburg 2003). As this short review indicates, safety-net hospitals operate in a competitive, price-sensitive market in which policy changes have a direct impact on their viability. Policy makers and providers must consistently be concerned and vigilant in evaluating how these hospitals are affected and whether any of these hospitals fall through the cracks.

Multihospital Systems and Networks

According to the American Hospital Association, multihospital systems are defined as two or more hospitals that are owned, leased, or contract managed by the same organization (AHA 1998). These systems can be either for profit or not for profit and may be limited to the local area or part of a national company. The AHA defines alliances as formal organizations that work for the benefits of their members to provide services and products as well as the promotion of activities and ventures. Though many hospitals participate in one or both of these activities, some hospitals remain independent and unaffiliated in any way.

Professionals Working in Hospitals

Historically, hospitals have been considered to be the "physician's workshop." As was discussed earlier in this chapter, the development of hospitals in the 20th century was closely tied to the development of a bioscientific model of medicine. Today, hospitals are a center of health care technology applied to disease and injury. As a result, a number of professions have sizable workforces in hospitals (see Table 9–1 ■).

Active Learning Exercise

On the World Wide Web, go to the Kaiser Family Foundation at http://www.statehealthfacts.org and get the most recent data on number of hospitals, admission outpatient visits, and more. You can also examine the data by state.

Table 9–1.   Characteristics of Professionals Employed by Hospitals

Profession	No. Employed	Education	Avg. Salary ($)
General Medicine	16,000	Post-Doctorate	147,000
Surgeons	4,920	Post-Doctorate	154,500
Registered Nurses	1,373,610	Associate's Degree	60,970
Respiratory Therapists	74,630	Associate's Degree	48,510
Occupational Therapists	23,340	Master's Degree	62,960
Physical Therapists	44,980	Master's Degree/ Doctoral Degree	67,210

Source: Bureau of Labor Statistics. 2006. Occupational Employment Statistics. http://www.bls.gov/oes/ (accessed September 16, 2007).

LEVELS OF CARE

Hospitals are capable of providing various levels of care. Some hospitals are known as tertiary facilities, while others are primary or secondary care hospitals. In this section, we focus on the three most common levels of care: primary, secondary, and tertiary. The main features of these levels of care are summarized in Table 9–2 ■.

Primary Care

The first level of care in the U.S. health care system is known as **primary care** and represents the main entry point by which most people come into contact with the health care delivery system. Primary care deals with illnesses that are general, episodic, common, and nonchronic in nature. In 1995, the Institute of Medicine offered a revised definition of primary care: "Primary care is the provision of integrated,

Table 9–2.   Characteristics of Primary, Secondary, Tertiary, and Quaternary Care

A. Primary care	Treats common, nonchronic, episodic disorders
	Provides care in the context of family and community
	Coordinator of care in managed care systems
B. Secondary care	Treats common, chronic-type disorders
	Long-term care required (e.g., management of diabetes or hypertension)
C. Tertiary care	Treats complex, acute, and chronic disorders
	Utilizes specialized diagnostic and treatment procedures
D. Quaternary Care	Treats uncommon acute and chronic disorders—for example, organ transplantation
	Associated with academic medical centers

accessible health care services by clinicians who are accountable for addressing a large majority of personal health care needs, developing a sustained partnership with patients, and practicing in the context of family and community." Central to this definition are the concepts of access, accountability, and integrated services, all of which are discussed throughout this text.

Primary care provides most of the health care that people usually need and is the vehicle used to integrate the delivery of health care services. Primary care physicians practice in family medicine, internal medicine, pediatrics, and obstetrics/gynecology.

Therapists Working in Primary Care

The development of direct access to therapy services and the growth of an outpatient model of therapy care have resulted in more therapists working in disease and injury prevention, triage in the emergency room, and in the assessment of patients without a physician referral. The best known model of direct access in primary care physical therapy is in the military. Moore, McMillian, Rosenthal, and Weishaar (2006) examined nearly 51,000 physical therapist direct-access encounters with patients over a 40-month period and found no adverse events. In 2006, over 48,000 physical therapists and 18,000 occupational therapists worked in an outpatient office model of care (Bureau of Labor Statistics 2007).

Secondary Care

Secondary care, like primary care, may be provided in an ambulatory setting or on an inpatient basis. Secondary care is more intense than primary care and often extends over a longer period. Unlike primary care, in which illnesses or injuries are acute, secondary care focuses on injuries or illnesses that are chronic and require continuing care. Examples of conditions that require secondary care include arthritis, diabetes, and hypertension.

Tertiary and Quaternary Care

The last level of care discussed here is **tertiary care**. This care is highly specialized, complex, and costly, and delivery takes place in an inpatient setting. Teaching hospitals or academic medical centers were once the main setting for tertiary care services. However, because of the advances being made and the fierce competition among health care providers, many community hospitals can now offer these services. Some examples of tertiary care include such procedures as coronary artery bypass grafting, truama care, transplants, burn care, and other specialized diagnostic devices. With the continual advances being made, an even higher level of tertiary care known as **quaternary care** is available and is provided predominantly at academic medical centers. Quaternary care facilities and services include burn units, trauma centers, transplant services, and so forth. Many physical therapists and occupational therapists work in tertiary and quaternary care settings to improve function and quality of life, enabling patients and clients to return to less restrictive and less medically intensive environments.

HOSPITAL INTEGRATION

During the 1990s, an increase in public awareness of the problems of the uninsured and the costs of health care services, coupled with the threat of government reform, set in motion a number of consolidation activities and other market responses from hospital organizations and other health care providers. These responses included outright mergers, vertical integration, and the formation of hospital alliances between various health care organizations (e.g., physician–hospital alliances).

The hospital industry has gone through significant restructuring over the past several decades, beginning with multihospital system growth in the 1970s and 1980s (Ermann and Gabel 1986; Shortell 1988; Alexander and Morrisey 1988) and shifting to local market consolidation in the 1990s (Luke 1991). The formation of local hospital collectives helped hospitals defend themselves against increasingly powerful competitors and improve their market positions relative to such rivals as managed care organizations, consolidating physician populations, active business coalitions, large businesses, and government agencies (Zelman 1996).

Efforts to reform the delivery of health care have emphasized the importance of offering cost-effective, comprehensive patient care. One mechanism that has the capability of providing this comprehensive care is the integrated delivery system (American Hospital Association 1992). Integrated delivery systems often consist of a variety of delivery components and payment mechanisms. Many players are involved in the creation of integrated delivery systems, including managed care organizations, which have been a major driving force behind hospital and physician integration (Shortell and Hull 1996; Advisory Board 1993; APM/University Hospital Consortium 1995). Thus, health care providers nationwide are finding themselves in increasingly complex systems that include such organizational structures as integrated delivery systems and strategic alliances (Luke, Olden, and Bramble 1998; Bazzoli, Shortell, Dubbs, Chan, and Kralovec 1999; Burns, Bazzoli, Dynan, and Wholey 1997). Many argue that by joining together, greater efficiency has been achieved.

There is a wide variety of integrated delivery system models. Integrated delivery systems are commonly formed through a process of horizontal or vertical integration (see Figure 9–6 ■). Many of these changes represent partial integration in organizations that are in the midst of transition. Horizontal integration occurs when two or more firms producing similar services join to become a single organization (or a strong interorganizational alliance). Hospitals merging or forming strategic hospital alliances (Luke, Olden, and Bramble 1998) and the consolidation of smaller solo practices into larger multispecialty group practices (see Kralewski et al. 2000) are examples of horizontal integration.

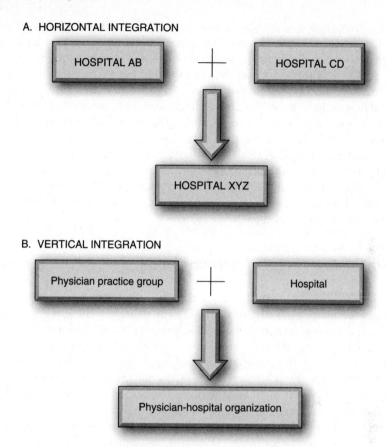

A. HORIZONTAL INTEGRATION

HOSPITAL AB + HOSPITAL CD

HOSPITAL XYZ

B. VERTICAL INTEGRATION

Physician practice group + Hospital

Physician-hospital organization

Figure 9–6. Integrated Delivery Systems

In the early 1990s, the American Hospital Association advocated the formation of local "integrated delivery systems" (American Hospital Association 1990). These systems were intended to improve the efficiency of care, increasing system accountability in both community needs and health outcomes (American Hospital Association 1992). Although some hospitals have begun to move toward a system that integrates a variety of providers, the most common activity is the horizontal combination of hospitals into local systems of networks within local markets.

There are many reasons organizations come together to form strategic partnerships. In health care, unique and specific reasons precipitate their formation (Luke, Olden, and Bramble 1998). Foremost was the threat of managed care in the market (Olden, Roggenkamp, and Luke 2002). As hospitals combine to form local hospital systems and networks, they collectively increase their geographic presence. By thus offering greater spatial coverage, they increase their leverage in negotiations for managed care contracts. Joining together at the local level also allows organizations to develop health care products that enhance their positions in the markets.

In addition to forming horizontal relationships, hospitals are joining vertically with physician organizations. Physician–hospital relationships are sometimes called **physician–hospital organizations** and represent a vertical integration strategy.

Vertical integration is the combination of two or more firms that were previously separate and whose products or services are inputs (or outputs) from the production of another service into a single firm. One possible advantage of this type of integration is transaction cost savings (D'Aunno and Zuckerman 1987). Combinations of clinical group practices and acute care facilities are examples of vertical integration and represent an essential feature of fully integrated delivery systems. These vertical combinations (i.e., physicians and hospitals) provide a mechanism that aligns incentives among the players and makes it possible to unify marketing efforts directed at managed care organizations (Burns and Thorpe 1995; Morrisey, Alexander, Burns, and Johnson 1999).

Physician–Hospital Relationships

Physician–hospital relationships are defined as the structural mechanism that facilitates the integration of physicians into the management and governance of a hospital, as well as the integration of management into the activities of the clinical–medical staff (Alexander, Morrisey, and Shortell 1986). The purpose of these relationships is to link patient-entry points to the health care delivery system, forming a continuum of services for the patient (Harris, Hicks, and Kelly 1992). Over the last five years, physician–hospital organizations have been cited with increased frequency. In the changing health care environment, physician groups are forging closer ties with hospitals as a means of lowering expenses and taking advantage of managed care contracting opportunities (Zajac, D'Aunno, and Burns 2006).

Having recognized the use of primary care physicians as gatekeepers to manage the entry of patients into the system (Burns and Thorpe 1993), hospitals are trying to establish linkages with physician groups to ensure a constant flow of patients. Linking up with physician groups increases hospitals' leverage over managed care firms by allowing the hospitals to pool their contracting activities with other providers to achieve economies and efficiencies of scale (Burns and Thorpe 1993). Hospitals are facing growing competitive threats to their market share and profitability. Large multispecialty group practices are one source of competition. In the face of this threat, hospitals have sought to gain control over the ambulatory care of physicians in the market, thus preempting possible competitive initiatives from physicians.

Physician–system integration and clinical integration include developing mechanisms for joint hospital–physician planning and patient care services. Many new organizations attempt to integrate physicians vertically with acute care facilities, using various mechanisms to achieve this goal. Hospital–physician organizations can be arranged in a variety of ways and with different types of governance structures in which one or another of the founding entities takes a leadership role. The simplest categorization of these organizations is the four-level model developed

Active Learning Exercise

On the World Wide Web, go to the Kaiser Family Foundation at http://www.commonwealthfund.org and search on "hospital" to read about specific issues facing hospitals today.

by Shortell and his colleagues. The integrated delivery system may be either hospital or health system led, physician or group practice led, insurance company led, or a hybrid model in which the hospital organization and the physician groups are codominant (Shortell, Gillies, and Anderson 1994).

Among the various models that have been developed for the integration of hospitals and physicians are the group practice without walls model (GPWW), the independent practice association (IPA), the management services organization (MSO), the physician–hospital organization (PHO), the salary staff models, the foundation model, and the physician equity model (Conners 1997). Although newer terms for these organizations have been introduced, such as "joint-operating agreements," "franchise agreements," "master affiliation agreements," "gain-sharing models," and "regional service organizations" (Zajac, D'Aunno, and Burns 2006), many of the goals and purposes of the organizations remain the same. These goals and purposes include increased leverage in negotiating managed care contracts, capital and information systems sharing, quality improvement and efficiency, creating a broad continuum of care, sharing administrative expenses, and increasing physician involvement in the process of managed care contracting (Coile and Grant 1997; Fine 1997; Burns and Thorpe 1993; Dowling 1995; Shortell and Hull 1996). In part to reduce uncertainty in a continually increasing complex and competitive environment, hospitals and physicians continue to engage in integration activities (Zajac et al. 2006). Thus, the trend of hospitals joining larger health systems continues to grow. Since 1999, approximately 100 additional hospitals participated in a health system, bringing the total number of hospitals to over 2,600 (AHA 2005). (This number includes all hospitals that are part of a corporate organization that either owns or manages health care facilities, health-related subsidiaries, or, possibly, non-health-related facilities.)

CONCLUSION

The 20th century saw the development of the hospital as the cornerstone of the acute medical care delivery system. Advances in biomedical science and policy decisions to fund hospital services were important catalysts in the development of the hospital. The provision of tertiary and quaternary care was the pinnacle of these 20th-century trends. However, the increasing utilization of hospital services and the high costs associated with hospital growth have factored into the move toward community-based primary care to prevent illness and injury. As a result, the acute medical care delivery system has seen the development of integrated health systems in many markets, as providers align with one another both vertically and horizontally to provide services in a more cost-effective manner. For therapists, the hospital represents an important workplace, primarily for persons experiencing acute illness or injury or long-term, complex medical problems.

CHAPTER REVIEW QUESTIONS

1. Describe the development of the U.S. hospital in three periods:
   a. pre-1900
   b. 1900 to 1945
   c. 1945 to the present
2. How are hospitals administratively organized?
3. Define patient-focused care, product-line teams, and matrix management in a hospital.
4. Identify common characteristic descriptors of a hospital.
5. Define primary care, secondary care, tertiary care, and quaternary care.
6. Describe the incentives for and process of development of integrated health systems in the United States.
7. Summarize the relationship of physicians and hospitals over the last century.

CHAPTER DISCUSSION QUESTIONS

1. Discuss how the administrative structure of hospitals enhances and limits the professional autonomy of occupational therapists and physical therapists. What are the historical reasons for this situation?
2. Clinical occupational therapists and physical therapists working on product-line teams may report directly to a nontherapist supervisor on a regular basis. Discuss the pros and cons of this form of hospital organization with regard to the role of physical therapists and occupational therapists in a hospital.
3. Integrated health delivery systems that coordinate and, in some cases, consolidate primary, secondary, and tertiary care in a community are a contemporary form of acute medical care delivery. What effect could you expect to observe on small, private-practice providers (e.g., physicians, therapists) in communities with large integrated health delivery systems? Discuss some strategies that would be necessary to compete with such systems.

REFERENCES

Advisory Board. 1993. *The Grand Alliance: Vertical Integration Strategies for Physicians and Health Systems.* Washington DC: Advisory Board.
Alexander, J. A., G. J. Bazzoli, L. R. Burns, and S. M. Shortell. 1999, June. Measures of physician system integration. Paper presented at the annual meeting of the Association for Health Service Research, Chicago.

Alexander, J. A., and M. A. Morrisey. 1988. Hospital-physician integration and hospital costs. *Inquiry* 25(4): 388–401.

Alexander, J. A., M. A. Morrisey, and S. M. Shortell. 1986. Effects of competition, regulation, and corporatization on hospital–physician relationships. *J Health and Soc Behav* 27: 220–35.

American Hospital Association. 2006. *TrendWatch Chartbook, 2006.* http://www.aha.org/aha/trendwatch/2006/cb2006chapter3.PPT#285,5,Slide5 (accessed September 2007).

American Hospital Association. 1990. *Renewing the U.S. Health Care System.* Washington DC: Section for Health Care Systems, Office of Constituency Sections.

———.1992. *Overview: AHA's National Reform Strategy.* Chicago: American Hospital Association.

———.1998. *AHA Guide, 1999–2000 Edition.* Chicago: American Hospital Association.

APM/University Hospital Consortium. 1995. *How Markets Evolve: Hospitals and Health Markets* 69(5): 60.

Bazzoli, G. J., R. Kang, R. Hasnain-Wynia, and R. C. Lindrooth. 2005. An update on safety-net hospitals: Coping with the late 1990s and early 2000s. *Health Affairs* 24 (4): 1047–56.

Bazzoli, G. J., S. M. Shortell, N. Dubbs, C. Chan, and P. Kralovec. 1999. A taxonomy of health networks and systems: Bringing order out of chaos. *Health Serv Res* 33(6): 1683–1717.

Boissoneau, R. 1983. Matrix management in the health care organization. *Health Care Sup.* 2(1): 22–36.

Bureau of Labor Statistics. 2007. Occupational Employment Statistics for Physical Therapists and Occupational Therapists. http://www.bls.gov/oes (accessed September 17, 2007).

Burns, L. R., G. J. Bazzoli, L. Dynan, and D. R. Wholey. 1997. Managed care, market stages, and integrated delivery systems: Is there a relationship? *Health Affairs* 16: 204–18.

Burns, L. R., and D. P. Thorpe. 1993. Trends and models in physician–hospital organization. *Health Care Management Rev* 18(4): 7–20.

———.1995. Managed care and integrated health care. *Health Care Management* 2(1): 101–08.

Coile, R. C., and P. N. Grant. 1997. Group practice affiliation structures. In *Integrating the practice of medicine,* ed. R. B. Conners, 307–331. Chicago: American Hospital Publishing.

Conners, R. B., ed. 1997. *Integrating the Practice of Medicine.* Chicago: American Hospital Publishing.

D'Aunno, T. A., and H. S. Zuckerman. 1987. The emergence of hospital federations: An integration of perspectives from organizational theory. *Med Care Rev* 44(2): 323–43.

Dowling, W. L. 1995. Strategic alliances as a structure for integrated delivery systems. In *Partners for the dance: Forming strategic alliances in health care,* ed. A. D. Kaluzny, H. S. Zuckerman, and T. C. Ricketts, 139–76. Ann Arbor: Health Administration Press.

Ermann, D., and J. Gabel. 1986. Investor-owned multihospital systems: A synthesis of research findings. In *For-profit enterprise in health care,* ed., 474–491 B. H. Gray. Washington DC: National Academy Press.

Fine, A. 1997. Integrated delivery systems. In *Integrating the practice of medicine*, ed. R. B. Conners, 273–87. Chicago: American Hospital Publishing.

Fishman, L. 1997. What types of hospitals form the safety net? Despite public financial support, safety-net hospitals are in a worse financial position than other hospitals are. *Health Affairs* 16(4): 215–222.

Freymann, J. G. 1974. *The American health care system: Its genesis and trajectory.* New York: Medcom Press.

Harris, C., L. L. Hick, and B. J. Kelly. 1992. Physician hospital networking: Avoiding a shotgun wedding. *Health Care Management Rev* 17(4):17–28.

Iglehart, J. K. 1993. The American health care system: Teaching hospitals. *N Engl J Med* 329(14): 1052–56.

Institute of Medicine. 1995. *Primary Care: America's Health in a New Era.* Washington DC: National Academy Press.

Kaiser State Health Facts. 2007. The Kaiser Family Foundation. http://www.statehealthfacts.org (accessed September 2007).

Kane, R. A., and R. L. Kane. 1987. *Long-term care: Principles, programs and policies.* New York: Springer Publishing Co.

Kovner, A. R. 1995. Hospitals. In *Health care delivery in the United States,* ed. A. R. Kovner, 162–83. New York: Springer Publishing.

Kralewski, J. E., E. C. Rich, R. Feldman, B. Dowd, T. Bernhardt, C. Johnson, and W. Gold. 2000. The effects of medical group practice and physician payment methods on costs of care. *Health Serv Res,* 35(3): 591–613.

Luke, R. D. 1991. Spatial competition and cooperation in local hospital markets. *Medical Care Review* 48(2): 207–237.

Luke, R. D., P. C. Olden, and J. D. Bramble. 1998. Strategic hospital alliances: Countervailing responses to restructuring health care markets. In *Handbook of health care management,* eds. W. J. Duncan, L. E. Swayne, and P. M. Ginter, 81–116. Cambridge MA: Blackwell Publishers.

Moore, J. H., D. J. McMillian, M. D. Rosenthal, and M. D. Weishaar. 2006. Risk determination for patients with direct access to physical therapy in military health care facilities. *J Orthop Sports Phys Ther* 35(10): 674–78.

Morrisey, M. A., J. Alexander, L. R. Burns, and V. Johnson. 1999. The effects of managed care on physician and clinical integration in hospitals. *Medical Care* 37(4): 350–61.

Moy, E., E. Valente, R. J. Levin, K. J. Bhak, and P. F. Griner. 1996. The volume and mix of inpatient services provided by academic medical centers. *Acad Med* 71(10): 1113–22.

Olden, P. C., S. D. Roggenkamp, and R. D. Luke. 2002. A post-1900s assessment of strategic hospital alliances and their marketplace orientation: Time to refocus. *Health Care Management Review* 27 (2): 33–49.

Shortell, S. M. 1988. The evolution of hospital systems: Unfulfilled promises and self-fulfilling prophesies. *Medical Care Review* 45(2): 177–214.

Shortell, S. M., R. Gillies, and D. Anderson. 1996. *The new American healthcare: Creating organized delivery systems.* San Francisco: Jossey-Bass.

Shortell, S. M., R. R. Gillies, and D. A. Anderson. 1994. The new world of managed care: Creating organized delivery systems. *Health Affairs* 13(5): 46–64.

Shortell, S. M., and K. E. Hull. 1996. The new organization of health care: Managed care integrated health systems. In *Strategic choices for a changing healthcare system*, eds. S. Altman and U. Reinhardt, 101–48. Chicago: Health Administration Press.

Starr, P. 1982. *The social transformation of American medicine.* New York: Basic Books.

Stevens, R. 1971. *American medicine and the public interest.* New Haven: Yale University Press.

Strunk, B. C., and P. B. Ginsburg. 2003. Tracking health care costs: Trends stabilize but remain high in 2002. Health Affairs 24 (W3): 266–74.

Sultz, H. A., and K. M. Young. 1999. *Health care USA: Understanding its organization and delivery.* Gaithersburg MD: Aspen.

Zajac, E. J., T. A. D'Aunno, and L. R. Burns. 2006. Managing Strategic Alliances. In *Health care management: Organization design and behaviors, eds.* S. M. Shortell and A. D. Kaluzney, 356–81. New York: Thomson Delmar Learning.

10

The Post-Acute Health Care System

CHAPTER OBJECTIVES

At the conclusion of this chapter, the reader will be able to:

1. Discuss the development of the post-acute health care system in the United States during the last quarter of the 20th century.
2. Define the main components of the post-acute health care system: informal care and formal care.
3. Discuss the size, importance, and function of the informal care system of post-acute health care.
4. Identify the components, discuss the services, define likely users, and relate the effectiveness of levels of the formal post-acute health care system.
   a. home health care
   b. hospice
   c. adult day services
   d. assisted living
   e. skilled nursing facilities
   f. subacute care
   g. inpatient rehabilitation facilities
5. Identify and characterize the sites of community-based mental health practice.
6. Define the role of occupational therapy and physical therapy in the post-acute health care system.

KEY WORDS: Custodial Care, Formal Care, Informal Care, Intermediate Care, Level of Care, Swing-bed Unit, Voluntary Agency

Case Example

Mr. Johnson is a 78-year-old man living at home. Since his wife died, he has become more dependent upon his daughter and son, who live nearby. His daughter checks on him regularly, takes him to physician appointments, and performs light housekeeping tasks. At his latest visit, Mr. Johnson was diagnosed with Type II diabetes and now needs to take insulin injections. His daughter did not feel comfortable giving Mr. Johnson his injections, so a home health agency was contacted to provide these injections. A nurse visited Mr. Johnson and noted that he was having increasing problems with walking and transferring from the toilet due to pain in his hip. She arranged for a physical therapist and occupational therapist to visit Mr. Johnson. The physical therapist provided Mr. Johnson with exercises and a cane to use at home. The occupational therapist arranged for a grab bar to be installed near his toilet to assist with transfers. Mr. Johnson is able to continue living in the community with the assistance of home health care.

Case Example Focus Question:

1. What types of patient situations are addressed in the post-acute health care environment?

INTRODUCTION

Occupational therapists and physical therapists are important providers of rehabilitation services in the post-acute care system. Patients who survive a serious medical illness or an injury often require a lengthy recuperative period. At one time, the post-acute care environment was limited to nursing homes and a small home health industry. Nursing homes focused on custodial care for persons with chronic disease and for persons with illnesses that gave them little chance for improvement.

The growth and development of the post-acute health care system parallels the policy changes in health care financing and the desire to move away from the hospital to a community-based care system. With the inception of Medicare Diagnosis-Related Groups prospective payment in 1983, the incentives for extended post-acute care increased. The world of post-acute care has created multiple alternatives for patient treatment after an acute illness or injury. Each **level of care** provides different services and has different costs. The complexity of the system has created the need for a case manager to assist the patient in navigating the system (see Chapter 6).

The development of the post-acute care continuum has not been consistent, complete, or without challenges. Problems include unequal access to care and an inability to finance care. Certain populations continue to lack access to necessary services that would permit full restoration of function. For example, fewer options for long-term care exist in many rural communities, and African Americans are less likely to utilize institutional care and are more likely to use informal care or receive no care at all (Wallace et al., 1998). Indeed, Clark (1997) reported that African Americans are experiencing increasing rates of disability and institutionalization compared with the majority population. Hispanic Americans and African Americans are more dependent upon informal care systems than formal long-term care services (Li and Fries 2005; Weiss Gonzalez, Kabeto, and Langa 2005).

The previous chapter introduced the acute health care system. For patients with chronic disease and disablement, the need for health care extends well beyond the acute health care system. In this chapter, we will explore the multiple levels of care that make up the post-acute care continuum. In a broad sense, the post-acute

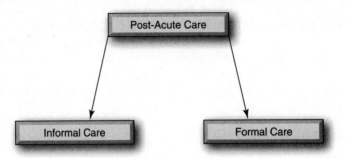

Figure 10–1.   The Post-acute Health Care

care continuum has two fundamental components: **informal care** and **formal care** (see Figure 10–1 ■). Informal care consists of the care provided by the family unit. Formal care is a continuum of services that begins with services to supplement informal care (e.g., home health care) and extends to services that replace informal care (e.g., skilled nursing care and intermediate care for persons with developmental disabilities). Formal care, then, consists of a mix of nonprofessional services, professional services, and residential care. Physical therapy and occupational therapy are critical professional services on many levels of the formal care continuum. The complexity of each individual patient's situation and the availability of services will dictate which level of care is most appropriate. This chapter explains the structure and services of each level of the post-acute care continuum, as well as their effectiveness. We will conclude with a brief discussion of the community-based mental health system, a small, but important, site of practice for occupational therapists.

INFORMAL CARE

Post-acute care is a system of formal and informal services that make up a continuum of rehabilitation and personal care for people with chronic disease and disabilities. The foundation of long-term care in the United States is the family, the earliest informal care system (Montgomery 1999; Wolf 1999; Robinson 1997). Recent estimates of older Americans with chronic disabilities living in the community place that population at 3.5 million people (Wolff and Kasper 2006). The combined prevalence of mental retardation and intellectual disabilities in the United States is 1.27 percent, or about 3.25 million Americans (Fujiura 2003). A conservative estimate is that at least 2 percent of the population is in need of, or is receiving, informal care. Wolff and Kasper (2006) found that the average person in need of informal care is older than age 75, is female, lives alone or with a spouse, rates his or her health as fair or poor, and needs help with instrumental activities of daily living (ADLs) or one or two basic ADLs. The national economic value of informal caregiving was estimated at $196 billion, which is more than all forms of formal long-term care combined (Arno, Levine, and Memmott 1999). This aspect of the informal care system has important social, cultural, and policy implications.

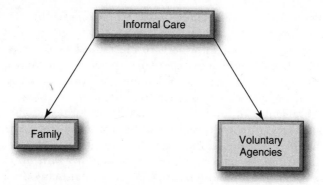

Figure 10–2. The Informal Care System

The informal care system (see Figure 10–2 ■) is inexpensive to the larger society and is a desirable alternative to formal care for many persons with chronic disease and disability (Chappell, Dlitt, Hollander, Miller, and McWilliam 2004; Charles and Sevak, 2005). Donelan et al. (2002) found that each year 23 percent of Americans provide informal care to other persons and 71 percent of the caregivers do not live with the recipient of the care. The presence of a spouse caregiver reduces formal long-term care costs by $28,840 per year (Yoo, Bhattacharya, McDonald, and Garber 2004). A child caregiver can reduce annual costs by up to $3,830.

Typical informal care activities include helping with household chores, preventing accidents, assisting with personal care, and dressing (McCann and Evans 2002). Informal care is heavily dependent on female spouses and adult female children for its implementation. In a study of informal versus formal care for patients with dementia, researchers found that if family labor costs were considered, nursing home care costs would actually be lower than the cost of informal care (Chiu, Tang, Liu, Shyu, and Chang 1999). One study describing the major values of elderly Americans who are facing the need for long-term care found that a sense of independence and participation in life decisions were important in determining whether to access post-acute care services (Forbes and Hoffart 1998). Among other concerns considered by persons potentially in need of informal or formal care were cost, stress on the family, personal preference, and premorbid attitudes about levels of care in the post-acute care continuum (Keysor, Desai, and Mutran 1999). Typically, older Americans prefer to stay at home, but this attitude changes if a significant illness will overburden the informal care system (Fried, van Doorn, O'Leary, Tinetti, and Drickamer 1999; Wielink and Huijsman 1999).

Boaz and Hu (1997) report that, depending on marital status, networks consisting of family members and friends of elderly persons with disabilities can typically provide 10 to 40 hours per week of informal assistance. The burden of informal caregiving typically falls on female spouses and the adult female children of aging relatives (Montgomery 1999; Lee and Tussing 1998). Informal caregivers are mainly older and female, rate their own health as poor or fair, are more likely to be living in poverty, and describe themselves as work disabled (Kennedy, Walls, Owens-Nicholson 1999). The family is the predominant source of care for persons with developmental disabilities. Nearly 90 percent of the nation's 3 million people with developmental disabilities are cared for by family members (Fujiura 1998). The experience of providing informal care affects the lives of the caregivers. Parents caring for children with disabilities experience anxiety and increased responsibility for the care of the child (McDermott, Valentine, Anderson, Gallup, and Thompson 1997).

The informal care system is also under pressure. Stewart (2006) reported a reduced availability of informal care. Wolff and Kasper (2006) found an increase in the number of primary caregivers without support and an increase in the number of disabilities reported in their sample population. A greater proportion of chronically ill or disabled elders live in the community with no informal care support. O'Keefe, Long, Liu, and Kerr (2001) found that many persons with multiple disabilities lived in the community and were supported by Medicare home care and informal care, but their informal care network was "overextended, stressed and vulnerable to breakdown." Long, Liu, Black, O'Keefe, and Molony (2005) found that persons living in these situations were more likely to enter a nursing home. Finally, it is important to recognize that informal care is not a static system; rather, the process of caregiving changes over time and is related to the social context, caregiver ability, and the often increasing burden of care (Szinovacz and Davey 2007).

The family frequently obtains information and referrals for problems in caregiving through **voluntary agencies** such as the American Heart Association and the National Multiple Sclerosis Society, which offer educational, support, and advocacy services for persons with chronic illness or disease and their families. Typically, these organizations provide health education and health maintenance activities to their constituencies, disease prevention and detection programs to the general public, and advocacy in the area of public and private policy to the government. By their nature, voluntary agencies are not-for-profit organizations that have primarily an educational purpose and provide limited direct patient-care services. It is important for occupational therapists and physical therapists to understand and be involved with these organizations in order to recognize the needs and concerns of people with disabilities and their informal care systems.

For society, the economic and social value of the informal care system is enormous. The development of formal long-term care services (e.g., home health care, skilled nursing facilities) can be traced to the need to bolster the family as primary caregiver for patients with chronic disease and disability. For occupational therapists and physical therapists, this need has applications to the design and implementation of intervention plans for patients with chronic disease and disability (e.g., the incorporation of family goals into treatment plans and the development of patient/family education programs).

FORMAL CARE

Formal care consists of a mix of residential and professional sites and types of care (see Figure 10–3 ■). Residential services range from facilities that provide supervision and minimal assistance (e.g., assisted living facilities) to facilities that provide multiple

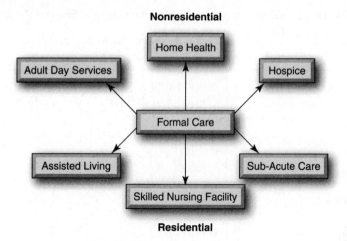

Figure 10–3. The Formal Care System

medical and rehabilitation treatments (e.g., skilled nursing facilities and subacute care units). As we will discover, the deterioration of a person's ability to perceive the environment, think, communicate, and perform basic activities of daily living is critical to determining the appropriate level of formal post-acute care.

There are a number of professionals that work in the formal care system. Table 10–1 ■ presents data on two of the most commonly used types of formal care: the skilled nursing facility and the home health agency. The professional most commonly working in these settings is the registered nurse. Physical therapists, occupational therapists, and social workers also commonly work in these settings.

There are two types of formal care: nonresidential and residential (see Tables 10–2 ■, 10–3 ■). Nonresidential types of formal care include home health agencies,

Table 10–1. Professionals Found in U.S. Skilled Nursing Facilities and Home Health Agencies (2006)

Profession	No. Employed	Education	Avg. Salary($)
Occupational Therapist	13,840	Bachelor's/ Master's	69,000
Physical Therapist	27,190	Master's/ Doctorate	72,500
Recreational Therapist	7,940	Bachelor's	31,000
Registered Nurses	247,370	Associate's	55,000
Social Worker	24,260	Bachelor's	44,000
Speech Language Pathologists	6,700	Master's	72,500

Source: Bureau of Labor Statistics. Occupational Employment Statistics. 2006. http://www.bls.gov/oes/ (accessed July 3, 2007).

Table 10–2. Common Services in Nonresidential Sites of the Post-acute Health Care System

	Skilled	*Nonskilled*
Home Health	Physical therapy Occupational therapy Nursing Speech/language pathology Dietetics Pharmacy Social work	Homemaking Personal Services
Hospice	Medicine Nursing Pastoral care Social work Counseling Rehabilitation therapy Dietetics Pharmacy	Homemaking Personal hygiene Volunteer companions
Adult Day Services	Nursing Social work Physical therapy Occupational therapy Recreational therapy	Transportation Meals Personal care

Table 10–3. Common Services in Residential Sites of the Post-acute Health Care System

	Skilled	*Nonskilled*
Assisted Living		Meals Transportation Social activities ADL assistance Security
Skilled Nursing Facility	Nursing Physical therapy Occupational therapy Social work Dietetics	Personal hygiene Restorative care
Subacute Care	Medicine Nursing Occupational therapy Physical therapy Speech-language pathology	Personal hygiene

hospices, and adult day services. In these situations, the informal care system is supported with targeted interventions based on the needs of the client. Much of the day-to-day care is provided by the person's family. Along with other services, residential care gives a person a place to live. Both types of formal care provide skilled and nonskilled services. The type of formal care and the exact mix of services provided depend on the needs of the patient. The type of care a person receives also depends upon the opinions of the professionals working with them. Kane et al. (2006) found that professionals favored the locations where they worked or with which they were more familiar. For example, registered nurses were likely to recommend home health care, assisted living, and adult day services, and primary care physicians favored rehabilitation and skilled nursing care. In the remainder of the chapter, we will explore the different types of nonresidential and residential formal care.

NONRESIDENTIAL FORMAL CARE

Home Health Care

Home health care is "provided to individuals and their families in their places of residence for the purpose of promoting, maintaining or restoring health or maximizing the level of independence while minimizing the effects of disability and illness, including terminal illness" (National Center for Health Statistics 2007). In the United States, home health care is a large industry. About 1.4 million Americans are receiving home health care services, and there are 7.2 million discharges from home health agencies annually (National Center for Health Statistics 2004) (see Table 10–4 ■). The average length of stay is 69 days. In 2005, there were 8,040 Medicare-certified home health care agencies in the United States (Centers for Medicare and Medicaid Services 2006).

Home health care is a set of health care services organized and delivered by nurses and rehabilitation professionals under medical supervision. Home health agencies provide a package of skilled services as well as nonskilled services intended for short-term, intermittent needs after an acute illness (see Table 10–2 ■). Skilled services include physical therapy, occupational therapy, nursing, speech-language pathology, dietetics, and pharmacy. Nonskilled services (i.e., homemaking and personal hygiene care) are provided when they are related to the care and recovery from a medical illness.

Table 10–4. Characteristics of Patient Discharges from Home Health Care (2000)

Total number of discharges: 7.2 million
Rate per 100,000 population: 258.2
Mean length of stay: 69 days
Gender: Female: 64%, Male: 36%
Age > 65: 69%
Most common medical problems: Circulatory System: 22%, Injuries and
Poisoning: 12%, Musculoskeletal and Connective Tissue System: 12%, Respiratory
System: 9%
Racial distribution: Caucasian/non-Hispanic: 79%, Black: 10%, Hispanic: 4%,
Other: 7%
Source of payment: Medicare: 67%, Private insurance/funds: 19%, Medicaid:
10%, Other: 4%
Has a primary caregiver: 85%
Discharge status: Community: 71%, Hospital or other institution: 21%, Deceased: 2%
Percent requiring assistance with basic Activities of Daily Living: 38%
Percent requiring assistance with instrumental Activities of Daily Living: 28%
Percent receiving physical therapy: 37%
Percent receiving occupational therapy: 9%
Percent using a mobility aid: 57%
Percent using a self-care aid: 30%

Source: National Center for Health Statistics. 2000. National Home and Hospice Care Data.
Data Tables. *Home Care Discharges.* http://www.cdc.gov/nchs/about/major/nhhcsd/nhhc-
shomecare3.htm (accessed June 27, 2007).

Home health care is most beneficial for individuals who need comprehensive
care to recover from an illness or injury, who desire to live in their home, and who
have some social support. Intrator and Berg (1998) found that patients who received home health care services after hip fracture were less likely to need rehospi-
talization or a nursing home admission and were more likely to survive the
following year without another Medicare claim. Penrod, Kane, Finch, and Kane
(1998) found that the effect of home health care on functional status was not significant, but nonetheless concluded that home health care does help maintain the
patient in the home.

Individuals receiving home health care services are homebound, meaning
that they are unable to leave their homes except for medical appointments or religious services. Persons most commonly needing home health care services are
older, female, and Medicare beneficiaries, have limited ability to perform activities
of daily living, and have another primary caregiver in the home (see Table 10–4 ■)
(National Center for Health Statistics 2007). The most common medical diagnoses
of persons utilizing home health care services are circulatory system disease, injuries, poisoning, and musculoskeletal/connective tissue system disorders. Falls are
a major concern with home health patients (Lewis, Moutoux, Slaughter, and Bailey

Table 10–5.   Common Mobility and Self-care Aids Used by Home Health Patients (2000)

Total number of discharges: 7,179,000
  Total number of patients with mobility aids: 4,080,800
  Walkers: 2,806,900
  Cane or crutches: 1,671,800
  Wheelchair: 1,138,500
  Transfer equipment: 232,500
  Orthotics, including braces: 108,000
Total Number of patients with self-care aids: 2,152,300
  Bedside commode: 946,400
  Shower chair or bath bench: 848,000
  Hospital bed: 662,300
  Grab bars: 404,600
  Elevated or raised toilet seat: 327,700
  Special mattress: 142,600
  Chairs: 95,000
  Overbed table: 90,900

Source: National Center for Health Statistics. 2000. National Home and Hospice Care Data. Data Tables. *Home Care Discharges.* http://www.cdc.gov/nchs/about/major/nhhcsd/nhhc-shomecare3.htm (accessed June 27, 2007).

2004; Carroll, Slattum, and Cox 2005). Patients who have neurological or cardiopulmonary impairments, who have a history of falling, and who take medications intended to prevent falling are at higher risk at home for falls (Lewis et al. 2004). About 4 in 10 patients receive physical therapy and 1 in 10 receives occupational therapy. A majority of home care recipients use a mobility aid (most commonly a walker) and about one-third use a self-care aid (most commonly a bedside commode) (see Table 10–5 ■).

Patients entering home health care services receive a comprehensive evaluation and a plan of care developed to meet their needs. The plan of care needs to be certified by the person's physician every 60 days. Discharge from the hospital raises many concerns for patients and their caregivers, including the procedures to be followed at home, communication with providers, and expectations for the future (Weaver, Perloff, and Waters 1998). A program of skilled and nonskilled services can ensure a smooth transition to the community after illness.

Home health care is provided by nonprofit, for-profit, and governmental agencies that are either freestanding organizations or components of an integrated health care system. Home health care agencies provide services to patients who are medically stable but cannot access other community-based resources. Home health care has filled in the gap created by the increasing orientation of medical physicians to high-technology practice environments. Historically a routine part of medical practice, a family physician today makes an average of 0.4 home visit per week (American Academy of Family Physicians 2006).

Overall, the services most commonly utilized by patients (85 percent) in home health care are provided by a nurse (National Center for Health Statistics 2007). Home health aides provide assistance with activities of daily living, light housekeeping, and basic medical procedures (e.g., wound-dressing changes). About one in four home health patients will receive personal care or companion services from a home health worker (National Center for Health Statistics 2007). Skilled nursing services are closely related to the need for a home health aide and the presence of significant disease (Diwan, Berger, and Manns 1997). Case management, patient education, intravenous therapy, wound care, and pain control are frequently employed nursing procedures (Montauk 1998). Nursing care is limited to no more than 8 hours per day, and less than 28 hours per week. Skilled nursing and physical therapy are the professional services most commonly utilized in home health care.

Physical therapy and occupational therapy services are important components of a home health care plan (Coke, Alday, Biala, Luna, and Martines 2005; O'Sullivan and Siebert 2004). Payne, Thomas, Fitzpatrick, Abdel-Rahman, and Kayne (1998) studied patterns of home health visit length and found that case management, functional limitations, and clinical instability affected the need for professional intervention. Limitations in performing activities of daily living are the strongest predictor of overall utilization of home health care, with bathing identified as the most common ADL limitation in the home health care population (Torrez, Estes, and Linkens 1998). Collins, Beissner, and Krout (1998) reported that patients with musculoskeletal conditions were treated most frequently by physical therapists, followed by patients with neurological and cardiopulmonary problems. Therapists spent an average of 74 minutes per visit, with 35 minutes of that period given over to direct treatment of the client. Patients with neurological problems needed longer visits. Travel and documentation were the most common activities performed by the physical therapists. In a study of goal achievement in home health care, O'Sullivan and Volicer (1997) reported that persons discharged after total hip replacement and who received physical therapy home care were more likely to be discharged with their goals achieved.

Hospice Care

Hospice services provide care for individuals with terminal illness and for their support systems during and after the dying process. The early development of hospice services can be traced to the efforts of volunteers interested in providing services to persons with terminal illness (Petrisek and Mor 1999). The first hospice organization was St. Christopher's Hospice, which opened in London in 1967 (Leland and Schonwelter 1997; Pickett, Cooley, and Gordon 1998). The first hospice in the United States opened in New Haven, Connecticut, in 1974. Today there are approximately 3,078 hospice organizations in the United States (Hospice Association of America 2007). In

2005, nearly 900,000 persons received services through a Medicare-certified hospice program (Centers for Medicare and Medicaid Services 2007).

Hospice is founded upon a philosophy of palliative care, not curative medicine. Palliative care focuses on pain management, emotional counseling, and social support (Petrisek and Mor 1999). Byock (1996) has summarized the philosophy of hospice care: "Beyond symptom management, hospice and palliative care intervention can be directed at helping the person to attain a sense of completion within the social and interpersonal dimensions, to develop or deepen a sense of worthiness, and to find their own unique sense of meaning in life"(p. 251). As Leland and Schonwelter (1997) succinctly state, hospice is about "dying well"(p. 381).

Persons in need of hospice care most frequently have cancer, heart disease, or pulmonary disease (Emmanuel, Fairclough, and Slutsman 1999; Rasmussen and Sanderson 1998; Haupt 1997). To qualify for hospice benefits, patients with terminal illness are usually expected to die within six months (Petrisek and Mor 1999; Gabel, Hurst, and Hunt 1998). Patient populations are usually older and are equally divided between males and females. The most common physical complaints of patients receiving hospice services include pain, fatigue, anorexia, dyspnea, nausea, confusion, and depression (Ng and von Gunten 1998; Friedrich 1999; Cleary and Carbone 1997). Hospice care ameliorates the social isolation faced by persons with terminal illness in the hospital (Rasmussen and Sanderson 1998). About two in three hospice patients need help with one basic activity of daily living and one instrumental activity of daily living. About 3 in 10 hospice patients need assistance with walking (Haupt 1997). Nearly 2 in 3 persons need help with transportation, over half with homemaking, and 1 in 4 with personal care (Emmanuel et al.).

The vast majority of hospice services are provided in private residences (Haupt 1997; Emmanuel et al.). Increasingly, skilled nursing facilities are offering hospice care (Petrisek and Mor 1999; Castle, Mor, and Banaszak-Hull 1997). Some hospice services, including respite care, are provided in special residential hospice facilities (Leland and Schonwelter 1997). The median length of stay in a hospice is 15 days (Hospice Association of America 2007).

Hospice services are characterized by a patient-focused, interdisciplinary, coordinated plan of care. Not only the family, but also physicians, nurses, clergy, social workers, home health aides, counselors, and volunteers make up the core of the hospice team. Occupational therapists, physical therapists, speech-language pathologists, dietitians, and pharmacists are other important contributing professions to hospice care. Hospice care benefits are typically inclusive of necessary prescription drug and durable medical equipment needs. A unique Medicare benefit for hospice services is follow-up bereavement care for family members after the patient's death.

Certain populations have less access to hospice services. For example, some patients do not have families to provide hospice care. Hispanic Americans are less likely than Caucasians or African Americans to utilize hospice services (Johnson et al. 2005). Personal factors can also affect the utilization of hospice services. Weggel (1999) found that patient and family resistance to the acceptance of terminal illness and their unwillingness to give up curative therapy were factors limiting the use of hospice care. In some cases, physicians do not provide hospice care as an option for terminally ill patients, primarily because they lack information about hospice services (Weggel 1999).

Adult Day Services

For the caregivers of adults with chronic disease and disability, the ongoing provision of informal care can be exhausting. A respite from providing care can alleviate this stress and allow for the continuation of informal care. For working caregivers, the ability of an agency to provide services during workday hours allows informal care to continue in the evening or during the weekend. One option in the post-acute care continuum designed to meet these needs is adult day services.

According to the National Adult Day Services Association (2007), adult day services consist of services based on two models of care: the social model and the medical model. The social model program provides a "variety of social and other related support services in a protective setting" in a "community based setting" to "meet the needs of functionally and/or cognitively impaired adults" (National Adult Day Services Association 2007). In the United States, there are over 3,500 adult day service providers, and the vast majority of them are not-for-profit agencies. Adult day services provide transportation, meals, social services, personal care, occasional nursing services, rehabilitation services, and activities, usually during normal day business hours, five days per week. Adult day services allow for the supervision and care of an adult while the primary caregiver works or is given a respite from daily care.

The National Adult Day Services Association (2007) reports that the typical adult day services client would be a 72-year-old female who lives with a spouse, family, or friends. One-half of the recipients of adult day services have a cognitive impairment, and 60 percent of persons served need help with at least two activities of daily living. The average daily fee for adult day care is $56, much less than the daily cost of skilled nursing facility care (National Adult Day Services Association 2007).

The Program of All-Inclusive Care (PACE) is a program designed to increase the availability of adult day care as an option to institutionalization. PACE is unusual in adult day services in that it has served a large minority, low-income population (Irvin, Massey, and Dorsey 1997). PACE originated in San Francisco's Chinatown in the early 1970s. Recent changes in Medicare law have created expanded opportunities for PACE programs across the country (Lee, Eng, Fox, and Etienne 1998). There are 36 PACE sites nationally (Centers for Medicare and Medicaid Services 2007).

PACE sites each serve 120 to 150 participants who come several times per week to adult day service centers for medicine, nursing, social services, occupational therapy, physical therapy, home care, and other services (Shannon and Van Reenen 1998). The typical PACE participant is female and has three to five limitations in activities of daily living (Mukamel, Temkin-Greener, and Clark 1998; Irvin, Massey, and Dorsey 1997).

Several studies have addressed the effectiveness of PACE. Persons using PACE services have fewer hospital admissions and emergency room visits (Kane, Homyak, Bershadsky, and Flood 2006). Specifically, older adults who had their unmet ADL limitations addressed by PACE were less likely to be admitted to a hospital (Sands et al. 2006) or to a nursing home (Friedman, Steinwachs, Rathouz, Burton, and Mukamel 2005).

RESIDENTIAL FORMAL CARE

Assisted Living

Assisted living "provides relatively independent seniors with assistance and limited health care services in a home-like atmosphere" (National Center for Assisted Living 2006). Unlike home health care, adult day care, and much hospice care, assisted living provides residential care in facilities outside of the home. About 900,000 Americans live in one of 36,000 assisted living facilities in the United States (National Center for Assisted Living 2006). The average length of stay is three years (Golant 2004).

The typical resident is "an 86-year-old woman who is mobile, but needs assistance with approximately two ADLs" (National Center for Assisted Living 2006). Most residents require assistance with bathing, housekeeping, and managing their medications, and many require help with dressing and transferring. This level of care is commonly called **intermediate care.** Assisted living facilities usually provide three meals per day, transportation, social activities, assistance with activities of daily living, medication monitoring, and security services (see Table 10–2 ■). Assisted living facilities may be freestanding buildings or, in some cases, part of a skilled nursing facility. According to the National Center for Assisted Living, the typical facility has 58 units and charges $87.50 per day. This is more than adult day services, but less than skilled nursing facility care. Payment is primarily by private funding, although state Medicaid programs are increasingly viewing assisted living facilities as a cost-effective alternative to expensive skilled nursing facility care (Mollica 1998). A study of the needs of the Veteran's Health Administration found that 19 percent of veterans in nursing homes were functioning at a status consistent with assisted living (Kinosian, Stallard, and Wieland 2007).

Sikorska (1999) interviewed 156 residents of 13 assisted living facilities and found higher rates of resident satisfaction in smaller facilities with limited activities and more personal space. Bishop (1999) reported that assisted living facilities were replacing skilled nursing facilities as the residential choice for persons with minimal disability or post-acute care needs. The goal of many assisted living admissions is to allow the person to "age in place" (Ball et al. 2004). Providing the appropriate mix of services for this to occur is difficult. Cognitive decline and an increased number and severity of medical conditions is common and is associated with transfer to more medically intensive facilities (Burdick et al., 2005; Sloane et al., 2005; Fonda, Clipp, and Maddox 2002). Exercise and walking programs have been found to be beneficial in this population (Taylor et al., 2003; Baum, Jarjoura, Polen, Faur, and Rutecki 2003).

Skilled Nursing Facilities

Skilled nursing facilities (SNFs), or nursing homes, are the oldest type of long-term care facility. They have been present in the United States in one form or another for over a century. Originally designed to provide long-term **custodial care,** skilled nursing facilities have been transformed in the last two decades into facilities that are a key part of a continuum of care for patients with complex illnesses (American Health Care Association 2000) (see Table 10–6 ■). An indication of this change is the development of specialized units in SNFs for Alzheimer's disease, AIDS, ventilator-dependent patients, and subacute care. Reschovsky (1998) classifies persons served by skilled nursing facilities into two types: post-acute and chronic (see Figure 10–4 ■). Post-acute patients receive subacute care or skilled services with the anticipation of a community discharge. Chronic patients receive skilled nursing and occasional skilled rehabilitation services to prevent the deterioration of function and health status, with the expectation of long-term residence in a skilled nursing facility.

About 1.4 million Americans reside in 16,000 skilled nursing facilities in the United States (American Health Care Association 2007). Nationally, occupancy is about 89 percent of capacity (American Health Care Association 2007). Most skilled nursing facilities (53 percent) are part of a multifacility chain, and two-thirds

Table 10–6.   Characteristics of U.S. Skilled Nursing Facilities

Type of ownership:	Multifacility/chain:	53%
	Independent:	47%
	Hospital:	8%
Sponsorship:	For Profit:	66%
	Not-for-profit:	27%
	Government:	7%
Medicare and Medicaid certified:		89%
Average number of beds:		108
Special beds designated:	Alzheimers:	5%
	Rehabilitation:	1%
	Ventilator:	0.5%
Average number of direct care staff per facility: 62		
Percentage of nursing homes with outside contracts for therapy services: 69%		

Sources: OSCAR Data Reports. 2007. *Operational Characteristics.* American Health Care Association. http://www.ahca.org/research/oscar_oper.htm (accessed June 29, 2007). National Nursing Home Survey. *2004 Facility Tables.* http://www.cdc.gov/nchs/about/major/nnhsd/Facilitytables.htm (accessed July 2, 2007).

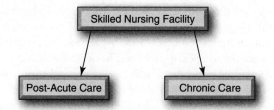

Figure 10–4.   Persons Served in Skilled Nursing Facilities (SNF)

are for-profit enterprises (see Table 10–6 ■). The average facility has 90 beds and consists of resident rooms, dining and activity areas, and therapy space. Skilled nursing facility care is the most expensive site of care in the post-acute care continuum. The average daily cost for a stay in a skilled nursing facility is $194 (American Association of Retired Persons 2006). The federal Medicaid program funds almost 7 in 10 persons residing in skilled nursing facilities (see Table 10–7 ■).

Skilled nursing facility care is for patients who have complex nursing or rehabilitation needs that cannot be provided in another environment (e.g., home health, assisted living). Persons in skilled nursing facilities typically need help with at least three activities of daily living, and three in four have cognitive problems (see Table 10–7 ■). Typically, these individuals have complex care needs, but are medically stable with regular nursing observation/treatment. Examples of care needs that

Table 10–7.   Characteristics of Residents in U.S. Nursing Homes

Average number of ADL limitations: 3.98
Percentage requiring assistance with bathing: 95.2%
Percentage requiring assistance with dressing: 89.0%
Percentage requiring assistance with transferring: 78.6%
Percentage requiring assistance with toileting: 82.7%
Percentage requiring assistance with eating: 51.9%
Percentage bed bound: 3.5%
Percentage restricted to a chair: 57.4%
Percentage ambulatory: 41.3%
Percentage physically restrained/with orders to be restrained: 6.2/1.3%
Percentage with dementia: 46.4%
Percentage with behavioral problems: 29.3%
Percentage experiencing depression: 48.6%
Percentage with pressure sores: 7.1%
Payer Source: Medicaid 64.4%
                     Medicare 13.6%
                     Other 22%

Source: OSCAR Data Reports. *Patient Characteristics.* American Health Care Association. http://www.ahca.org/research/oscar_patient.htm (accessed June 29, 2007).

would qualify an individual for skilled nursing care include daily injections, wound care, tube feedings, needing the assistance of more than one person for mobility tasks, needing help with all personal hygiene care, and significant confusion.

Four basic services are provided in skilled nursing facilities: nursing and rehabilitation, personal care, residential services, and medical care (see Table 10–2 ■). Each resident receives an individualized plan of care developed by a multidisciplinary team. All facilities have 24-hour nursing services staffed by nurse's aides for personal care, with supervision by licensed practical nurses and registered nurses. Nurse's aides assist with feeding, bathing, dressing, walking, and transfers. Professional nurses provide examination, evaluation, and technical nursing interventions.

Occupational therapists and physical therapists provide evaluation and intervention to improve function and prevent secondary conditions in this population. For patients with short-term, post-acute care needs, nursing homes have become important sites for receiving rehabilitation therapy services (Murray, Singer, Fortinsky, Russo, and Cebul 1999). Over half of the residents in a study of Ohio nursing homes were receiving physical therapy, occupational therapy, or speech-language pathology services (Murray et al. 1999). Rehabilitation in a nursing home typically takes longer, and the post-acute care patients served have more severe deficits. However, one study of nursing home rehabilitation reports that nearly two in three patients ultimately return to the community (Kosasih, Borca, Wenninger, and Duthie 1998). A younger age, fewer limitations in ADL performance, and rehabilitation therapy are associated with a greater likelihood of community discharge (Mehr, Williams, and Fries 1997). Kauh, Polak, Hazelett, Hua, and Allen (2005) found that persons treated in a geriatric rehabilitation unit within a skilled nursing facility had a shorter length of stay, a greater likelihood of community discharge, and greater improvement in ADLs and mobility. Jette, Warren, and Wirtalla (2005) found that higher physical therapy and occupational therapy intensities were associated with shorter lengths of stay and greater functional gains for patients receiving care in a skilled nursing facility.

Restorative care is an important component of rehabilitation services for persons with long-term chronic disease in nursing homes. Porell, Caro, Silva, and Monane (1998) describe how the slow rate of decline in functional task performance among nursing home residents with chronic conditions is exacerbated by serious medical illness (e.g., congestive heart failure, chronic obstructive pulmonary disease, cancer). Restorative care is commonly implemented by a specially trained nursing aide. Training usually encompasses, at a minimum, basic range-of-motion exercise and ambulation training. Restorative care services are usually overseen by a nursing supervisor. Restorative aides can help with the completion of rehabilitation protocols established by physical and occupational therapists and with providing maintenance therapy, which is not reimbursable as a professional service. An initial evaluation by an occupational therapist or a physical therapist to establish a maintenance program in a skilled nursing facility is a Medicare-reimbursable service (see Chapter 7). Katz, Karuza, Kolassa, and Hutson (1997) found that, while medical direction is required in skilled nursing facilities, relatively few physicians spend time caring for residents of nursing homes.

The experience of nursing-home living is life changing. The decision to place a family member in a nursing home is usually not preplanned, is often rushed, and is made at a time of emotional stress for the informal care system (Rodgers 1997). Nearly three in four nursing home admissions are prompted by a hospitalization after a major event, most commonly stroke, hip fracture, congestive heart failure, pneumonia, cancer, or diabetes (Ferruci, Guralnik, Pahor, Corti, and Havlik 1997). Wilson (1997) describes the adjustment to nursing home life for new residents in three phases: overwhelmed, adjustment, and initial acceptance. Fiveash (1998) found that some residents experienced satisfaction with living in a nursing home, but others described the experience as limiting and "dehumanizing." The patient's experience of residential life is very important. Residents place importance on choice and control over bedtime, waking time, food, roommates, care routines, outside trips, the use of money, and the telephone (Kane et al. 1997). Residents who are active, have a positive attitude, and believe that they have control over their environment make better adjustments to life in a nursing home (Johnson, Stone, Altmaier, and Berdahl 1998).

Concerns regarding the quality of care in nursing homes have been addressed within the health care community. In the past, nursing homes were criticized for excessive use of restraints. Currently, the use of restraints is restricted and must be well documented (Sullivan-Marx, Strumpf, Evans, Baumgarten, and Maislin 1999). Another chronic problem in skilled nursing facilities is absenteeism and turnover among nursing home workers (Cohen-Mansfield 1997; Parsons, Parker, and Ghose 1998). The Nursing Home Reform Act of 1987 initiated the development of a standardized assessment tool for evaluating the health status and care needs of nursing home residents. The Resident Assessment Instrument (RAI) has resulted in several improvements in nursing home quality. Researchers have found improved patient care documentation, better patient care planning, a lower use of restraints, fewer hospital admissions from nursing homes, and improvements in ADL function, social interactions, and cognition among nursing home residents after implementation of the RAI (Mor et al. 1997; Phillips et al. 1997; Hawes et al. 1997).

The RAI (see Table 10–8 ■) represents a process of problem recognition and care planning designed to improve, prevent, or slow the decline in function of nursing home residents. As can be seen in Table 10–7, most nursing home residents have a number of impairments and functional limitations. The RAI process has three components: assessment, Resident Assessment Protocols (RAPs), and utilization guidelines. Patient assessment is performed with the Minimum Data Set (MDS), the same instrument used for determining payment (see Chapter 7). Information from the MDS may "trigger" the identification of a problem area that will require a more formal assessment. These problem areas fall into one of 18 categories of common challenges faced by nursing home residents. A "trigger" takes one of four forms: potential problem, broad screen, prevention of problem, or rehabilitation potential. The outcome of a RAP is to investigate, identify, document, and address the problem, after which a plan of care is developed to address the problem. The plan includes an intervention and a method for evaluating the outcome of the care.

Table 10–8.   Components of the SNF Resident Assessment Instrument (RAI)

Assessment

Minimum Data Set (MDS)

Resident Assessment Protocols

Problem Areas Identified By Analysis of MDS Data

1. Delirium	7. Psychosocial wellbeing	14. Dehydration/
2. Cognitive loss	8. Mood state	fluid maintenance
3. Visual function	9. Behavior symptoms	15. Dental care
4. Communication	10. Activities	16. Pressure ulcers
5. ADL function/rehab potential	11. Falls	17. Psychotropic drug use
6. Urinary incontinence and indwelling catheter	12. Nutritional status	18. Physical restraints
	13. Feeding tubes	

Utilization Guidelines

Instructions on how to implement the Resident Assessment Instrument

Source: Center for Medicare and Medicaid Services. 2002. *Resident Assessment Instrument Manual.* http://www.cms.hhs.gov/nursinghomequalityinits/20_nhqimds20.asp (accessed July 3, 2007).

Active Learning Exercise

To learn more about the use of the Resident Assessment Instrument in nursing homes, visit the CMS training website at http://www.mdstraining.org/upfront/u1.asp

---

Subacute Care

Subacute care is defined as a "comprehensive, cost effective inpatient level of care for patients who have had an acute event . . ., have a determined course of treatment and though stable, require diagnostics or invasive procedures, but not intensive procedures requiring an acute level of care" (National Association of Subacute/Post Acute Care 2005). Subacute care is intended for the short-term recuperation of a person after a significant illness or injury. Subacute care units have developed both in nursing homes and hospitals. The units in hospitals are sometimes termed **swing bed** units. Other locations for subacute care units include rehabilitation hospitals and freestanding subacute care units. Subacute care facilities are licensed as skilled nursing facilities and provide a level of care between those of a hospital and a skilled nursing facility.

Subacute care units tend to be organized around patient types (e.g., medically complex, respiratory/ventilator care, postsurgical, stroke or orthopedic rehabilitation, oncology). In contrast to acute hospital care patients, subacute care patients receive a lower level of physician and nursing care. Physicians typically do not visit on a daily basis; occasionally they visit only weekly. Nursing time is closely monitored and is typically four to seven contact hours per day. In general, physical therapy and occupational therapy services are provided on a daily basis. In contrast to therapy time in inpatient rehabilitation facilities, subacute rehabilitation total therapy time is less than three hours per day. The goal is to move the patient to a less intense level of care (perhaps home or long-term care) as soon as possible. About 50 percent of patients in subacute care facilities are discharged to their homes (American Health Care Association 2000).

Inpatient Rehabilitation Facilities

Inpatient rehabilitation facilities are either independent, stand-alone institutions or dedicated units within hospitals or nursing homes that provide intensive inpatient rehabilitation. Inpatient rehabilitation facilities provide care for patients recovering from serious illness and injury in preparation for reentry into the community. Typically, these programs provide rehabilitation care for patients with the most complex conditions (e.g., traumatic brain injury and spinal cord injury survivors); at least 60 percent of a facility's admissions must come from patients with complex illnesses and injuries (see Chapter 7). Consistent with Medicare rules, patients in these facilities need to be able to tolerate at least three hours of therapy per day in order to be admitted. Occupational therapy, physical therapy, speech-language pathology, therapeutic recreation, rehabilitation nursing, psychological and counseling services, and rehabilitation medicine (physiatric) services are common to these centers.

COMMUNITY-BASED MENTAL HEALTH PRACTICE

About one in four Americans will experience a diagnosable mental illness in a year, and 6 percent of the population has a serious and persistent mental illness (National Institute of Mental Health 2006). To provide care for these persons, a mental health system has been created. Occupational therapists provide a small, but important, component of the mental health service team. This system consists of both medical and human services. Medical services include psychiatric care and pharmacologic therapy. Human services include vocational training and supported employment, the justice system, and education. The system has been criticized for poor integration between the medical and human services (Horvitz-Lennon, Kilbourne, and Pincus 2006). The number of persons receiving mental health treatment is increasing, but the system is still meeting the needs of only half of the persons who require care (Kessler et al. 2005).

In Chapter 9, we mentioned the organization of inpatient mental health care in specialty hospitals (i.e., psychiatric hospitals). The delivery of health care to persons with mental illness has changed from an institution-centered approach to providing services in community clinics and centers. About 10 percent of the mental

Table 10–9.   Components of the U.S. Mental Health System (2000)

Total number of mental health organizations:	4,546
Outpatient clinics, partial care organizations, multiservice mental health organizations:	2,068
General hospitals with psychiatric units	1,373
Residential treatment centers for emotionally disturbed children	474
Private psychiatric hospitals	269
State and county mental hospitals	220
VA medical centers	142

Source: National Mental Health Statistics. Table 1. *Number of Mental Health Organizations by type of organization, United States, selected years, 1970–2000.* http://mentalhealth.samhsa.gov/publications/allpubs/SMA04-3938/chp18table1.asp (accessed July 18, 2007).

health care system is centered in an inpatient facility devoted to mental or psychiatric conditions (see Table 10–9 ■). Increasingly, mental health care is being delivered in community health centers, assisted living facilities, adult day care environments, "clubhouse" or supported employment models, and the justice system (e.g., in prisons and schools) (Farmer, Burns, Phillips, Angold, and Costello 2003). With the development of more effective pharmacologic agents, treatment is moving from "care" toward "cure" (Gruhl 2005). A new challenge to providers in mental health practice is an increasing number of persons with "dual diagnoses" (i.e., a mental health condition and a substance abuse problem) (Kessler 2004).

Community Health Centers

Community health centers are a type of multiservice mental health organization. Community health centers developed because of the Community Mental Health Act of 1963 and are the largest treatment provider for people with mental illness (Punwar 1994). These facilities receive federal and state funding and therefore may receive guidance from community citizen boards (Richert and Gibson 1993). The goal of community health centers is to maintain people with mental health concerns in the community in their contextual surroundings rather than in hospitals (Mosey 1986). Table 10–10 ■ lists required and optional mental health services for community health centers, based on the Community Mental Health Act. If a community health center offers all 10 services and is located in a community with a population between 75,000 and 200,000, it is titled a "comprehensive community mental health center" (Barry 2002).

Programs in community health centers are becoming more consumer driven than professionally driven, and this emphasis helps to empower the clients (Feder 1998). Services offered by these centers address all age groups and may include outpatient therapy, medication supervision, chemical-dependency services, health prevention, and crisis intervention. Programming may occur during the day or evening. Occupational therapists employed by these facilities work with

Table 10–10. Basic and Optional Services in a Community Mental Health Center (Services Based on the Community Mental Health Act)

Basic Services	Optional Services
Comprehensive Community Health Center	
Inpatient	Diagnostic
Outpatient	Rehabilitation
Partial hospitalization	Precare and aftercare
Emergency services	Professional and staff training programs
Consultation and education to community, organizations, groups, and residents	Research and evaluation

Adapted from: Barry 2002.

clients on community-living skills and social skills, and may perform case-management roles (Richert and Gibson 1993). Usually, far fewer people actually receive interventions from community health centers than the number who need such interventions (Abrams, Beers, and Berkow 1995).

Clubhouse Models

Clubhouse models, or community rehabilitation programs, are another interesting mental health alternative. These programs focus on skill acquisition for reentry into society and are based on a social, rather than a medical, model. Thus, programming may include vocational skills, independent living skills, social skills, and stress-reduction skills (Richert and Gibson 1993; Norman 2006). Supported employment has been found to be more effective than prevocational training for persons with severe mental illness (Crowther, Marshall, Bond, and Huxley 2001). Schoenebaum, Boyd, and Dudek (2006) found that 60 percent of clubhouse participants were in a job after 30 months of treatment. Clients adapting to community living may learn shopping skills, money-management skills, and transportation skills.

Adult Day Care Programs

Adult day care programs service people who require supervision during the day but can spend their evenings with supervised help in the community (Abrams, Beers, and Berkow 1995). Adult day care programs offer highly structured environments providing group and individual interventions (Hooper 1998). Some adult day care programs focus specifically on community-dwelling persons with mental illness, especially elders (Coveinsky and Buckley 1993). Day hospital programs have been found to improve mental state, but not social function, at less cost than inpatient hospital facilities (Marshall et al. 2001).

Nursing Homes

Some elders with mental illness (often deinstitutionalized elders) are found in nursing home settings. Regrettably, for many elderly persons with mental illness who have been reinstitutionalized in nursing homes, there are no structured programs to address many of their mental health concerns. This could be a growth area for occupational therapy mental health practice.

Another growing population found in nursing homes is elders with Alzheimer's disease. About 1 in 4 residents in a nursing home has a mental illness as his or her primary diagnosis (National Center for Health Statistics 1999). These individuals require specialized services, often offered in nursing home programs. Some programs focus on the continuum of specialized care designed to accommodate the residents' changing needs as they progress through the stages of dementia. For clients with Alzheimer's disease, Medicare will reimburse for therapy if there is a change in status or a skilled need (e.g., if a client falls and breaks a hip). Practitioners can assume consultative roles in these units. Therapists have the kinds of skills required to adapt activities and address activities of daily living at the client's functional level, to develop or provide group programming, and to consult about environmental adaptations and behavioral concerns.

Nontraditional Settings

Occupational therapists have now begun to branch out into nontraditional community settings. Nontraditional settings include part of the human services system—specifically, the justice and school systems (Armbruster 2002; Provident and Joyce-Gaguzis 2005)—and the workplace. Examples of nontraditional mental health settings are correctional centers, residential settings for people with mental illness, community programs for people on Medicaid (Kautzmann 1998; Wilberding 1993) and health-promotion programs in community businesses (Maynard 1993). Provident and Joyce-Gaguzis (2005) have reported that prisoners in the Allegheny County Jail Project benefited from occupational therapy intervention, which yielded an improvement in employment rates and reduced recidivism. Rai (2002) found that occupational therapists may have a role in reducing violence in the workplace.

CONCLUSION

In this chapter, we have explored the range of care options for persons in need of rehabilitation and recuperation after serious illness or injury (see Figure 10–5 ■). Given these options, the informal care system remains the largest and most important component of the post-acute care system. The experience of disablement increases the need for formal post-acute care services, a fact that bears relevance to both physical therapists and occupational therapists. Therapists make important contributions to reducing the risk of disablement. Rehabilitation services exist to promote and restore the ability of patients with chronic disease and disability to live in

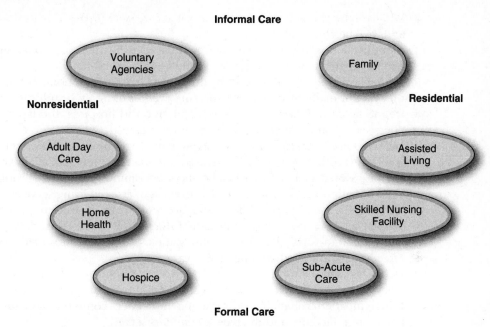

Figure 10–5. The Post-acute Health Care System

the community. For most of these patients, community living will depend on the strength of their informal care system that is, the care provided by parents, female spouses, and adult female children.

The formal care system consists of professional services, nonprofessional services, and residential care to either support or replace the informal care system. The majority of the residents in formal post-acute care sites are older women, a fact that reflects both the longer life span of women and the disproportionate share of informal care provided by women. Home health care and adult day services support the informal care system, both professionally and nonprofessionally. Assisted living facilities, skilled nursing facilities, subacute care facilities, and inpatient rehabilitation facilities provide a continuum of residential, professional, and nonprofessional services for the short-term or long-term care of persons with chronic disease and disability. Finally, the majority of mental health practice is provided in community environments and, increasingly, in nontraditional settings (e.g., schools, the justice system, and the workplace).

CHAPTER REVIEW QUESTIONS

1. Consider how the post-acute care continuum has evolved over the last 20 years. What are the reasons for these changes?
2. Identify the two components of the post-acute care continuum. How are they related to each other?

3. What are the characteristics of the informal care system? Describe its strengths and weaknesses.

4. Identify the levels of the formal care system. Identify the professional services and residential features, if any, of each level of care.

5. Define home health care. Describe the services common to home health care, the types of patients served, and the effectiveness of home health care.

6. Define hospice. Describe the services common to hospices, the types of patients served, and the effectiveness of hospice care.

7. Define adult day services and the PACE program. Describe the services common to adult day care, the types of patients served, and the effectiveness of adult day care.

8. Define assisted living. Describe the services common to assisted living, the types of patients served, and the effectiveness of assisted living services.

9. Define skilled nursing facilities. Compare and contrast post-acute care services and chronic care services in skilled nursing facilities. Describe the services common to skilled nursing facilities, the types of patients served, and the effectiveness of skilled nursing facility care.

10. Define subacute care. Describe the services common to subacute care, the types of patients served, and the effectiveness of subacute care services.

11. Define inpatient rehabilitation. Describe the services common to inpatient rehabilitation facilities and the types of patients served.

CHAPTER DISCUSSION QUESTIONS

1. Consider and discuss how societal gender roles have influenced the development of the post-acute care system.

2. Consider the development of the post-acute care continuum in light of the medical and social models of disablement. Which model has been most influential in the development of the system to date? Why?

3. A primary purpose of occupational therapy and physical therapy is to promote independence in the patient's living environment. Compare and contrast the settings in the post-acute continuum as they affect the ability of physical therapists and occupational therapists to fulfill their roles.

REFERENCES

American Academy of Family Physicians. 2006. Average number of family physician visits per week and average number of patients in various settings. http://www.aafp.org/online/en/home/aboutus/specialty/facts/5.html (accessed June 27, 2007).

American Association of Retired Persons. 2006. Average daily cost for nursing home care by state, 2006. http://www.aarp.org/bulletin/longterm/Articles/a2003-10-30-dailycost.html (accessed June 29, 2007).

American Health Care Association. 1999. Today's nursing facilities and the people they serve. *www.ahca.org/who/profile3.htm* (accessed April 18, 2000).

————. 1999. National data on nursing facilities. *www.ahca.org/who/profile4.htm* (accessed April 18, 2000).

————. 1999 Nursing facilities. *www.ahca.org/info/pubthink.htm* (accessed April 18, 2000).

Armbruster, P. 2002. The administration of school-based mental health services. *Child Adolesc Psychiatr Clin N Am* 11(1): 23–41.

Arno, P. S., C. Levine, and M. M. Memmott. 1999. The economic value of informal caregiving. *Health Affairs* 18(2): 182–88.

Assisted Living Federation of America. 2000. What is assisted living? *www.Alfa.org/Whats AL.htm* (accessed April 17, 2000).

Ball, M. M., M. M. Perkins, F. J. Whittington, B. R. Connell, C. Hollingsworth, S. V. King, C. L. Elrod, and B. L. Combs. 2004. Managing decline in assisted living: The key to aging in place. *J Gerontol B Psychol Sci Soc Sci* 59(4): S202–12.

Baum, E. E., D. Jarjoura, A. E. Polen, D. Faur, and G. Rutecki. 2003. Effectiveness of a group exercise program in a long term care facility: A randomized pilot trial. *J Am Med Dir Assoc* 4(2): 74–80.

Bishop, C. E. 1999. Where are the missing elders? The decline in nursing home use.1995. *Health Affairs* 18(4): 146–55.

Boaz, R. F., and J. Hu. 1997. Determining the amount of help used by disabled elderly persons at home: The role of coping resources. *J Gerontol B* 52(6): S317–24.

Brannen, J. J., and E. R. Griemel. 1997. Professional burnout among nursing home personnel: Effects of a training intervention. *Abst Book Assoc Health* 14: 352.

Burdick, C. J., A. Rosenblatt, Q. M. Samus, C. Steele, A. Baker, M. Harper, L. Mayer, J. Brandt, P. Rabins, and C. G. Lysetsos. 2005. Predictors of functional impairment in residents of assisted-living facilities: The Maryland assisted living study. *J Gerontol A Biol Sci Med Sci* 60(2): 258–64.

Byock, I. 1996. The nature of suffering and the nature of opportunity at the end of life. *Clin Geriatr Med* 12: 237–52.

Carroll, N. V., P. W. Slattum, and F. M. Cox. 2005. The cost of falls among the community-dwelling elderly. *J Manag Care Pharm* 11(4): 307–16.

Castle, N. G., V. Mor, and J. Banaszak-Hull. 1997. Special care hospice units in nursing homes. *Hosp J* 12(3): 59–69.

Centers for Medicare and Medicaid Services. 2006. Other Medicare suppliers and providers. Selected years. Data compendium. http://www.cms.hhs.gov/DataCompendium/18_2006_Data_Compendium.asp#TopOfPage (accessed June 26, 2007).

————. 2007. List of PACE provider organizations. http://www.cms.hhs.gov/PACE/LPPO/list.asp?listpage=4 (accessed June 29, 2007).

Chappell, N. L., B. H. Dlitt, M. J. Hollander, J. A. Miller, and C. McWilliam. 2004. Comparative costs of home care and residential care. *Gerontologist* 44(3): 389–400.

Charles, K. K., and P. Sevak. 2005. Can family caregiving substitute for nursing home care? *J Health Econ* 24(6): 1174–90.

Chiu, L., K. Y. Tang, Y. H. Liu, W. C. Shyu, and T.P. Chang. 1999. Cost comparisons between family-based care and nursing home care for dementia. *J Adv Nurs* 29(4): 1005–12.

Clark, D. O. 1997. U. S. trends in disability and institutionalization among older blacks and whites. *Am J Pub Health* 87(3): 438–40.

Cleary, J., and J. Carbone. 1997. Palliative medicine in the elderly. *Cancer* 80(7): 1335–47.

Cohen-Mansfield, J. 1997. Turnover among nursing home staff. A review. *Nurs Manage* 28(5): 59–62, 64.

Coke, T., R. Alday, K. Biala, S. Luna, and P. Martines. 2005. The new role of physical therapy in home health care. *Home Healthc Nurse* 23(9): 594–99.

Collins, J., K. L. Beissner, and J. A. Krout. 1998. Home health physical therapy: Practice patterns in western New York. *Phys Ther* 78(2): 170–79.

Crowther, R., M. Marshall, G. Bond, and P. Huxley. 2001. Vocational rehabilitation for people with severe mental illness. *Cochrane Database Syst Rev* 2: CD003080.

Diwan, S., C. Berger, and E. K. Manns. 1997. Composition of the home care service package: Predictors of type, volume, and mix of services provided to poor and frail older people. *Gerontologist* 37(2): 169–81.

Donelan, K., C. A. Hill, C. Hoffman, K. Scoles, P. H. Feldman, C. Levine, and D. Gould. 2002. Challenged to care: Informal caregivers in a changing health care system. *Health Aff* 21(4): 222–31.

Emmanuel, R. J., D. L. Fairclough, J. Slutsman, H. Alpert, D. Baldwin, and L. L. Emmanuel. 1999. Assistance from family members, friends, paid caregivers and volunteers in the care of terminally ill members. *N Engl J Med* 341(13): 956–63.

Farmer, E. M., B. J. Burns, S. D. Phillips, A. Angold, and J. Costello. 2003. Pathways into and through mental health services for children and adolescents. *Psychiatr Serv* 54(1): 60–66.

Ferruci, L. K., J. M. Guralnik, M. Pahor, M. C. Corti, and R. J. Havlik. 1997. Hospital diagnoses, Medicare charges, and nursing home admissions in the year when older persons become severely disabled. *JAMA* 277(9): 728–34.

Fiveash, B. 1998. The experience of nursing home life. *Int J Nurs Prac* 4(3): 166–74.

Fonda, S. J., E. C. Clipp, and G. L. Maddox. 2002. Patterns of functioning among residents of an affordable assisted living housing facility. *Gerontologist* 42(2): 178–87.

Forbes, S., and N. Hoffart. 1998. Elders' decision making regarding the use of long-term care services: A precarious balance. *Qual Health Res* 8(6): 736–50.

Fried, T. R., C. van Doorn, J. R. O'Leary, M. E. Tinetti, and M. A. Drickamer. 1999. Older persons' preferences for site of terminal care. *Ann Intern Med* 131(2): 109–12.

Friedman, S. M., D. M. Steinwachs, P. J. Rathouz, L. C. Burton, and D. B. Mukamel. 2005. Characteristics predicting nursing home admission in the program of all-inclusive care for elderly people. *Gerontologist* 45(2): 157–66.

Fujiura, G. T. 1998. Demography of family households. *Am J Ment Ret* 103(3): 225–35.

Fujiura, G. T. 2003. Continuum of intellectual disability: Demographic evidence for the "forgotten generation". *Ment Retard* 41(6): 420–29.

Gabel, J. R., K. M. Hurst, and K. A. Hunt. 1998. Health benefits for the terminally ill: Reality and perception. *Health Affairs* 17(6):120–27.

Golant, S. M. 2004. Do impaired older persons with health care needs occupy U.S. assisted living facilities? An analysis of six national studies. *J Gerontol B Psychol Sci Soc Sci* 59(2): S68–79.

Gruhl, K. L. 2005. Reflections on . . . the recovery paradigm: Should occupational therapists be interested? *Can J Occup Ther* 72(2): 96–102.

Haupt, B. J. 1997. Characteristics of hospice care discharges. *Adv Data* 25(287): 1–14.

Hawes, C., V. Mor, C. D. Phillips, B.E. Fries, J.N. Morris, E. Steele-Friedlob, A. M. Greene, and M. Nennstiel. 1997. The OBRA-87 nursing home regulations and implementation of the Resident Assessment Instrument: Effects on process quality. *J Am Ger Soc* 45(8): 977–85.

Horvitz-Lennon, M., A. M. Kilbourne, and H. A. Pincus. 2006. From silos to bridges: Meeting the general health needs of adults with severe mental illnesses. *Health Aff* 25(3): 659–69.

Hospice Foundation of America. 1999. What is hospice? *www.hospicefoundation.org/virtual_html/whatis.htm* (accessed March 31, 2000).

Intrator, O., and K. Berg. 1998. Benefits of home health care after inpatient rehabilitation for hip fracture: Health service use by Medicare beneficiaries, 1987–1992. *Arch Phys Med Rehabil* 79(10): 1195–99.

Irvin, C. V., S. Massey, and T. Dorsey. 1997. Determinants of enrollment among applicants to PACE. *Health Care Fin Rev* 19(2): 135–53.

Jette, D. U., R. L. Warren, and C. Wirtalla. 2005. The relation between therapy intensity and outcomes of rehabilitation in skilled nursing facilities. *Arch Phys Med Rehabil* 86(3): 373–79.

Johnson, B. D., G. L. Stone, E.M. Altmaier, and L. D. Berdahl. 1998. The relationship of demographic factors, locus of control and self-efficacy to successful nursing home adjustment. *Gerontologist* 38(2): 209–16.

Johnson, K. S., M. Kuchibhatala, R. J. Sloane, D. Tanis, A.N. Galanos, and J. A. Tulsky. 2005. Ethnic differences in the place of death of elderly hospice enrollees. *J Am Geriatr Soc* 53(12): 2209–15.

Kane, R. A., A. L. Caplan, E. K. Urv-Wong, I. C. Freeman, M. A. Aroskar, and M. Finch. 1997. Everyday matters in the lives of nursing home residents: Wish for and perception of choice and control. *J Am Ger Soc* 45(9): 1086–93.

Kane, R. L., P. Homyak, B. Bershadsky, and S. Flood. 2006. Variations on a theme called PACE. *J Gerontol A Biol Sci Med Sci* 61(7): 689–93.

Kane, R. L., B. Bershadsky, and J. Bershadsky. 2006. Who recommends long term care matters? *Gerontologist* 46(4): 474–82.

Katz, P. R., J. Karuza, J. Kolassa, and A. Hutson. 1997. Medical practice with nursing home residents: Results from the National Physician Professional Activities Census. *J Am Ger Soc* 45(8): 911–17.

Kauh, B., T. Polak, S. Hazelett, K. Hua, and K. Allen. 2005. A pilot study: Post-acute geriatric rehabilitation versus usual care in skilled nursing facilities. *J Am Med Dir Assoc* 6(5): 321–26.

Kennedy, J., C. Walls, and D. Owens-Nicholson. 1999. A national profile of primary and secondary household caregivers: Estimates from the 1992 and 1993 surveys on income and program participation. *Home Health Care Serv Q* 17(4): 39–58.

Kessler, R. C., O. Demler, R. G. Frank, M. Olfson, H. A. Pincus, E. E. Walters, P. Wang, K. B. Wells, and A. M. Zaslavsky. 2005. Prevalence and treatment of mental disorders, 1990–2003. *New Engl J Med* 352(24): 2515–23.

Kessler, R. C. 2004. The epidemiology of dual diagnoses. *Biol Psychiatry* 56(10): 730–37.

Keysor, J. J., T. Desai, and E. J. Mutran. 1999. Elders' preferences for care setting in short- and long-term disability scenarios. *Gerontologist* 39(3): 334–44.

Kinosian, B., E. Stallard, and D. Wieland. 2007. Projected use of long term care services by enrolled veterans. *Gerontologist* 47(3): 356–64.

Kosasih, J. B., H. H. Borca, W. J. Wenninger, and E. Duthie. 1998. Nursing home rehabilitation after acute rehabilitation: Predictors and outcomes. *Arch Phys Med Rehab* 79(6): 670–73.

Lee, M., and A. D. Tussing. 1998. Influences on nursing home admissions: The role of informal caregivers. *Abstr Book Assoc Health* 15: 55–56.

Lee, W., C. Eng, N. Fox, and M. Etienne. 1998. PACE: A model for integrated care of frail older patients. *Geriatrics* 53(6): 62, 65–66, 69, 73.

Leland, J. Y., and R. S. Schonwelter. 1997. Advances in hospice care. *Clin Geriatr Med* 13(2): 381–401.

Lewis, C. L., M. Moutoux, M. Slaughter, and S. P. Bailey. 2004. Characteristics of individuals who fell while receiving home health services. *Phys Ther* 84(1): 23–32.

Li, L. W., and B. E. Fries. 2005. Elder disability as an explanation for racial differences in informal home care. *Gerontologist* 45(2): 206–15.

Long, S. K., K. Liu, K. Black, J. O'Keefe, and S. Molony. 2005. Getting by in the community: Lessons from frail elders. *J Aging Soc Policy* 17(1): 19–44.

Marshall, M., R. Crowther, A. Almaraz-Serrano, F. Creed, W. Sledge, H. Kluiter, C. Roberts, E. Hill, D. Wiersma, G. R. Bond, P. Huxley, and P. Tyrer. 2001. Systematic reviews of the effectiveness of day care for people with severe mental disorders: 1) acute day hospital vs. admission; 2) vocational rehabilitation; 3) day hospital vs. outpatient care.

McCann, S., and D. S. Evans. 2002. Informal care: The views of people receiving care. *Health Soc Care Community.* 10(4): 221–28.

McDermott, S., D. Valentine, D. Anderson, D. Gallup, and S. Thompson. 1997. Parents of adults with mental retardation living in home and out of home: Caregiving burdens and gratifications. *Am J Orthopsychiatr.* 67(2): 323–29.

Medicare Payment Advisory Commission. 1998. Home health utilization. In *Medicare Payment Policy. Report to the Congress: Context for a Changing Medicare Program,* 107–15.

———. 1998. Program of all-inclusive care for the elderly. In *Report to Congress: Medicare Payment Policy, Vol. 2,* 111–20

Mehr, D. R., B. C. Williams, and B. E. Fries. 1997. Predicting discharge outcomes of VA nursing home residents. *J Aging Health* 9(2): 244–65.

Meyer, G. S., and R. V. Gibbons. 1997. House calls to the elderly: A vanishing practice among physicians. *N Engl J Med* 337(25): 1815–20.

Mollica, R. L. 1998. Managed care and assisted living: Trends and future prospects. *J Health Hum Serv Adm* 20(3): 264–80.

Montauk, S. L. 1998. Home health care. *Am Fam Physician* 58(7): 1608–14.

Montgomery, R. J. 1999. The family role in the context of long-term care. *J Aging Health* 11(3): 383–416.

Mor, V., O. Intrator, B. E. Fries, C. Phillips, J. Teno, J. Hiris, C. Hawes, and J. Morris. 1997. Changes in hospitalization associated with introducing the Resident Assessment Instrument. *J Am Geri Soc* 45(8): 1002–10.

Mukamel, D. B., H. Temkin-Greener, and H. Clark. 1998. Stability of disability among PACE enrollees: Financial and programmatic implications. *Health Care Fin Rev* 19(3): 83–100.

Murray, P. K., M. E. Singer, R. Fortinsky, L. Russo, and R. D. Cebul. 1999. Rapid growth of rehabilitation services in traditional community-based nursing homes. *Arch Phys Med Rehabil* 80(4): 372–78.

National Adult Day Services Association. 2007. Adult day services: The Facts. http://www.nadsa.org/adsfacts/default.asp (accessed June 29, 2007).

National Center for Assisted Living. 2006. Resources and Publications. http://www.ncal.org/resource/index.cfm (accessed June 29, 2007).

National Center for Health Statistics. 2007. Home Health Definition of Terms. http://www.cdc.gov/nchs/about/major/nhhcsd/nhhcsdefhomehealth.htm (accessed June 26, 2007).

————. 1999. Mental Health Disorders. http://www.cdc.gov/nchs/fastats/mental.htm (accessed July 18, 2007).

National Institute of Mental Health. 2006. The numbers count: Mental illness in America. http://www.nimh.nih.gov/publicat/numbers.cfm (accessed July 18, 2007).

Ng, K. and C. F. von Gunten. 1998. Symptoms and attitudes of 100 consecutive patients admitted to an acute hospice/palliative care unit. *J Pain Symptom Manage* 16(5): 307–16.

Norman, C. 2006. The Fountain House movement, an alternative rehabilitation model for people with mental health problems, members' descriptions of what works. *Scand J Caring Sci* 20(2): 184–92.

O'Keefe, J., S. K. Long, K. Liu, and M. Kerr. 2001. How do they manage? Disabled elderly persons in the community who are not receiving Medicaid long term care services. *Home Health Care Serv Q* 20(4): 73–90.

O'Sullivan, A., and C. Siebert. 2004. Occupational therapy and home health. A perfect fit. *Caring* 23(5): 10–16.

O'Sullivan, M. J., and B. Volicer. 1997. Factors associated with achievement of goals for home health care. *Home Health Care Serv Q* 16(3): 21–34.

Parsons, S., K. P. Parker, and R. P. Ghose. 1998. A blueprint for reducing turnover among nursing assistants: A Louisiana study. *J La State Med Soc* 150(11): 545–53.

Payne, S. M., C. P. Thomas, T. Fitzpatrick, M. Abdel-Rahman, and H. L. Kayne. 1998. Determinants of home health visit length: Results of a multisite prospective study. *Med Care* 36: 1500–14.

Penrod, J. D., R. L. Kane, M. D. Finch, and R. A. Kane. 1998. Effects of post-hospital Medicare home health and informal care on patient functional status. *Health Serv Res* 33(3 pt.1): 513–29.

Petrisek, A. C., and V. Mor. 1999. Hospice in nursing homes: A facility level analysis of the distribution of hospice beneficiaries. *Gerontologist* 39(3): 279–90.

Phillips, C. D., J. N. Morris, C. Hawes, B. E. Fries, V. Mor, M. Nennstiel, and V. Iannacchione. 1997. Association of the Resident Assessment Instrument with changes in function, cognition and psychosocial status. *J Am Ger Soc* 45(8): 986–93.

Pickett, M., M. E. Cooley, and D. B. Gordon. 1998. Palliative care: Past, present and future perspective. *Sem Oncol Nurs* 14(2): 86–94.

Porell, F., F. G. Caro, A. Silva, and M. Monane. 1998. A longitudinal analysis of nursing home outcomes. *Health Serv Res* 33(4 pt. 1): 835–65.

Provident, I. M., and K. Joyce-Gaguzis. 2005. Creating an occupational therapy Level II fieldwork experience in a county jail setting. *Am J Occup Ther* 59(1): 101–16.

Rai, S. 2002 Preventing workplace aggression and violence—a role for occupational therapy. *Work* 18(1): 15–22.

Rasmussen, B. H., and P. O. Sanderson. 1998. How patients spend their time in a hospice and in an oncological unit. *J Adv Nurs* 28(4): 818–28.

Reschovsky, J. D. 1998. The demand for post-acute and chronic care in nursing homes. *Medical Care* 36(4): 475–90.

Robinson, K. M. 1997. The family's role in long term care. *J Gerontol Nurs* 23(9): 7–11.

Rodgers, B. L. 1997. Family members' experiences with the nursing home placement of an older adult. *Appl Nurs Res* 10(2): 57–63.

Sands, L. P., Y. Wang, G. P. McCabe, K. Jennings, C. Eng, and K. E. Covinsky. 2006. Rates of acute care admissions for frail older people living with met versus unmet activity of daily living needs. *J Am Geriatr Soc* 54(2): 339–44.

Schonebaum, A. D., J. K. Boyd, and K. J. Dudek. 2006. A comparison of competitive employment outcomes for the clubhouse and PACT models. *Psychiatr Serv* 57(10): 1416–20.

Sikorska, E. 1999. Organizational determinants of resident satisfaction with assisted living. *Gerontologist* 39(4): 450–56.

Sloane, P. D., S. Zimmerman, A. L. Gruber-Baldini, J. R. Hebel, J. Magaziner, and T. R. Konrad. 2005. Health and functional outcomes and health care utilization of persons with dementia in residential care and assisted living facilities: Comparison with nursing homes. *Gerontologist* 45 Spec 1(1): 124–32.

Stewart, K. 2006. Perspectives on the recent decline in disability at older ages. *Policy Brief (Cent Home Care Policy Res)* 27: 1–6.

Stillman, M. J., and K. L. Syrjala. 1999. Differences in physician access patterns to hospice care. *J Pain Symptom Manage* 17(3): 157–63.

Sullivan-Marx, E. M., N. E. Strumpf, L. K. Evans, M. Baumgarten, and G. Maislin. 1999. Predictors of continued physical restraint use in nursing home residents following restraint reduction efforts. *J Am Geri Soc* 47(3): 342–48.

Szinovacz, M. E., and A. Davey. 2007. Changes in adult child caregiver networks. *Gerontologist* 47(3): 280–95.

Taylor, L., F. Whittington, C. Hollingsworth, M. Ball, S. King, V. Patterson, S. Diwan, C. Rosenbloom, and A. Neel, Jr. 2003. Assessing the effectiveness of a walking program on physical function of residents living in an assisted living facility. *J Community Health Nurs* 20(1): 15–26.

Wallace, S., L. Levy-Storms, R. Kingston, and R. Anderson. 1998. The persistence of race and ethnicity in the use of long term care. *J Gerontol B Psychol Sci Soc Sci* 53(2): S104–112.

Weggel, J. M. 1999. Barriers to the physician decision to offer hospice as an option for terminal care. *WMJ* 98(3): 49–53.

Weiss, C. O., H. M. Gonzalez, M. U. Kabeto, and K. M. Langa. 2005. Differences in amount of informal care received by non-Hispanic whites and Latinos in a nationally representative sample of older Americans. *J Am Geriatr Soc* 53(1): 146–51.

Wielink, G., and R. Huijsman. 1999. Elderly community residents' evaluative criteria and preferences for formal and informal in-home services. *Int J Aging Hum Dev* 48(1): 17–33.

Williams, J., B. Lyons, and D. Rowland. 1997. Unmet long term care needs of elderly people in the community: A review of the literature. *Home Health Care Serv Q* 16(1–2): 93–119.

Wilson, S. A. 1997. The transition to nursing home life: A comparison of planned and unplanned admissions. *J Adv Nurs* 26(5): 864–71.

Wolf, D. A. 1999. The family as provider of long-term care: Efficiency, equity and externalities. *J Aging Health* 11(3): 360–82.

Wolff, J. L., and J. D. Kasper. 2006. Caregivers of frail elders: Updating a national profile. *Gerontologist.* 46(3): 344–56.

Yoo, B. K., J. Bhattacharya, K. M. McDonald, and A. M. Garber. 2004. Impacts of informal caregiver availability on long term care expenditures in OECD countries. *Health Serv Res* 39(6 Pt2): 1971–92.

11

Special Education, Public Health, and Complementary/Alternative Medicine

CHAPTER OBJECTIVES

At the conclusion of this chapter, the reader will be able to:

1. Define special education and the role of the Individual Education Plan team.
2. Relate the needs of special education children and the role of occupational therapists and physical therapists in meeting those needs.
3. Define public health and discuss the role of public health services within the overall health care system.
4. Describe the levels of organization of public health services:
   a. international
   b. federal
   c. state
   d. local
5. Describe the delivery of public health services:
   a. assessment
   b. policy development
      1. Healthy People 2010
   c. assurance of access to health care services
6. Discuss the opportunities for physical therapist and occupational therapist involvement in public health activities.
7. Identify and define alternative medicine, complementary medicine, and conventional medicine providers and practices.

KEY WORDS: Alternative Medicine, Complementary Medicine, Conventional Medicine, Epidemiology, Public Health Model, Special Education

Case Example

A number of assisted living and retirement facilities have been built in the city where Sally, a physical therapist, works for a home health agency. While seeing patients at these sites, Sally notices that many of the residents are sedentary and have mobility limitations. She understands that a regular exercise program can improve mobility and reduce disability in a community-living, older population. She contacts her local public health agency and learns that a grant program exists to provide resources for these types of programs. Sally applies for and receives the grant. She develops a program for the residents of these facilities, and everyone notices that falls are decreasing and health status has increased.

Case Example Focus Question:

1. What types of health problems in the community do you think physical therapists and occupational therapists should address?

INTRODUCTION

In the previous two chapters, we discussed the acute medical care system and the post-acute health care system. The organizations in these two systems are the location of work for many therapists. In this chapter, we conclude with a discussion of other parts of the health care system affecting therapy practice: special education, public health, and complementary/alternative medicine. For pediatric therapists in the schools, the special education system is the site of their work. Work in schools is structured differently from work in medical environments. In Chapter 4, we discussed the Individuals with Disabilities Education Act, the law that mandates therapy services in schools. In this chapter, we will explore the needs and opportunities of public health. Public health is an increasingly important area of health care for therapists, given the increasing incidence of chronic disease and the known effects of lifestyle and environment on health status. Finally, some therapists employ procedures and techniques that are considered alternative medicine. In this chapter, we will define alternative, complementary, and conventional medicine and introduce several alternative medicine providers.

SPECIAL EDUCATION

Special education is provided in the public schools as "specially designed instruction, at no cost to the parents, to meet the unique needs of a child with a disability including instruction conducted in the classroom, in the home, in hospitals, in institutions and in other settings, and in physical education" (U.S. Department of Education 2006, p. 46761). Occupational therapy and physical therapy services are provided to children in school systems, which are the top employer of occupational therapists. Therapy services are a "related service"(U.S. Department of Education 2006, p. 46760). A related service is "transportation, and such developmental, corrective, and other supportive services as are required to assist a child with a disability to benefit from special education . . ." (U.S. Department of Education 2006, p. 46760). Related services are provided to children as a component of the Individualized Education Plan (see Chapter 4), the plan that defines the educational and related services a child will receive in his or her school. The required members of the team developing the annual plan are listed in Table 11–1 ∎.

Table 11–1. Members of the Individualized Education Plan Team

Parents of the Child
At least one regular education teacher of the child
At least one special education teacher of the child
A representative of the school or other special education provider

- who is qualified to provide or supervise special education services
- who is knowledgeable about the regular education curriculum
- who is aware of the resources of the school or other special education provider

A person who can interpret the educational evaluation results
At the discretion of the parents or school/other special education provider, related service providers
The child with the disability

Source: U.S. Department of Education. 2006. 34 CFR Parts 300 and 301. Assistance to the States for Education of Children with Disabilities and Preschool Grants for Children with Disabilities; Final Rule. *Federal Register* 46540–46845.

Table 11–2 ■ lists the available related services and the utilization rates for high school students in special education. As shown, about 40 percent of special education students do not utilize a related service from the school, primarily because they do not need such a service. About 16 percent of students need a related service but are unable to access it. The most common reasons for lack of access to related services are found in Table 11–3 ■. The school is the primary source of information for parents about needed and available services. Psychological services are the most common related service utilized by special education students. Speech-language pathology is the most common related service provided by the school. Twelve percent of special education students utilize occupational therapy services. Less than 10 percent of special education students are receiving physical therapy. As can be seen in the table, for most services, many students are receiving a related service from a source outside the school, typically in the medical environment. This is especially true for physical therapy, with an equal number of students receiving services from outside the school as in the school.

All children are eligible for a "free and appropriate public education" from age 3 to age 21 in the "least restrictive environment," with few exceptions (e.g., state law specifically precludes funding for all students receiving preschool education or education after age 18). This requirement includes the responsibility to provide comparable services to children in private schools. The states are free to decide whether to organize their special education services as a state responsibility, a local public school responsibility, or as a cooperative, interschool responsibility (termed an *educational service agency*). Indeed, this organization may vary within a state. For example, metropolitan school districts may provide special education and related services as a local responsibility, whereas small, rural districts will more typically provide services through an educational service agency or a statewide mechanism.

Table 11–2. **Secondary School Student Utilization of Related Services in Special Education**

Service	% Receiving from Any Source/from the School
Psychological services	31.6/15.5
Speech-language pathology	25.7/25.3
Medical and diagnostic services	23.5/7.5
Counseling services, including rehabilitation counseling Vocational services	19.8/17.6
Social work services	12.8/7.7
Occupational therapy	12.1/10.8
Transportation	10.8/10.7
Physical therapy	9.2/4.1
Assistive technology/services	6.7/4.9
Audiology	3.4/2.3
School health services Nursing care	1.5/1.1
None of these services	28.4/41.1
Therapeutic recreation	Not Reported
Early identification of disabilities	Not Reported
Parent counseling and training	Not Reported

Source: SRI. 2004. National Longitudinal Transition Study 2. *Services and Supports for Secondary School Students with Disabilities.* Office of Special Education Programs. U.S. Department of Education. http://www.eric.ed.gov/ERICDocs/data/ericdocs2sql/ content_storage_01/0000019b/80/28/0c/7d.pdf (accessed July 9, 2007).

Table 11–3. **Barriers to Receiving Related Services in Special Education**

Lack of information	24%
Services not available	23%
Poor quality	20%
Scheduling conflicts	18%
Cost of services	17%
Youth ineligibility for services	17%
Location of services	16%
Lack of time	15%
Transportation barriers	12%
Language barriers	5%
Other	4%

Source: SRI. 2004. National Longitudinal Transition Study 2. *Services and Supports for Secondary School Students with Disabilities.* Office of Special Education Programs. U.S. Department of Education. http://www.eric.ed.gov/ERICDocs/data/ericdocs2sql/content_storage_01/0000019b/80/28/0c/7d.pdf (accessed July 9, 2007). Exhibit 2–5, p. 2–8.

Table 11–4.   **Characteristics of Preschool Students with Disabilities**

Race:	White: 67%, Hispanic: 22%, Black: 11%	
Household income:	<$20,000: 27.2% $20,000–$50,000: 38.8%	>$50,000: 34%
Living with two parents:	67%	
Primary disability:	Speech/language impairment:	46%
	Developmental delay:	28%
	Autism:	7%
Mean age for start of special education and related services: 31 months		
Types of services received:		
Speech-language pathology:		93%
Special education:		42%
Occupational therapy:		34%
Physical therapy:		21%
Tutoring:		19%
Respite care, behavior therapy, vision care:		5%

Source: National Center for Special Education Research. 2006. Preschoolers with disabilities: Characteristics, services and results. NSCER 2006–3003. http://www.eric.ed.gov/ERICDocs/data/ericdocs2sql/content_storage_01/0000019b/80/28/04/14.pdf (accessed July 9, 2007).

Depending on the type of organization, a therapist may serve children in one school district or in several school districts.

Table 11–4 ■ identifies the common characteristics of preschool students with disabilities who are served in special education. The racial, household income, and parental status distributions approximate those of the general population. The most common reason a child is receiving special education is for a speech or language impairment or a developmental delay. Speech-language pathology is the most common therapy provided in special education (see Table 11–2 ■). About one in three preschool children with disabilities receive occupational therapy, and one in five children receive physical therapy. Occupational therapy is most commonly provided to preschool children with autism and to secondary school students with multiple disabilities (e.g., mental retardation and an orthopedic impairment) (see Table 11–5 ■). Physical therapy is most commonly provided to preschool children with other health impairments (e.g., a health condition, such as diabetes, resulting in diminished strength, vitality, or alertness) and secondary school children with orthopedic impairments or multiple disabilities (see Table 11–6 ■).

The model for the delivery of occupational therapy and physical therapy services in special education varies. Services may be provided either directly by the therapist individually, as part of a monitoring program, or as part of a collaborative consultation with the parents at school (King et al. 1999). Oriel (2003) found that physical therapists in schools perceived their role to be different from that of their colleagues in the medical environment. In the same study, physical therapists stated that they worked in an interdisciplinary and integrated service delivery model and that the majority of their interventions were delivered by aides. Kemmis and Dunn

Table 11–5.   **Percentage of Preschool Children with Disabilities Who Are Receiving Occupational Therapy and Physical Therapy Services, by Type of Disability**

	Occupational Therapy	*Physical Therapy*
Autism:	77	25
Developmental delay:	43	39
Emotional disturbance:	47	NA
Learning disability:	29	19
Mental retardation:	54	51
Other health impairment:	62	54
Speech-language impairment:	12	6

Source: National Center for Special Education Research. 2006. Preschoolers with disabilities: Characteristics, services and results. NSCER 2006–3003. http://www.eric.ed.gov/ERICDocs/data/ericdocs2sql/content_storage_01/0000019b/80/28/04/14.pdf (accessed July 9, 2007).

(1996) found that collaboration between occupational therapists and teachers facilitated student success. Nolan, Mannato, and Wilding (2004) studied therapy practices in school settings in New York State and found that about half of the children received treatment in therapy-only settings and one in four received services in integrated environments.

Table 11–6.   **Percentage of Secondary School Students Receiving Occupational Therapy and Physical Therapy Services, by Type of Disablement**

	Occupational Therapy		*Physical Therapy*	
	From Any Source	*From School*	*From Any Source*	*From School*
Learning disability	6.9	5.8	7.1	1.4
Speech-language impairment	5.5	5.1	5.6	2.2
Mental retardation	25.1	23.9	12.5	9.3
Emotional disturbance	13.6	11.8	6.0	2.2
Hearing impairment	14.5	13.5	8.2	4.9
Vision impairment	28.0	25.6	19.2	15.7
Orthopedic impairment	41.7	37.3	56.6	43.6
Other health impairment	13.3	10.6	8.5	3.3
Autism	49.0	46.4	17.3	13.7
Traumatic brain injury	32.3	26.0	23.2	13.2
Multiple disabilities	60.4	50.2	46.9	42.9
Deaf/blindness	52.8	49.1	33.7	30.3

Source: SRI. National Longitudinal Transition Study 2. *Services and Supports for Secondary School Students with Disabilities.* Office of Special Education Programs. U.S. Department of Education. 2004. http://www.eric.ed.gov/ERICDocs/data/ericdocs2sql/content_storage_01/0000019b/80/28/0c/7d.pdf (accessed July 9, 2007). Exhibit 2–6, p. 2–10.

The results as to which model works best are mixed. Karnish, Bruder, and Rainforth (1995) noted that practice in a natural environment (e.g., a classroom) was superior to therapy provided in a separate therapy room. Nolan et al. (2004) found that the integrated model was no more effective than stand-alone therapy services. Sekerak, Kirkpatrick, Nelson, and Propes (2003) found that multiple models are needed for treatment to be effective. King et al. (1999) noted that focusing on communication, productivity, and mobility improved student performance in the educational setting. Scott (1997) found that teachers benefited from a collaborative practice model.

WHAT IS PUBLIC HEALTH?

Today's world confronts people with new and emerging threats to their health. Terrorism, pandemic influenza, obesity, and antibiotic-resistant infections are among the emerging and current threats to populations. Public health services exist to identify, describe, understand, and address these issues. Public health services differ from personal health care primarily in their emphasis on populations, not individuals. The effect of public health on personal health, however, has been phenomenal. Many of the major achievements in individual health and longevity can be traced to improvements in public health practices (see Table 11–7 ■). Bunker, Frazier, and Mosteller (1994) calculated that 25 years of the 30-year gain in age longevity during the 20th century could be attributed to improved public health practices. This accomplishment is all the more remarkable given that expenditures on public health in 2005 were $57 billion out of total health care expenditures of $2 trillion (less than 3 percent of total spending) (Catlin et al. 2007).

Public health is a system of surveillance and services that are intended to identify and reduce mortality, morbidity, and disability due to illness, injury, and disease in a population. Table 11–8 ■ defines public health and lists 10 essential public health

Table 11–7.   20th-Century Achievements in Public Health

1. Vaccination
2. Motor vehicle safety
3. Safer workplaces
4. Control of infectious diseases
5. Decline in deaths from coronary heart disease and stroke
6. Safer and healthier foods
7. Healthier mothers and babies
8. Family planning
9. Fluoridation of drinking water
10. Recognition of tobacco as a health hazard

Source: Centers for Disease Control. 1999. Ten great public health achievements: United States, 1900–1999. http://www.cdc.gov/od/oc/media/tengpha.htm (accessed July 12, 2007).

Table 11–8. What Is Public Health?

Public Health

1. Prevents and mitigates epidemics and the spread of disease.
2. Protects against environmental hazards.
3. Prevents injuries.
4. Promotes and encourages healthy behaviors.
5. Responds to disasters and assists communities in recovery.
6. Assures individuals of their quality of life and of the accessibility of health services.

Essential Public Health Services

Assessment

1. Monitor health status to identify community health problems.
2. Diagnose and investigate health problems and health hazards in the community.
3. Evaluate the effectiveness, accessibility, and quality of personal and population-based health services.
4. Research for new insights into, and innovative solutions to, health problems.

Policy Development

5. Develop policies and plans that support individual and community health efforts.
6. Mobilize community partnerships to identify and solve health problems.
7. Ensure the existence of a competent public health and personal health care workforce.

Assurance

8. Inform, educate, and empower people about health issues.
9. Enforce laws and regulations that protect health and ensure safety. Link people to needed personal health services, and ensure the provision of health care when it would otherwise be unavailable.

Adapted from: Public Health in America. 1994. www.health.gov/phfunctions/public.htm (accessed June 12, 2000).

services that have been identified by the Public Health Functions Steering Committee (1994), a coalition of public health and governmental agencies. As can be seen from this definition of public health, the emphasis is on community action, prevention, and health promotion. These 10 public health services have been further subdivided into the three major roles of public health agencies as defined by the Institute of Medicine (1988): assessment, policy development, and assurance. We will explore these functions of public health agencies in more detail later in the chapter.

ORGANIZATION OF PUBLIC HEALTH SERVICES

Public health services are organized and delivered by different levels of government. Internationally, the World Health Organization is the public health agency of the United Nations. On the national level, the Public Health Service is a major component of the United States Department of Health and Human Services. Each state has a public health department. Many counties and cities have their own public health organizations. Rural or poor communities may lack a local public health organization. Sometimes, certain responsibilities of public health are integrated within other governmental agencies. For example, the management of toxic wastes may be the responsibility of an environmental department.

The World Health Organization (WHO) was created as a branch of the United Nations in 1948 (WHO 2007). The responsibilities of the WHO are listed in Table 11–9 ■ and include the surveillance of disease, development of policy, and implementation of basic health procedures for persons around the world, especially in Third World countries. In addition, the WHO has an important consultative function with governments. Among its major accomplishments are the worldwide eradication of smallpox and the near-eradication of poliomyelitis and leprosy through extensive immunization programs. In Chapter 1, we discussed the International Classification of Functioning, Disability, and Health (ICF). The ICF is a major contribution of the WHO towards the development of a common understanding of disablement.

Active Learning Exercise

Learn about how WHO is addressing disablement worldwide. Go to http://www.who.int/topics/disabilities/en/to learn more.

Table 11–9. The World Health Organization Core Functions (2006–2015)

1. Providing leadership on matters critical to health and engaging in partnerships where joint action is needed;
2. Shaping the research agenda and stimulating the generation, translation, and dissemination of valuable knowledge;
3. Setting norms and standards, and promoting and monitoring their implementation;
4. Articulating ethical and evidence-based policy options;
5. Providing technical support, catalyzing change, and building sustainable institutional capacity; and
6. Monitoring the health situation and assessing health trends.

Source: World Health Organization, The Role of WHO in Public Health http://www.who.int/about/role/en/index.html (accessed July 12, 2007).

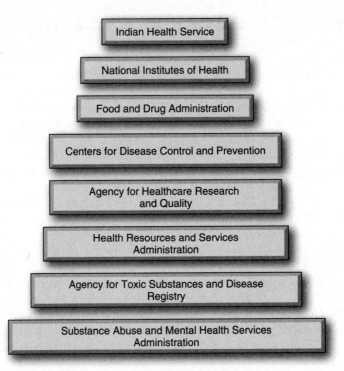

Figure 11–1.   Agencies of the U.S. Public Health Service

The U.S. Department of Health and Human Services is the primary federal agency with responsibilities for public health (U.S. Department of Health and Human Services 2007). We already have discussed in detail the function of one of its agencies: the Center for Medicare and Medicaid Services. The largest operating division of the U.S. Department of Health and Human Services is the Public Health Service, with eight agencies of its own (see Figure 11–1 ■). These agencies are involved in the support and delivery of a significant portion of the nation's agenda for health care research, education, and services to vulnerable, underserved communities. The Administration on Aging and the Administration on Children and Families completes the structure of the Department of Health and Human Services.

The National Institutes of Health (NIH), with a budget of $28 billion, is the largest medical research organization in the world. NIH has 27 "centers" of research on major public health problems (e.g., neurological diseases, stroke, aging). The National Center of Child Health and Human Development includes the National Center for Medical Rehabilitation Research, an important source of federal research planning and funding for occupational therapy, physical therapy, and rehabilitation research. The Food and Drug Administration (FDA) has primary public health responsibilities for the safety of food, pharmaceuticals, and medical devices.

The FDA assesses and develops policy for ensuring safety in many everyday products used by most Americans, including medical devices and equipment used by occupational therapists and physical therapists. The Centers for Disease Control

---

Active Learning Exercises

1. Therapy equipment (e.g., modalities) is approved and monitored by the FDA Center for Devices and Radiological Health. Equipment failures in the clinic must be reported to this agency. To learn more, go to http://www.fda.gov/cdrh/index.html.
2. The Centers for Disease Control and Prevention are interested in more than infectious diseases. The epidemiology of disablement is also studied at CDC. To learn more, go to http://www.cdc.gov/ncbddd/disabilities.htm.
3. To learn more about NIH support for rehabilitation research, go to http://www.nichd.nih.gov/. This is the website for the National Center for Medical Rehabilitation Research.

---

and Prevention is the primary federal epidemiological research organization and is responsible for the surveillance and control of communicable disease and, more recently, chronic disease, injuries, and disablement. The CDC maintains extensive laboratories for the identification of these conditions.

The Indian Health Service and the Health Resources Services Administration have important responsibilities in helping to improve the health of disadvantaged communities. The Indian Health Service provides primary health care services, including occupational therapy and physical therapy, for 1.9 million American Indians and Alaskan natives in both rural reservations and urban environments (Indian Health Service 2007). The Health Resources and Services Administration provides grants to establish educational programs that will improve access to health services for people in underserved communities. Federal agencies offer direct services to the public and grants to state and local public health departments, universities, tribes, and other organizations to address public health problems in communities.

States have the primary constitutional responsibility for the health of their populations. Policy development is an important function of each state's public health agency. In some states that agency is an independent department, and in others its public health functions are integrated within other state agencies (e.g., an agency for environmental quality). Many counties and cities have public health agencies that perform assurance and assessment functions at the local level. Some large local public health organizations participate in policy development.

This multilevel system of public health provides for the development and employment of extensive resources to battle public health problems. It also creates a complicated bureaucracy that has been criticized for being ineffective, excessively political, and unreactive to public needs. The resources provided to public health agencies, however, are generally viewed as inadequate to manage the problems faced by such organizations (Institute of Medicine 2003). In the next section, we will discuss how public health organizations manage these challenges by functioning in their assessment, policy development, and assurance roles.

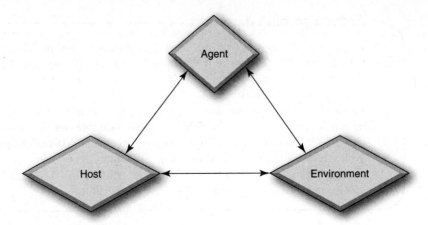

Figure 11–2.   Public Health Model

ASSESSMENT

Epidemiology is the foundational science of public health. The purpose of epidemiology is to identify the threats to a population and to devise a control strategy to reduce them. This is done by routine surveillance, which includes gathering vital statistics (birth and death records), analyzing water quality, investigating outbreaks of disease, and determining the incidence of disablement.

The purpose of epidemiological assessment is to identify the cause of a problem. This is done by investigation, using the **public health model** (see Figure 11–2 ■). This classic epidemiological model is widely utilized to identify the cause of communicable diseases and develop effective control strategies. It has been applied to the problems of chronic disease and disability (Verbrugge and Jette 1994). In this model, the agent is the factor that is causing the problem. For example, the human immunodeficiency virus (HIV) is the agent causing AIDS. The host is the person who is the target of the agent and who is afflicted by the disease or injury process. The environment is the third factor. The environment can beneficially or detrimentally modify the disease process by affecting either the host or the agent. Removing the agent, quarantining the host, and modifying the environment are fundamental strategies in managing public health problems.

POLICY DEVELOPMENT

Policy development is the second purpose of public health agencies. The identification of public health problems and strategies to control them requires planning, coordination, and education. Policy development begins with analysis and interpretation of the data. After this phase is completed, a strategic plan can be developed to address the identified problem areas in order to shape state public health policy in the 21st century.

Table 11–10.   Healthy People 2010 Focus Areas

Access to quality health services	Injury and violence prevention
Arthritis, osteoporosis, and chronic back conditions	Maternal, infant, and child health
	Medical product safety
Cancer	Mental health and mental
Chronic kidney disease	disorders
Diabetes	Nutrition and overweight
Disability and secondary conditions	Occupational safety and health
Educational and community-based programs	Oral health
Environmental health	Physical activity and fitness
Family planning	Public health infrastructure
Food safety	Respiratory diseases
Health communication	Sexually transmitted diseases
Heart disease and stroke	Substance abuse
HIV	Tobacco use
Immunization and infectious diseases	Vision and hearing

Source: Healthy People 2010. Healthy people in healthy communities. *http://www.health.gov/ healthypeople/About/hpfactsheet.pdf* (accessed June 12, 2000).

The Healthy People Initiative is an excellent example of public health policy. The initiative began after the release of the surgeon general's report in 1979 and has had several iterations over the last 20 years. The newest version, Healthy People 2010, is a "prevention agenda for the nation" (Department of Health and Human Services 1999). Healthy People 2010 was developed by a coalition of 600 governmental and private organizations that established goals in 28 "focus areas" (see Table 11–10 ■). The overall goals of Healthy People 2010 are to (1) increase quality and years of healthy life and (2) eliminate health disparities among groups in the population. The Healthy People Initiatives include measurement and reporting of progress of the status of these national public health goals. Ten percent of specific objectives in each focus area have already been achieved, and progress had been made on 50 percent more by 2005 (Healthy People 2010 2006). As we will discuss later, the Healthy People Initiative has ramifications for the practice of physical therapy and occupational therapy.

ASSURANCE

Assurance, the third role of public health organizations, is the primary function of local and state public health agencies. Assurance activities measure and determine whether policy standards and goals are being achieved. In some policy areas, public health agencies have enforcement power. A good example is the regular inspection of restaurants by local public health agencies. A restaurant that does not maintain a clean food-preparation environment can be closed by a public health agency. In

another example, the regulatory actions of state licensing boards restrict the professional practice of physical therapy and occupational therapy to qualified practitioners.
Licensing boards have enforcement power to revoke the licenses of practitioners
who harm patients or otherwise endanger public health.

Public health organizations also act to provide basic health care services to
their communities. On the local level, many public health organizations provide
immunization and emergency mental health and dental health screening programs. Some local governments provide health care services to indigent persons
through hospitals or long-term care facilities. As mentioned earlier, the Indian
Health Service is a federal effort to provide primary health care services to American Indians. Many public health agencies have active health promotion and disease-
prevention education programs.

PUBLIC HEALTH AND THERAPY SERVICES

Today, the increased incidence of chronic disease is creating new public health
challenges in preventing and controlling disablement. This situation is creating
population-based practice opportunities for occupational therapists and physical
therapists in such areas as reducing repetitive workplace injuries (Keller, Corbett,
and Nichols 1997), developing fall-prevention programs (Gillespie, Gillespie, Cumming, Lamb, and Rowe 2000; Harada et al. 1995), and designing health-promotion
interventions for persons with disabilities (Rimmer 1999; Buning 1999). Hageman
et al. (2005) found that middle-aged and older rural women were not meeting activity and fitness goals set by Health People 2010. Brach and VanSwearingen (2002)
found that mobility/fall risk, coordination, fitness, and flexibility were strongly coordinated with performance of ADL in community-living elderly men. The increasing level of obesity, especially in children, is a new concern (Bjornson 2005).

At least 11 target areas of the Healthy People 2010 Initiative have applicability
to occupational therapy and physical therapy practice (see Table 11–10 ■). Move-
ment-, fitness-, and physical activity-related public health issues are serious national
problems. Therapists do not consistently integrate these vital public health efforts
into their everyday practice. Rea, Hopp Marshak, Neish, and Davis (2004) found
that physical therapists are addressing health promotion topics at lower rates than
the goals set in the Healthy People 2010 initiative. Occupational therapists have
also been challenged to adopt new roles as health educators in public health and
health promotion (Filiatrault and Richard 2005).

The need to consider significant change in practice in light of the pressing
public health goals in the area of chronic disease and disability has been advocated.
Erikssen et al. (1998) found that even small improvements in physical fitness resulted in lower death rates for healthy middle-aged men. Finlayson and Edwards
(1995), noting the shift to primary care away from specialty services, encourage occupational therapists to utilize the concept of occupation as a useful template for
health-promotion and disease-prevention activities. As an example, Finlayson and
Edwards (1995) reported on the Canadian Seniors' Health Promotion Project. This

public health effort was implemented in two provinces by occupational therapists and resulted in active therapist involvement in advocacy for transportation services, the development of health-promotion videotapes, and a regular health-promotion column in a newsletter for seniors. Finally, Jette et al. (1999) demonstrated that a community-based, resistance-exercise program for elderly persons could achieve high rates of compliance, improved lower-extremity strength, and lower rates of disability. This Strong for Life program was advocated as an effective public health strategy.

COMPLEMENTARY AND ALTERNATIVE MEDICINE

More than one-third of Americans utilize complementary or alternative medical procedures each year (Institute of Medicine 2005), with annual expenditures exceeding $27 billion. The National Center for Complementary and Alternative Medicine (NCCAM) of the National Institutes of Health (2007) has defined seven categories of complementary and alternative medicine:

- whole medical systems
- mind–body medicine
- biologically based practices
- manipulative and body-based practices
- energy medicine
- biofield therapies
- bioelectromagnetic-based therapies

Occupational therapists and physical therapists are considered to be *conventional* medical providers. This means that most therapy practices are grounded in the allopathic, bioscientific model. Therapists, however, do occasionally utilize alternative medicine techniques to supplement a conventional procedure. When they do so, they are using *complementary* techniques. Other providers, however, employ these procedures instead of conventional procedures. When they do so, these persons are termed *alternative* medicine providers. In this section, we will explore four providers who can be considered practitioners of complementary or alternative medicine: chiropractors, massage therapists, homeopathic physicians, and naturopathic physicians.

Chiropractic medicine (see Table 11–11 ■) is defined as a manipulative and body-based practice of alternative medicine (NCCAM 2007). Chiropractic treatment "focuses on disorders of the musculoskeletal system and the nervous system, and the effects of these disorders on general health. Chiropractic care is used most often to treat neuromusculoskeletal complaints, including but not limited to back pain, neck pain, pain in the joints of the arms or legs, and headaches" (American Chiropractic Association 2007). There were 53,000 practicing chiropractors in the United States in 2004 (Bureau of Labor Statistics 2004). Chiropractic education is provided in 17 educational institutions in the United States.

Table 11–11.   Characteristics of Selected Alternative Medicine Providers

Provider	Education	Role
Chiropractor	Clinical doctorate	Assess and treat, using the manipulative model of treatment
Massage therapist	High School diploma/certificate	Use manual techniques to improve health
Naturopathic physician	Clinical doctorate	Assess and treat, using naturopathic model of treatment
Homeopathic physician	Clinical doctorate	Assess and treat, using homeopathic model of treatment

The philosophy of chiropractic medicine centers on self-healing of the body and the use of natural approaches to healing (Mootz and Phillips 1997). Similar to naturopathy and contrary to the allopathic philosophy, chiropractic treatment or medicine does not emphasize the identification of external agents causing disease, but instead focuses on strengthening the body's capabilities to maintain and restore normal function. The importance of the nervous system to maintaining good health is at the core of chiropractic practice. Manipulation of individual spinal segments to alleviate misalignment of the spine and abnormal pressure on spinal nerves is intended to maintain and restore good health. Chiropractors who use only manipulation procedures are called "straights." Chiropractors who incorporate modality treatment, nutrition, and lifestyle counseling into their practices are commonly referred to as "mixers" (Mootz and Phillips 1997).

Massage therapy is a type of manipulative body-based system of alternative medicine (NCCAM 2007). Massage therapy is "a profession in which the practitioner applies manual techniques, and may apply adjunctive therapies, with the intention of positively affecting the health and well-being of the client" (American Massage Therapy Association 2007). Massage therapy is regulated in 33 states and the District of Columbia (Bureau of Labor Statistics 2007). A typical educational requirement is 500 hours of classroom preparation or experiential training.

Homeopathic and naturopathic physicians are other examples of alternative medicine providers. **Homeopathy** can be traced to the late 18th- and early 19th-century advocacy of Samuel Hahnemann (Gevitz 1993). Homeopathic physicians employ strategies to restore the homeostasis of the whole person who is ill or injured. The philosophy of homeopathy holds that substances which create symptoms in normal persons can be used to treat similar symptoms in persons with disease. Small doses of these substances are used to treat illness and disease (Frey 1999a). Naturopathic providers emphasize prevention, patient education, and the body's natural healing capabilities (vitalism) in treatment (Frey 1999b). Nutrition, herbalism, detoxification, and acupuncture are common treatment modalities employed by naturopaths.

In the 19th century, manipulative medicine, homeopathy, and **naturopathy** were competing systems with allopathic medicine. The successes of the bioscientific model in diagnosing and treating illness and injury (e.g., the development of microbiology) led to the rapid growth of allopathic medicine and the slow growth or decline of these other systems. (Chiropractic is a notable exception.) Today, the limitations of the allopathic model in treating some forms of chronic disease have brought about a renewed interest in complementary and alternative medicine models.

CONCLUSION

In this chapter, we explored three areas of the system where therapists find work. In the special education system, therapists provide related services so that children with disabilities may access education. In public health, therapists are challenged to meet the demands of achieving and maintaining a healthy population. Finally, in complementary and alternative medicine, therapists need to understand the contributions and limitations of these procedures and the roles of these providers.

CHAPTER REVIEW QUESTIONS

1. Define special education and a "related service."
2. Identify the common related services utilized by a child in the school setting and the barriers to a child's receiving these services.
3. Describe the most common conditions addressed by occupational therapists and physical therapists in the school setting.
4. Define public health and its purpose in the health care system.
5. Describe the role and function of the following organizations:
   a. World Health Organization.
   b. U.S. Public Health Service.
   c. State and local public health organizations.
6. Define epidemiology and its use in the public health model.
7. What is the Healthy People Initiative?
8. Identify and describe three assurance functions of public health organizations.
9. Describe the involvement of physical and occupational therapists in the public health care system.
10. Define alternative, complementary, and conventional medicine.

CHAPTER DISCUSSION QUESTIONS

1. Compare and contrast the settings of the acute or post-acute care system with the school system as a site of therapist work. How are they similar? How are they different?
2. Do you agree or disagree with current policy decisions regarding the allocation of money for personal health care versus public health care services. Why do you believe this discrepancy exists? What, if anything, should be done about it?

3. Many occupational therapists and physical therapists do not regularly provide health-promotion or disease-prevention information to their patients. What are the reasons for this problem? How can you ensure that each of your patients receives this necessary information?
4. Have you seen therapists perform complementary medicine? What procedures have you observed? What was their effect?

REFERENCES

American Chiropractic Association. 2007. What is chiropractic? http://www.amerchiro .org/level2_css.cfm?T1ID=13&T2ID=61 (accessed July 13, 2007).

American Massage Therapy Association. 2007. Glossary of terms. http://www.amtamas-sage.org/about/terms.html (accessed July 13, 2007).

Bjornson, K.F. 2005. Physical activity monitoring in children and youths. *Pediatr Phys Ther* 17(1): 37–45.

Brach, J.S., and J.M. VanSwearingen. 2002. Physical impairment and disability: Relationship to performance of activities of daily living in community-dwelling older men. *Phys Ther* 82(8): 752–61.

Buning, M.E. 1999. Physical activity and fitness for persons with disabilities: A call to action. *OT Practice* 4(8): 26–31.

Bunker, J.P., H.S. Frazier, and F. Mosteller. 1994. Improving health: Measuring the effects of medical care. *Milbank Q* 72: 225–58.

Bureau of Labor Statistics. 2007. Chiropractors. Occupational Outlook Handbook. http://www.bls.gov/oco/ocos071.htm (accessed July 13, 2007).

———. 2007. Massage Therapists. *Occupational Outlook Handbook*. http://www.bls.gov/ oco/ocos295.htm (accessed July 13, 2007).

Catlin, A., C. Cowan, S. Hefflin, and B. Washington, and The National Health Expenditures Account Team. 2007. National health spending in 2005: The slowdown continues. *Health Affairs* 26(1): 142–53.

Centers for Disease Control. 1999. Ten great public health achievements: United States, 1900–1999. *MMWR* 48(12): 241–43.

Erikssen, G., K. Liestol, J. Bjornholt, E. Thaulow, L. Sandvik, and J. Erikssen. 1998. Changes in physical fitness and changes in mortality. *Lancet* 352(9130): 759–62.

Filiatrault, J., and L. Richard. 2005. Theories of behavior change through preventive and health promotion interventions in occupational therapy. *Can J Occup Ther* 72(1): 45–56.

Finlayson, M., and J. Edwards. 1995. Integrating the concepts of health promotion and community into occupational therapy practice. *Can J Occup Ther* 62(2): 70–75.

Fisher, T.F. 1998. Preventing upper extremity cumulative trauma disorders: An approach to employee wellness. *AAOHN J* 46(6): 296–301.

Gillespie, L.D., W.J. Gillespie, R. Cumming, S.E. Lamb, and B.H. Rowe. 2000. Interventions for preventing falls in the elderly. *Cochrane Library* (Oxford), 1–35.

Hageman, P.A., S.N. Walker, C.H. Pullen, L.S. Boeckner, and M.K. Oberdorfer. 2005. Physical activity and fitness among midlife and older rural women. *J Aging Phys Act* 13(3): 327–42.

Harada, N., V. Chiu, J. Damron-Rodriguez, E. Fowler, A. Siu, and D. Reuben. 1995. Screening for balance and mobility impairment in elderly individuals living in residential care facilities. *Phys Ther* 75(6): 462–69.

Healthy People 2010. 2006. Healthy People 2010 Midcourse Review. http://www.healthypeople.gov/data/midcourse/html/execsummary/introduction.htm (accessed July 13, 2007).

Indian Health Service. 2007. Indian Health Service Year 2007 in Profile. http://info.ihs.gov/ (accessed July 13, 2007).

Institute of Medicine. 1988. *The Future of Public Health.* Washington DC: National Academy Press.

————. 2003. *The Future of the Public's Health in the 21st Century.* Washington DC: National Academy Press.

————. 2005. *Complementary and Alternative Medicine in the United States.* Washington DC: National Academy Press.

Jette, A.M., M. Lachman, M.M. Giorgetti, S.F. Assman, B.A. Harris, C. Levenson, M. Wernick, and D. Krebs. 1999. Exercise: It's never too late: The Strong for Life program. *Am J Pub Health* 89(1): 66–72.

Karnish, K., M.B. Bruder, and B. Rainforth. 1995. A comparison of physical therapy in two school based treatment contexts . . . an isolated therapy room or a natural education setting. *Phys Occup Ther Pediatr* 15(4): 1–25.

Keller, K., J. Corbett, and D. Nichols. 1998. Repetitive strain injury in computer keyboard users: Pathomechanics and treatment principles in individual and group intervention. *J Hand Ther* 11(1): 9–26.

Kemmis, B.L., and W. Dunn. 1996. Collaborative consultation: The efficacy of remedial and compensatory interventions in school contexts. *Am J Occup Ther* 50(9): 709–17.

King, G.A., J. McDougall, M.A. Tucker, J. Gritzan, T. Malloy-Miller, P. Alambets, D. Cunning, K. Thomas, and K. Gregory. 1999. An evaluation of functional, school-based therapy services for children with special needs. *Phys Occup Ther Pediatr* 19(2): 5–29.

National Center for Complementary and Alternative Medicine. 2007. What is CAM? http://nccam.nih.gov/health/whatiscam/ (accessed July 13, 2007).

Nolan, K.W., L. Mannato, and G.E. Wilding. 2004. Integrated models of pediatric physical and occupational therapy: Regional practice and related outcomes. *Pediatr Phys Ther* 16(2): 121–28.

Oriel, K.N. 2003. The scope of physical therapy practice in Idaho public school systems. Unpublished Ed.D. dissertation, Idaho State University.

Public Health Foundation. 2000. Where do the dollars go? Measuring local public health expenditures, 6. *www.phf.org/Reports/Expend1/loclexpn.pdf* (accessed July 12, 2000).

Public Health Functions Steering Committee. 1994. Public health in America. *www.health.gov/phfunctions/public.htm* (accessed June 12, 2000).

Rea B., H. Hopp Marshak, C. Neish, and N. Davis. 2004. The role of health promotion in physical therapy in California, New York and Tennessee. *Phys Ther* 84(6): 510–23.

Rimmer, J. H. 1999. Health promotion for people with disabilities: The emerging paradigm shift from disability prevention to prevention of secondary conditions. *Phys Ther* 79(5): 495–502.

Scott, S.B. 1997. Comparison of service delivery models influencing teachers' use of assistive technology for students with severe disabilities. *Occup Ther Health Care* 11(1): 61–74.

Sekerak, D.M., D.B. Kirkpatrick, K.C. Nelson, and J.H. Propes. 2003. Physical therapy in preschool classrooms: Successful integration of therapy into classroom routines. *Pediatr Phys Ther* 15(2): 93–104.

U.S. Department of Education. 2006. 34 CFR Parts 300 and 301. Assistance to the States for Education of Children with Disabilities and Preschool Grants for Children with Disabilities; Final Rule. *Federal Register* 46540–845.

U.S. Department of Health and Human Services. 2007. HHS What We Do. http://www.hhs.gov/about/whatwedo.html/ (accessed July 13, 2007).

———. 2000. Healthy People 2010. *www.health.gov/healthypeople* (accessed June 12, 2000).

Verbrugge, L.M., and A.M. Jette. 1994. The disablement process. *Soc Sci Med* 38(1): 1–14.

World Health Organization. 2007. History of WHO. http://www.who.int/about/history/en/index.html (accessed June 13, 2007).

12
Effecting Policy Change: Therapist as Advocate

CHAPTER OBJECTIVES

At the conclusion of this chapter, the reader will be able to:

1. Recognize the role of the occupational therapist and physical therapist as an advocate.
2. Discuss the ethical responsibilities of the therapist as a patient advocate.
3. Relate the basic skills of effective advocacy.
    a. self-reflection/attitude
    b. knowledge
    c. assertive communication
4. State the responsibilities of the therapist in client advocacy.
5. State the responsibilities of the therapist in advocating in professional organizations.
6. Discuss methods of effective advocacy in the health care environment.
    a. policy analysis
    b. lobbying
    c. legislative process

KEY WORDS: Advocacy, Coalitions, Empowerment, Lobbying, Reflection, Testimony

Case Example

John was very frustrated. He had no idea that he would become involved in advocacy, but because of his frustration about a client's situation, he had become an advocate. John worked in an outpatient physical and occupational therapy clinic. One Medicaid client who was referred to both services was able to be followed up only with physical therapy, as occupational therapy was not reimbursed in the client's state. As a result, the client did not get much-needed occupational therapy. This client's situation motivated John to network and get involved with his state therapy association's legislative and reimbursement committees. John presented his client's story to them and explained how it exemplified a powerful rationale for why the state association should become involved with getting occupational therapy covered by Medicaid. He learned that the battle to improve coverage would be difficult, as Medicaid in his state was experiencing funding cuts and priorities were given to other programs. However, members of the state legislative committee decided to methodically take on the challenge. First, they networked with the State Affairs group at the American Occupational Therapy Association (AOTA) for guidance. From there, the state legislative committee, with assistance from AOTA, developed a plan to change the law—a plan that involved support from state agency officials and key legislators. From networking with State Affairs at AOTA, the committee received names of other state therapy associations that were working on similar issues. So the members of the committee began their campaign to have occupational therapy funded by Medicaid in their state. Part of the campaign involved e-mails and letter writing.

Recognizing the need to get support from outside the occupational therapy field, John worked closely with physical therapists on his job, as well as with the physical therapy state legislative committee, to solicit letters for this cause. In addition, the occupational therapy legislative committee met several times with Medicaid representatives and with key legislators. John found that telling the story of his client seemed to have an emotional impact on the audiences. The audiences were especially affected by the fact that the client's failure to receive much-needed therapy ultimately led to increased costs for the health care system. John was asked to present this story as formal testimony in front of the Medicaid committee and to staff at legislative offices.

As a result of all of these efforts, positive changes occurred in John's state for getting occupational therapy reimbursed under Medicaid. The following year, John received an award from his state association for his advocacy efforts. John's comments when he got his award were that he would encourage all therapists to become advocates and that he would never hesitate to advocate in the future, as one client's story can plant the seed for creating real changes.

Case Example Focus Questions:

1. What motivated John to get involved in advocating policy change?
2. What methods did John utilize to advocate for policy change?
3. Why, in your opinion, was John successful in effecting a policy change?

As you read this chapter, consider ways that you might become an advocate.

INTRODUCTION

Thus far, the material in this book has focused on policy and systems. This final chapter takes these discussions one step further by emphasizing **advocacy** skills. Therapy practitioners often encounter situations in which they can make a difference through the use of advocacy skills. Advocacy involves standing up for clients and advising clients and their caregivers about their rights. It also involves advancing legislation, public policy, and social awareness (Sachs and Linn 1997). To be effective in today's health care system, therapists must develop and use advocacy skills.

There has been very little research on the impact of client advocacy in the rehabilitation fields. Sachs and Linn (1997) studied client advocacy to determine when occupational therapists advocated and what affected their advocacy behavior. From their qualitative research, they identified three advocacy themes. The first advocacy theme was that therapists viewed themselves as "guardians of morals" for individual, professional, and social misbehavior aimed at their clients. The second advocacy theme involved representing the client's functional abilities to health and community agencies. This kind of representation allowed the therapists to increase public awareness about helping people with disabilities. The third theme was working with the interdisciplinary team, in either resulted in either support of advocacy efforts or restriction. Thus, as this research study illustrates, advocacy is multileveled.

Advocacy is an important professional skill. It can help clients, be used with peer professionals to advance one's profession, and can bring about changes in public policy. In this chapter, we will consider advocacy within all of these areas. First, we will discuss the linkage between advocacy and ethics, and then we will provide an overview of the advocacy skills necessary for therapists.

ADVOCACY AND ETHICS

The advocacy process is closely tied to professional ethics. Therefore, it is important to understand ethical principles and ethical reasoning and how they can be applied to public policy (Lohman, Gabriel, and Furlong 2004). Both the Physical Therapy Code of Ethics (APTA 2002a) and the Occupational Therapy Code of Ethics (SEC & Peloquin, 2005) address advocacy. The Physical Therapy Code of Ethics (APTA 2000a) and the Guide for Professional Conduct (APTA 2002b), which expands on the code, highlight advocacy in several principles. Principle 1 of the Physical Therapy Code of Ethics states that physical therapists should respect the rights and dignity of all individuals (APTA 2002a, p. 1). This means that "physical therapists shall recognize that each individual is different from all other individuals and shall respect and be responsible to those differences" (APTA 2002b, p. 1). Thus, physical therapists should not force advocacy on anyone who does not want it and shall respect personal differences in approaching advocacy. Furthermore, "physical therapists are to be guided at all times by concern for the physical, psychological, and socioeconomic welfare of those individuals entrusted to their care" (APTA 2002b, p. 1). This statement empowers physical therapists to advocate for clients. Principle 4 states that "physical therapists accept responsibility for the exercise of sound judgement" (APTA 2002a, p. 1). This includes referring the client to an appropriate practitioner "if the diagnostic process reveals findings that are outside the scope of the physical therapist's knowledge, experience, or expertise" (APTA 2002b, p. 2) and communicating findings to that practitioner (APTA 2002b). In addition, the Code of Ethics clearly states that physical therapists should address reimbursement concerns by informing patients of any known limitations on reimbursement. This role implies advocacy. Principle 7 states that "physical therapists seek remuneration for their services that is deserved and reasonable (APTA 2002a, p. 1). Therefore, on behalf of patients, physical therapists do not "place their own financial interest above the welfare of individuals under their care" or charge unreasonable fees (APTA

2002b). Therapists should not underutilize therapy services because of constraints by third-party insurers. Finally, Principle 10 implies that physical therapists should render pro bono (reduced or no-fee) services to patients who lack the ability to pay for services, as each physical therapist's practice permits (APTA 2002b). Helping people who do not have the means to pay is a strong example of professional advocacy.

The Occupational Therapy Code of Ethics (SEC and Peloquin 2005) also emphasizes advocacy and even mentions the word "advocate" in Principle 1 and its accompanying subprinciples. Principle 1 states that "occupational therapy personnel shall demonstrate a concern for the well-being of the recipients of their services (beneficence) (SEC and Peloquin 2005). A subprinciple discussed under this category is that "occupational therapy personnel shall make every effort to *advocate* for recipients to obtain needed services through available means" (SEC and Peloquin 2005, p. 639). Advocacy also involves respecting the rights of the client, which is clearly stated in Principle 3: "Occupational therapy personnel shall respect the recipients to assure their rights (autonomy, confidentiality)" (SEC and Peloquin 2005, p. 640). Principle 4 mentions that "occupational therapy personnel shall achieve and continually maintain high standards of competence (duty)" (SEC and Peloquin 2005, p. 649). Therefore, providing current and good patient care is a form of advocacy. Principle 5 states that "occupational therapy personnel shall comply with laws and the Association policies guiding the profession of occupational therapy (procedural justice)" (SEC and Peloquin 2005, p. 640). Principle 5 clearly refers to policy on the association, local, institutional, state, and federal levels. By being aware of policy on all levels, therapists can be advocates. Finally, Principle 7 states that "occupational therapy personnel shall treat colleagues and other professionals with fairness, discretion, and integrity (fidelity)" (SEC and Peloquin 2005, p. 641). This principle refers to professional relationships. Being an advocate involves respecting other professionals, as well as exposing breaches of the Code of Ethics to the proper boards.

THERAPIST SKILLS FOR ADVOCACY

In order to advocate, therapists need to have a correct attitude and self-understanding. Without a proper attitude, advocacy efforts by therapists will not be successful. A proper attitude involves embracing the idea of being capable of making changes and being proactive with changes. Proactivity, rather than reactivity, is a very important skill in today's ever-changing health care environment. In addition, therapists need to understand their personal perspectives and motivations for approaching client advocacy. Are they concerned about the client's well-being? Are they concerned about quality of care? Are they advocating because of concerns for the profession? Understanding one's self-motivation requires **reflection.** Perhaps, from self-reflection, the therapist discovers that the motivation for advocacy comes from a personal reason, such as meeting an unfulfilled need, rather than from a client-centered or professional reason. In that case, the therapist will need to further reflect about his or her motivation for advocacy. Consider the questions in Table 12–1 ■ to better understand personal motivation and advocacy.

Table 12–1. Reflective Questions for Advocacy

I advocate because of
  Concern for client's well-being
  Concern for quality of care
  Concern for the profession
  Concern for the health care environment
  Personal reasons
  Other reasons (please list)

In addition to possessing self-understanding, therapists need to be knowledgeable about different systems. For example, to advocate successfully with the legislature, therapists need to understand the legislative process. (Advocacy with the legislature will be discussed later in the chapter.) Furthermore, assertive communication skills are imperative for successful advocacy. Therefore, it is beneficial to review these skills.

Assertive Communication

Assertive communication is empowering. It allows people to speak up for their own rights without stepping on others. To understand what assertive communication is, one must understand what it is not. On the one hand, assertive communication is not aggressive communication. Aggressive communication is acting out or being angry in order to get one's way. Aggressive communication does not respect the rights of others. On the other hand, assertive communication is also not being quiet or passive. Being quiet about what is important allows others to achieve what they want to achieve at the expense of one's own position. Assertive communication is not passive–aggressive communication or undermining others, such as talking about a person without the person being present.

Assertive communication involves clearly expressing one's feelings, beliefs, and attitudes. Different methods for assertive communication are presented in

---

Example of DESC Methodology with Professional-level Advocacy

Description: I observed Mr. C. in room 210 eat lunch. He was noted to pocket food in his right cheek and not fully chew his food. In addition, I noted that he coughed with each bite.

  Expression: I feel that Mr. C. might have an aspiration risk.

  Specification of change: Mr. C. would benefit from a swallowing study.

  Consequences: Such a study may prevent him from being an aspiration risk.

the literature (Alberti and Emmons 1978). Davis (1998) provides one option: the DESC communication model. DESC is an acronym for *describing* the circumstance, *expressing* feelings, *specifying* the change, and identifying the *consequences*. The example of communication between a therapist and a physician in the accompanying box illustrates how a therapist uses the DESC method to advocate for a client who is an aspiration risk.

Assertive communication skills accompany advocacy skills and can be used with various levels of advocacy for clients. Clients in the medical system are often in a dependent role and have minimal control over their situation. Therapists can advocate, using assertive communication skills, for clients who are vulnerable. Therapists can also encourage family members and caregivers to advocate assertively for the client. In addition, assertive skills can be used on the professional level. Therapists can advocate for appropriate referrals to help patients when therapy is not being utilized. Assertive communication skills can be used with the legislature to articulate professional concerns. Let us now examine advocacy skills on these different levels.

Patient/Client Advocacy Skills

A traditional view of advocacy involves helping vulnerable people who cannot effectively help themselves (Namerow 1982; Carpenter 1992). Advocacy in this sense involves helping people who lack the ability to advocate on their own behalf, such as children, people with disabilities, or people who are unaware of available resources (Carpenter 1992). Therapists develop a rapport with clients that allows them to learn about situations that may require advocacy. Reporting someone for elder abuse is an example of advocating for a vulnerable client (Foose 1999).

As discussed, advocacy should be a reflective process. Reflection involves utilizing an in-depth problem-solving or clinical-reasoning process. Therapists may ask themselves the following questions:

- Is it necessary that I intervene?
- Does the person want me to intervene?
- Can the client self-advocate without my help?
- Can the client's caregiver advocate for the client?
- What resources are available to help the person?
- What would empower the person to self-advocate?

These reflective questions bring up an important topic: When should a therapist intervene, and how can therapists empower clients to be their own self-advocates? Sachs (1989, as cited by Sachs and Linn 1997) found in her study that very few therapists helped patients or families by giving them the necessary information to self-advocate. Sometimes therapists or others may jump in when a person is perfectly capable of self-advocating on his or her own behalf. Allowing people to do their own advocating is empowering, and just providing the resource information may be

Table 12–2. Areas Where Therapists Can Help Clients Through Advocacy

1. Suggesting that a client seek legal advice and where to get it.
2. Providing an explanation of insurance plans.
3. Suggesting that a client seek counseling and where to get it.
4. Providing information to help the client make an informed decision (Sachs and Linn 1997).
5. Providing information about services offered from public policies that can help the client.
6. Suggesting that a client get a referral to a specialist for better medical care.
7. Referring a client to social services for different types of help (e.g., with housing).
8. Suggesting resources that will enable a client to remain in his or her home.
9. Educating clients on how to write Congress about key issues.
10. Educating clients how to appeal a denial of coverage.
11. Educating and communicating with managed care organizations (MCOs) on behalf of clients.
12. Educating a potential client who has a consumer-directed health care plan about the value of paying for and receiving therapy.
13. Acting as an expert witness in court.

all that the therapist will have to do. However, advocacy is important for clients who are incapable of self-advocating. Sometimes, for a person who is sick and vulnerable in the hospital or in some other institution, it is beneficial to suggest having a caregiver present to advocate for that person's needs. Table 12–2 ■ addresses some of the areas in which therapists can help with client advocacy. The list is not all-inclusive, and the reader may identify other areas.

The American Occupational Therapy Association (AOTA) and the American Physical Therapy Association (APTA) have government affairs departments that can help practitioners with client advocacy. Through the Trialliance of Health Rehabilitation Professions, consisting of the presidents of AOTA, APTA, and the American Speech-Language-Hearing Association (ASHA), advocacy efforts, such as advocacy for the Americans with Disabilities Act (ADA), have been made to influence health care policy (Evert 1995). Ultimately, these health policies benefit client care. In addition, both associations have pledged their support for outcome or efficacy studies that also improve client care. Informal collaboration between these associations is often done at the staff level.

Professional Level of Advocacy

On the professional level, therapists advocate with peer professionals and others, such as insurers. A basic form of advocacy is knowledge about what gets reimbursed, as well as how therapy gets reimbursed, so that clients do not end up with unnecessary out-of-pocket expenses. Simply documenting clients' visits according to insurance standards often enables appropriate reimbursement. Advocacy with payers may also include appealing a denial of therapy coverage, which involves understanding an insurance company's appeal policies. Providing excellent treatment so that clients choose to pay for therapy out of pocket or pay from the deductible of a consumer-based health care plan is a form of advocating for the profession. Contributing to the research for evidence-based treatment is another means of advocating for the profession.

Another key area for professional advocacy is with employers, to improve insurance coverage for therapy benefits. Sometimes employers who self-insure do not understand the benefits and cost savings of therapy and may decide not to include it in their employee insurance plan. In such cases, meeting with key employers can make a difference for insurance coverage. In addition, professional advocacy may involve educating other professionals, such as the staff of a managed care organization (MCO), about the benefits of therapy services. Communication and education can make a difference with case managers or other MCO representatives.

In employment settings, therapists identify concerns about peer professionals that could involve advocacy. Sometimes, a therapist will identify unethical conduct in the way a peer professional deals with clients. Perhaps a peer professional has acted rudely toward a client, or a peer professional has made the wrong treatment decision. Working in an environment that allows open communication and the disclosure of issues such as errors encourages a reduction in errors, better client care (Joint Commission on Accreditation of Healthcare Organizations 2007), and better advocacy on behalf of the clients. When appropriate, such matters should be reported internally or to an outside agency (e.g., the state licensure board) for review. In some cases, states require the reporting of harmful behaviors through "mandatory reporting" laws. In other cases, a therapist may learn that therapy is not being given to a client who could benefit from physical or occupational therapy services. In that scenario, the therapist will need to advocate for a referral with the client's physician. Handling situations with peer professionals involves diplomacy and as-

---

Active Learning Exercise

Answer the following questions as a self-reflecting individual or in a group:

1. Describe how you would handle a situation in which a physician has ordered a treatment that is contraindicated. You are aware that this physician does not like to ever be seen as wrong.
2. Describe how you would handle a situation in which you feel that a patient being reviewed on a treatment team would benefit from your therapy services.
3. Describe how you would handle a situation in which you observe a peer therapist not providing the best treatment or providing an inappropriate treatment.
4. Describe how you would demonstrate client advocacy after making a practice error.
5. Describe how you would handle a situation in which you observe a peer engaging in unethical behavior.

sertive communication skills. Complete Exercise 12–1 to reflect about how you would handle advocacy situations involving peer professionals.

Advocacy with Professional Organizations

Both APTA and AOTA have legislative bodies that allow professional members to voice their opinions and influence the positions of the organization. The APTA House of Delegates is the organization's deliberative policymaking body. It meets annually to discuss and debate professional issues and to state policy positions of physical therapists to the outside community. AOTA has a legislative body called the representative assembly (RA). It is the governing and policy-making part of the association. "The RA consists of three standing commissions: Education, Practice, and Standards and Ethics and six Standing Committees: Agenda, Bylaws, Policies & Procedures, Credentials Review and Accountability, Nominating, Recognitions, and Strategic Plan" (AOTA 2000f, p. 1). Just as in Congress, state representatives debate and vote on important issues at the national AOTA conference. It is important for therapists to communicate their stance on resolutions that are up for discussion to their state representative prior to the national conference.

Both the APTA and the AOTA have government affairs departments to help lobby for issues. The APTA Department of Government Affairs maintains web-based legislative action centers for both federal and state legislative affairs (APTA 2000c). At the federal level, APTA maintains a Congressional Affairs and Federal Regulatory Affairs division that advocates for the profession in the Congress and in the Executive Branch of the federal government. The Federal Regulatory Affairs division of APTA's Department of Government Affairs "is responsible for Medicare policy and advocacy issues affecting physical therapists" (APTA n.d.). At the state level, the State Government Affairs division monitors and advocates for state-level issues affecting physical therapists (e.g., licensure). Government Affairs sponsors an annual State Government Affairs Forum, an Advocacy Academy, and PT Day on Capitol Hill to allow members to meet, discuss, and mobilize for legislative action. A federal government affairs committee advises the department on critical legislative and regulatory issues facing the profession. The Physical Therapy Political Action Committee (PT-PAC) is the political fundraising arm of the profession and makes contributions to the political campaigns of candidates running for public office. Finally, the division supports a grass roots advocacy network, the PTeam, to develop and implement local advocacy efforts at both the state and federal levels.

The AOTA has a Public Affairs Division that includes a State Affairs Group, a Federal Affairs Group, and a Reimbursement and Regulatory Affairs Group. Overall, the Public Affairs Division "supplies research, policy analysis, and supports State Affiliates and individual members on public policy issues" (AOTA n.d., p. 1). Through the State Affairs Group, AOTA works closely with individual members and state associations on state legislative and regulatory issues pertaining to occupational therapy practice. This group also works with OT regulatory boards. The Federal Affairs group is involved with monitoring current federal legislation and with lobbying the

U.S. Congress and other Federal agencies. The lobbyists act as liaisons to the American Occupational Therapy Political Action Committee, or AOTPAC. The Reimbursement and Regulatory Policy Group analyzes federal regulations and policies affecting occupational therapy practice, such as Medicare. They also act as advocates with federal agencies, payers, and external organizations, and they educate AOTA members about reimbursement and regulatory issues (AOTA, n.d).

AOTA has an AOTAction Network as well. This network, consisting of contacts in each state, provides a local person to distribute critical information and spur political action. Recently, AOTA launched the Alpha Advocates. This program has therapists serve as key contacts with identified members of the Congress and their staffs. AOTA sponsors a Capitol Hill Day, which involves occupational therapy practitioners coming to the AOTA headquarters for a legislative briefing. In addition, therapists learn the logistics of how to meet with members of Congress and/or their staffs about issues relevant to occupational therapy. This briefing is followed by actual meetings with members of the legislature. AOTA also serves as a year-round resource for occupational therapy practitioners interested in going to Washington, DC, to meet with their Congressional representatives and senators and offers educational activities on issues when needed.

In addition, AOTA has a political action committee, called AOTPAC, or the American Occupational Therapy Political Action Committee. This legally sanctioned committee "influences or attempts to influence the selection, nomination, election, or appointment of any individual to any Federal public office" (AOTA n.d., p. 1) who supports occupational therapy. AOTPAC also provides support to occupational therapy practitioners or students who are seeking public office. Overall, AOTPAC helps ensure the visibility of occupational therapy in Washington and in politics.

Finally, all the major rehabilitation associations in the Trialliance (APTA, AOTA, and ASHA) maintain websites with up-to-date information about legislative and advocacy issues relevant to the members of their associations. These websites are a great way to receive updates and calls for action about important political issues. AOTA, for example, has an Issues and Advocacy Section, which is a great resource for information about current issues. APTA has a similar Legislative Action Center. These websites contain information about how to network with members of Congress by e-mailing them about important issues or simply to identify whether a member of Congress supports a legislative issue. In the associations' professional magazines (e.g., *OTPractice*, *PTMagazine*) one can find articles related to legislative issues. At professional conferences, the associations provide workshops related to legislative and reimbursement issues.

Advocacy with the Health Care Environment

In the United States, the state and federal legislatures allow citizens to advocate for their concerns. As Scott-Lee (1999, p. 5) states, "The framers of the Constitution believed so strongly in the people's right to participate in government, that they preserved that right, among others, for themselves, their fellow colonials, and the future generations of Americans." Today, therapists advocate by **lobbying** for concerns that have an impact on therapy practice. Advocacy occurs in both the legislative process and the regulatory process. Legislative advocacy involves being informed about legislative issues, lobbying through personal visits or letters, and being involved in political campaigns.

Sometimes, physical and occupational therapists take on direct roles as hired lobbyists. As Amy Lamb (2004), an occupational therapist and a state lobbyist, reflects, "On the surface, being a lobbyist may seem unusual for an occupational therapist; however, I see it as a natural fit. . . . In the discussion of our field, occupational therapists and occupational therapy assistants are the experts" (p. 1).

Regulatory advocacy means being involved with providing input when the rules that implement legislation are written. A good example of the legislative advocacy process and the impact that advocacy can have involves the efforts that AOTA, APTA, and ASHA put forth for their members and for other consumer groups to avoid the implementation of the Medicare Part B outpatient therapy cap, which passed with the Balanced Budget Act of 1997 [P.L. 105–33]. Since 1997, the monetary limit established for therapy Part B ($1,780 for 2007) has been widely recognized as inadequate for providing necessary therapy services. Massive lobbying efforts by the professional organizations, along with individual efforts by therapists and clients, managed to successfully place a moratorium or alternative to the cap several times. Always at issue are finances and limited funding for Medicare. AOTA, APTA, ASHA and other provider and consumer groups have consistently worked with Congress and the Centers for Medicare and Medicaid Services (CMS) to find an appropriate long-term solution to the cap. Congress most recently (2006 and 2007) passed legislation that instructed CMS to develop an exceptions process to the cap, enabling those beneficiaries who need services costing more than the cap allows to receive those services. The exceptions process resulted from the large amount of feedback from therapists and clients, as well as lobbying efforts by the therapy associations. This example illustrates several points. First, therapists must stay aware of what happens in the larger health care environment that affects practice, and they do need to advocate for client concerns. Second, sometimes advocacy efforts partially work, but if none are made, then compromises like the exceptions process for certain diagnoses would not happen. Lastly, therapists need to pay close attention to regulations related to public policy, such as the exceptions process, as changes will be made in the future for an appropriate permanent fix.

Now let us consider a regulatory advocacy example. One of the authors of this book (H.L.) made a difference on the state level by successfully advocating for legislative changes in the state worker's compensation law to increase therapy coverage. After reviewing the state law, she went to the billing officer of the hospital to express her concerns about limitations in therapy payment for key codes for worker's compensation clients. The billing officer immediately connected her with the lawyer for the State Worker's Compensation Court so that she could voice her concerns. From this communication, she learned about an upcoming hearing. Along with a representative from the state occupational therapy organization, she prepared and presented testimony that resulted in increased payment for therapy services. Thus, successful changes because of advocacy can and do occur on the state and national levels, and behind every successful advocacy effort are the power of motivation, passion about issues, and the desire to make changes.

Therapists can advocate with representatives of the state and federal governments to promote issues that help therapy practice. Advocacy is most effective when done in **coalitions**—groups of people with similar concerns. Although first attempts at advocacy may seem very overwhelming, sometimes just making the effort results in successful changes. Even if the effort at change is unsuccessful, just getting involved is a learning experience. Therapists should know the positions of the stakeholders and the majority and minority parties on important health care issues (Callahan 2000). Timing is essential. Obviously, a legislator will be most interested in learning the various viewpoints before a vote is taken. The next section highlights one method for promoting advocacy with state and federal legislatures (Vermithrax 2000). As noted in this discussion, there are many points in the sequence of events where therapists will need to critically analyze the political process.

SEQUENCE FOR ADVOCACY

Step I: Knowledge

Therapists should become aware of key issues that concern state or national therapy practice. Knowledge comes from state and national professional associations, professional news bulletins, professional Internet sites, state agencies, and the media.

Step II: Research

From doing research, therapists determine the key issues involved in the identified legislation so as to develop a clear understanding of the intent of a bill. It helps to have an understanding of the full history of the bill, including any previous legislative history (Callahan 2000). This understanding also involves being able to critically analyze the state of society at the time that the bill was introduced, as well as with the current bill. Some considerations are the status of the economy, who is in the majority party in the legislature, and the overall priorities of society. For example, one consideration might be the priorities for spending of the national budget: Is more money being spent on war efforts or international affairs over domestic issues, such as health care?

It helps to understand whether the bill is addressing a feature of a problem or the actual problem (Callahan 2000) and what may be missing from the current legislation. It is also interesting to consider how the issue is being presented by the media (Callahan 2000). Are the real facts being presented, or are biases being presented? Reading the actual legislative language of bills and comparing similar bills helps to clarify the different opinions. It also helps to be able to understand and articulate the reasons for opposing viewpoints. Therapists need to determine who (i.e., a professional organization, a coalition, or a political party) is behind the proposed legislation

Table 12–3. Questions to Consider When Researching a Bill

What is the history of this bill?

What is the current state of society at the time that the bill is introduced?

Does the bill address a feature of a problem or the entire problem?

What content is in the current bill and what is missing from the current bill?

What facts or biases about the bill are being presented by the media?

What is the opposing viewpoint on this bill?

Who (i.e., a professional organization, a coalition, or a political party) is behind this bill, and who is against the proposed legislation?

What is the future impact of this bill on society if the bill is passed?

Callahan 2000; Lohman 2003.

and who is against the proposed legislation, as well as their viewpoints. This involves identifying the key people involved with the proposed legislation and networking with them. Securing their cooperation as allies helps to make successful changes. Attending coalition meetings with allies can be highly beneficial in clarifying the political picture about the legislation. Some members of a coalition may share research about the legislation, and that research may benefit all members. Networking is also done with other rehabilitation professionals. For example, an occupational therapist in charge of legislative issues for a state occupational therapy organization may network with the legislative representative in the state physical therapy association about an issue of common concern. Therapists will also need to do additional journal or Internet research to better understand a bill. Internet sites often provide analyses of legislation. However, critical readers will need to consider the source of the information: Is the source supportive of one's viewpoints, and even if it is supportive, does it provide accurate information? Finally, one must contemplate the impact of a bill, if passed, on future generations. (Lohman 2003). Step I is completed when therapists are ready to take positive action because they clearly understand and have critically thought through all the issues related to a bill, for a "key means for understanding public policy is by using a critical analysis approach" (Lohman 2003). Table 12–3 ■ lists some questions to consider when doing this research.

Step III: Implementing Political Action

In order to implement political action, therapists must identify their state and national legislative representatives and the stances of those representatives regarding the legislation. If they do not have this information, they can get it from many sources, including various coalitions, the library, newspaper articles, and Internet sites. The APTA, AOTA, and ASHA sites, as well as other Internet sites, have links that make it possible to find out who one's legislative representatives are. Or one can call the U.S. Capitol switchboard at (202) 224–3121 and ask for the office of one's senator and/or representative. Newspaper articles will quote the key players and their stances on the legislation, as well as public opinions. Internet sites for the

Washington Post or the *New York Times* are helpful resources (see the appendix of this chapter). The Internet site www.Thomas.org features current legislation in the House and Senate and key sponsors. The Internet site of one's senator and representative can also help in determining their position on an issue.

A key to successful advocacy and implementing political action involves communicating with the appropriate legislative personnel and working with the staff people of the legislator. These people are the gatekeepers for the legislative representative and should be treated with respect. Furthermore, therapists should network with representatives from their own constituency.

Writing a letter is a popular method and can be highly effective in communicating with legislators, especially if the letter is well timed, relevant, and well written. Most members of Congress are very interested in knowing the opinions of their constituents. An understanding of where a bill is in the legislative process is helpful. To influence the legislative process, write a detailed letter to a member of a committee, as much of the actual work on developing legislation takes place in committees. If an issue is being discussed for a vote on the floor, a brief message sent to one's representative with a suggested stance on the vote may be all that is necessary (Weingarten 1996). Since 2001, it is considered to be quicker to send letters via fax than through regular mail, as letters sent by regular mail are held for inspection. Table 12–4 ■ lists hints for writing about a specific act or bill.

A Legislative Visit

Another highly successful advocacy technique is scheduling a visit with one's federal or state legislator. Ideally, it is helpful to visit someone who supports a bill or who is undecided about an issue, yet sometimes meeting with a person who opposes a bill can provide a clearer picture of another perspective, which is important for critical analysis of the bill. This meeting may result in changing the legislator's opinion or, at the very minimum, making the persons aware of your concerns. Visiting legislative offices is very important, as legislators are quite sensitive to public opinion, especially from their constituents. Often, therapists end up meeting with staff members rather than legislators themselves. However, as stated earlier, never underestimate the power of a staff member. Table 12–5 ■ provides hints for talking with legislative personnel. Legislators on the federal level will always have staff personnel. On the state level, legislators may or may not have a staff representative.

Appearing at Hearings and Preparing Testimony

Table 12–6 ■ summarizes the legislative process. Prior to appearing at hearings and providing **testimony**, therapists should review the legislative process, noting the many points where a bill can be killed. Therapists should also be aware that there can be key testimonial times during the process, unless the bill is directly marked up to the floor. In addition, legislation can change quickly. Bills can be reintroduced with changes. Therefore, it is important to find out if any last-minute changes have occurred. Table 12–7 ■ provides hints for preparing and presenting testimony.

Table 12–4. Writing a Letter to a Legislator About a Specific Act or Bill

1. Use a professional letterhead. Use a personal letterhead if your home is in the legislator's district and the address is in a district different from that of your work.
2. Addressing correspondence:

To a Representative

The Honorable (full name)
__(Rm.#)__(name of)House Office Building
United States House of Representatives
Washington, DC 20515
Dear Representative:

To a Senator

The Honorable (full name)
__(Rm.#)__(name of)Senate Office Building
United States Senate
Washington, DC 20510
Dear Senator:

To a Committee Chair or Speaker

Dear Mr. Chairman or Madam Chairwoman (Or Dear Mr. Speaker):

3. Clearly state in the first paragraph the number and name of the bill and your position with respect to it.
4. Clearly state who you are (a constituent, a stakeholder, someone directly affected by an issue, an expert about an issue, or a representative of an organization) and what perspective you are representing.
5. Make the letter clear and concise, usually no longer than one page. Limit issues presented, and present facts, as your credibility is important. If the purpose of the letter is to influence a vote, clearly describe what you want the person to do.
6. Use specific examples to support your views. If applicable, provide examples or a story from your practice area. Discuss any new information that may help the Congressperson form a viewpoint or provide information that is relevant to his or her interests.
7. Try to use your own words and not copy a form letter. Accessing a form letter can be a good beginning resource, but go on from there.
8. In representing an organization, it is important that everyone have the same stated stand.
9. Be constructive and provide solutions, not just complaints.
10. Thank the person for his or her time and attention.
11. Include your contact information (name, address, phone number, and e-mail address).
12. Double-check grammar and spelling before sending the letter.
13. The same guidelines apply for writing e-mails to congressional representatives as with writing letters. Remember to keep the e-mails original.
14. Faxes are the most expedient and preferred method for communication. Especially since 2001, they are recommended as a more efficient method for getting a letter to a congressional office. Fax numbers can be obtained from the same sources that provide legislative and congressional telephone numbers. These sources are given at the end of the chapter.

Sources: The American Occupational Therapy Association, 2000d; *www.learn2.com,* http://*www.propeople* .*org/advocate.htm,* http://*www.apha.org/legislative/Writingtips.htm;* Dodge 2005; Weigarten 1996.

Table 12–5.   Communicating with Legislators or Staff Members

1. Make an appointment by letter or phone, clearly stating the reason for the visit. If telephoning, after identifying yourself, briefly state your position on the specific bill.
2. If you receive an appointment with a staff member, ask to meet with the staff person who handles the issue that you are addressing, such as health care public policy.
3. Ask for the legislator's position on an issue if you do not know it.
4. Be aware of the timing of congressional recesses, as members often return to their home states during that period, and it may be easier to make an appointment then.
5. Work as part of the state and/or national therapy association (APTA or AOTA). As discussed, coalitions are more powerful. If going on your own, advise the state and/or national organization, because it can provide valuable resources. Also, members of the organization can advise you on how to present your case if your stance differs from that of the legislator with whom you are meeting.
6. Sometimes it helps to attend a meeting along with a coalition of other professionals in order to coordinate efforts.
7. Be prompt and dress professionally.
8. Be patient and flexible. It is not unusual for a meeting to be interrupted with other business.
9. Have the facts clearly outlined on a handout to provide to the legislator or staff member. It is best to research the literature and have clear facts rather than an emotionally based handout.
10. Be prepared to provide an explanation of physical or occupational therapy. Consider bringing an additional fact sheet about the profession.
11. Stick with the key points on the handout, so that the information will be presented clearly. Communicating different stories can undermine the power of a coalition.
12. Bring educational materials to the meeting. Often, a legislator or staff member is not familiar with the nuances of a situation. Therapy practitioners are experts on the impact of legislation on patient care.
13. Keep the meeting as an equal discussion, not as a lecture. Allow time for questions.
14. Remember the bigger picture by articulating the linkage between your position and the interests of the legislator's constituency.
15. Describe how you or your professional group can be of help to the legislator.
16. If appropriate, ask for a commitment to your stance.
17. If relevant, share a patient story that relates to the issues included in the bill.
18. Be polite and respectful. Consider the visit as the beginning of an ongoing relationship, so keep communication channels open.
19. Do not monopolize the legislator's time. Plan on taking 15 minutes, as legislators and their staff members are busy people.
20. Provide a prompt thank-you letter clearly restating the key points covered in the meeting. Include any requested materials with the letter.

Sources: (AOTA 2000d; AOTA 2000e; Vermithrax 2000)

Table 12–6.   Legislative Process: How a Federal Bill Becomes a Law

House	*Senate*
1. Bill is introduced in the House Bill is titled HR_____.	**1. Bill is introduced in the Senate** Bill is titled S_____. (Senate follows the same steps as House, with exception of the "rules" step.)
2. Bill is referred to committee Bill is carefully analyzed. If the committee takes no action, the bill is killed.	**2. Bill is referred to committee**
3. Bill is referred to a subcommittee At this point, therapists and others can provide testimony at a scheduled hearing. The specialized subcommittee may "mark up" the bill, or make changes to it, prior to recommending it back to the full committee. If the subcommittee votes not to report legislation to the full committee, the bill is killed.	**3. Bill is referred to a subcommittee**
4. Bill is reported by full House committee After obtaining the subcommittee's report, the full committee may do further study and hearings, which is again a time to testify. The full committee votes, or "orders a bill to be reported," on its recommendations.	**4. Bill is reported by full Senate committee**
5. Publication of Written Report After the full committee votes favorably to have a bill reported, the chairperson allocates staff to prepare a written report that includes the intent and scope of the legislation, its influence on existing laws, the position of the executive branch, and dissenting views.	**5. Publication of Written Report**
6. Rules Committee Action Many bills go to this committee for a "rule" to accelerate floor action and set conditions for discussion and amendments on the floor. Some "privileged" bills go directly to the floor for debate.	**6. Rules Committee Action** In the Senate, the "rules" step is skipped. In addition, some bills may skip committee discussions and go to the Senate floor for debate.
7. Debate/Floor Vote The bill is debated, is often amended, or can be killed. If passed, it goes on to the Senate to follow the same route.	**7. Debate/Floor Vote** The bill now goes on to the next step: conference action.

Table 12–7.   Preparation of Testimony

- Testimony involves research and clear, credible facts. As when studying for an examination, therapists need to know their subject.
- Type the testimony and have others review it.
- Role-play, presenting and timing the testimony. Be aware that usually there is a time limit to provide testimony, and stick to the key points of the testimony. Practice presenting the testimony in a calm and friendly tone.
- Prepare to answer questions or provide supplementary knowledge. Have someone role-play an adversarial stance in order to practice answering difficult questions. Know the opposition's position so that you are prepared with counterarguments.
- Know the names of all the legislators on the committee and something about their positions on the topic. Do your research!
- Address committee chairpersons as Mr. Chairman, Madam Chairwoman, Mr. Speaker, etc., depending on the person.
- Be clear and to the point. Do not use vague terminology such as "it seems" or "it appears."
- If possible, include relevant patient stories to make the testimony meaningful.
- Present what the committee might want to hear, such as fiscal issues. Clearly define any medical jargon.
- Complete a prehearing briefing to determine that everything is organized.
- Make sufficient copies of the testimony to bring to the hearing, and provide copies to members of the committee before the hearing actually takes place.

Presentation of Testimony

- Dress professionally.
- Address comments to the members of the committee.
- In your introduction, identify yourself, your professional background, and the organization you represent. Relate the importance of the issue, and thank the members of the committee for allowing you time to present your case. Always be very polite.
- Ask that your testimony be included in the record of the hearing.
- Articulate loudly and clearly. Do not read your testimony word for word; rather, provide a presentation.
- Do not repeat information that has already been stated in prior testimony.

Answering Questions and Conclusion of the Testimony

- Close the testimony with a brief summary of your position, and offer to answer any questions.
- Be clear and consistent, and not evasive, in your answers to questions.
- If you do not know the answer to a question, admit it, but offer to provide the answer in writing at a later date.
- Do not appear intimidated.
- Promptly follow up with members of the committee. Be sure to write thank-you letters. In the letters, include key points covered in the testimony and any requested materials.

Sources: Vermithrax 2000; Dodge 2005;

CONFERENCE ACTION

After the Senate and House have passed related bills, a conference occurs with representatives from both divisions to reconcile any differences between the bills.

If the conference does not reach a compromise, the bill is killed. If differences are reconciled, a written conference report is prepared, which both divisions must approve. The bill is then sent to the president.

PRESIDENTIAL ACTION

The president has four options:

Option 1: Sign the bill and it becomes law.
Option 2: Take no action for 10 days while Congress is in session, and the bill automatically becomes law.
Option 3: Veto the bill. If the bill is vetoed, Congress can override the veto by a two-thirds vote in both houses.
Option 4: Take no action after the Congress has adjourned for its second session, and the bill is killed.

Source: APTA. 2002c. *PT advocacy;* AOTA. 2000g. *OT Advocate Packet.*

Advocacy on the State Level

Most of what we have discussed applies to advocacy on both the federal and state levels. What is unique about advocacy on the state level is that oftentimes it is easier to get in contact with state personnel about issues and to maintain ongoing relationships. Also unique on the state level is that some public policies, such as Medicaid, are combined federal–state laws that are regulated at the state level. Therefore, state departments will have the responsibility for determining the particular state law. Therapists can have a strong impact when they advocate with these state-level agencies.

Step IV: Reflection

This step involves carefully evaluating what was and was not successful in the advocacy effort. Based on this step, alternative strategies may be tried if the initial effort was unsuccessful (Callahan 2000). Although reflection is written into the advocacy sequence as a final step, therapists should be critically analyzing the advocacy process throughout. Table 12–8 ■ presents some questions to ponder.

Table 12–8.   Reflective Questions After an Advocacy Effort

1. Were we proactive rather than reactive with our advocacy efforts?
2. Did we follow the steps for successful advocacy?
3. Which of our efforts worked?
4. Which didn't work and why?
5. What would we do differently next time?
6. Who are the key people that we will stay in contact with? Did we properly and promptly thank them for their help?

CONCLUSION

Advocacy is an essential skill that therapists should develop and be prepared to use on many levels, whether with clients, various professional and other organizations, the state legislature, or the U.S. Congress. Even if one does not get involved on a state or national level, advocacy can be done in one's own workplace by helping clients and promoting therapy. Essential to the advocacy process is an understanding of one's own motivation and having assertive communication and critical thinking skills to consider the public policy. Finally, advocacy involves personal strength, for, as Lohman, Gabriel, and Furlong (2004) state, "Being an advocate for change . . . may be difficult. It may put the practitioner in conflict with the prevailing political climate that seems focused on the bottom line and costs, rather than quality of life for people with disabilities. Such advocacy requires moral courage. . . ."

Active Learning Exercise

Advocacy Scenarios: Identify What You Would Do to Advocate in Each Situation.

Scenario 1: Mark works in an outpatient therapy clinic for a private company. He treats a large population of elderly people, particularly with orthopedic concerns. Mark's main concern is client care, and he does an adequate job rehabilitating the clients. He is, however, ignorant of the changes in the outer health care environment. If asked, he states, "I assume that the company I work for will keep me aware." Therefore, Mark is caught totally unaware when health care changes result in a prospective payment system with outpatient elders. Subsequently, when the prospective payment system is instituted, his hours are cut back due to decreases in reimbursement. What could Mark have done differently?

Scenario 2: Melissa works in acute care practice with people who have a variety of diagnoses. On the oncology floor, she is working with a middle-aged woman who seems very depressed. This woman indirectly hints of suicide. What should Melissa do?

Scenario 3: Mimi works in an interdisciplinary rehabilitation department. She is the only certified hand therapist employed there and has over 10 years working with that population, more than anyone else in her department. Lately, a new secretary in the department has been assigning the clients as the orders are processed. The secretary is now assigning clients with hand concerns to all the therapists, not primarily to Mimi. Mimi would like to follow more of the hand patients. What should she do?

Scenario 4: Melvin is the director of a small outpatient clinic. Lately he has noticed that his client load has decreased. He ignores the situation, thinking that it is temporary. Finally, he attempts to figure out what is wrong. By then it is too late, because he didn't realize that his primary admitting physician was unhappy with the care provided by one of the therapists in the department and is now admitting elsewhere. How should Melvin have handled the situation differently?

Scenario 5: You are the administrator of a therapy department. You find out that Medicaid is not reimbursing for a key therapy service in your state. Describe the steps that you will take to obtain reimbursement.

Scenario 6: You become aware that one of your state senators is supporting some Medicare concerns of elders, but not concerns related to therapy. Describe the steps that you would take to work with this senator.

Active Learning Exercise

Self-Reflection

Identify a situation in which you were an advocate. Reflect about the following questions:

Were you successful? Why or why not?

Did you take a proactive stance in the advocacy effort? Why or why not?

What did you learn from the experience? What would you do differently?

Source for some of the above resources: *http://www.apha.org/legislative/advocacylinks.htm*

Active Learning Exercise

- Utilizing the letter-writing guidelines provided in this chapter, write a letter to a senator or representative based on a bill relevant to therapy.
- Utilizing the information provided in this chapter on how to present testimony, simulate giving testimony about a bill relevant to therapy. Research and develop a "fact sheet" to include with the testimony. Then, in front of a mock committee, present a three-minute testimony. Be prepared to address opposing arguments. Or have someone prepare and present opposing testimony or supporting testimony from another perspective. Critique the testimony and fact sheet on the basis of the guidelines presented in the chapter.
- As a group, identify a bill relevant to therapy. Have each member of the group develop a persuasive argument based on different perspectives about the bill. Examples of these perspectives could be a constiuent's viewpoint, a health care provider's viewpoint, a senator's viewpoint, and a payer's perspective.
- Referring to the advocacy resources provided at the end of the chapter, identify an advocacy group that services clients who are also followed by physical and occupational therapy. Interview the lobbyist of the association. Prepare a list of five to six questions to find out how he or she advocates for the members of the organization.
- Interview a representative from your state association legislative committee. Find out what motivated him or her to become involved with the state committee. Identify the public policy issues relevant to therapy in your state. Find out about the background of your state lobbyist.

ADVOCACY RESOURCES

GENERAL INTERNET SITES RELATED TO HEALTH CARE PUBLIC POLICY:

The Bureau of National Affairs, Inc.   http://www.bna.com   This site provides material on a wide variety of news items, including health policy.

Duke University: Center for Health Policy   http://www.hpolicy.duke.edu   This site is a resource to much information about health policies. It also contains a large variety of Internet links.

FamiliesUSA   http://www.familiesusa.org   This national nonprofit organization advocates for high-quality affordable health care for all Americans. It focuses on the following health care policies: Medicaid, managed care, Medicare, children's health, and the uninsured. The site contains a link to information about advocacy.

HillWatch   http://subscript.bna.com/PIC/hillwatch.nsf   This subscription service provides detailed information about current health care public policies.

Kaiser Family Foundation   http://www.kaisernetwork.org   This organization deals with health-related policies and trends. The site contains health webcasts about current issues, and one can get on their e-mail list to receive health care policy updates.

The Moving Ideas: The Electronic Policy Network   http://www.movingideas.org/ This site offers a *comprehensive* list of policy resources.

GOVERNMENT PUBLIC POLICY RESOURCES AND BILL LANGUAGE:

To obtain free copies of up to six federal bills, contact Senate Document Room, Rm. B-04 Hart Bldg., Washington, DC 20510–7106 or House Document Room, Rm. B18 Ford Bldg., Washington, DC 20515–6620.

To contact a Website for the U.S. Capitol, call 202–224–3121 (number to get contact phone numbers of senators) FAX 202–456–246, or visit http://www2.Whitehouse.gov/site.

Congress Website: http://www.congress.org/—Provides information about what is happening in Congress.

The Dirksen Congressional Center: http://www.congresslink.org/—An educational site that provides information about Congress and public policies.

Federal Disability Laws: http://www.usa.gov/Topics/Reference_Shelf.shtml—This site contains the full text of the federal disability laws.

House Website: http://www.house.gov—This site contains many resources pertaining to the U.S. Congress. For example, one can find out who is on committees and what the different committees address. Representatives specifically involved with health policy often have statements on their sites.

Senate Website: http://www.senate.gov/—This site contains many resources pertaining to the U.S. Senate. Senators specifically involved with health or disability public policy often have statements on their sites.

Thomas: http://thomas.loc.gov—This site has all the bills listed in abbreviated and completed forms. From this site, one can identify the status of different bills.

Centers for Medicare and Medicaid: http://www.cms.hhs.gov—This is the site for the Centers for Medicare and Medicaid Services, the agency that governs Medicare, Medicaid, and child health insurance programs.

PROFESSIONAL ORGANIZATIONS WITH PUBLIC POLICY RESOURCES:

Agency for Health Care Policy and Research (AHCPR): http://www.ahcpr.gov Part of the Public Health Service in the U.S. Department of Health and Human Services, this agency supports efficacy and cost research.

American Association of Retired Persons (AARP): http://www.aarp.org This site has many resources for Americans age 50 and older and is strongly involved in policymaking.

American Chiropractic Association: http://www.amerchiro.org

American Health Care Association (AHCA): http://www.ahca.org This group deals with the concerns of those in the long-term care community.

American Medical Association: http://www.ama-assn.org/

American Medical Student Association: http://www.amsa.org This site has many advocacy resources, including an advocacy tool kit.

American Occupational Therapy Association: http://www.aota.org

American Physical Therapy Association: http://www.apta.org

American Psychological Association: http://www.apa.org

American Public Health Association: http://www.apha.org This site has advocacy resources.

Center for Medicare Advocacy: http://www.harp.org This private nonprofit organization focuses on Medicare and other issues for those with chronic conditions.

Health Administration Responsibility Project: http://www.harp.org This site helps with advocacy issues related to managed care.

Joint Commission on Accreditation of Healthcare Organizations: http://www.jcaho.org This agency evaluates and accredits health care organizations.

National Conference of State Legislatures: http://www.ncsl.org This site helps legislatures and staffs of state legislatures with information about resources.

National Information Center for Children and Youth with Disabilities (NICHCY): http:// www.nichcy.org

National Rehabilitation Organization: http://nationalrehab.org

National Senior Citizens' Law Center: www.nclc.org The center helps with advocacy for people with low incomes.

Quackwatch, Inc.: http://www.quackwatch.com This site provides resources for dealing with medical quackery.

NATIONAL ORGANIZATIONS FOR DISEASE AND DISABILITY CONDITIONS

Most of these organizations have policy sections. Consider networking with them about mutual concerns.

Alzheimer's Disease

Alzheimer's Association: http://www.alz.org

Arthritis

Arthritis Foundation: www.arthritis.org

Brain-injured

Family Caregiver Alliance: http://www.caregiver.org

Brain Injury Association: http://www.biausa.org/

Cerebral Palsy

United Cerebral Palsy (UCP): http://www.ucpa.org/

Diabetes

American Diabetic Association: http://www.diabetes.org/

Emphysema

National Emphysema Foundation: http://www.emphysemafoundation.org/

Epilepsy

Epilepsy Foundation: http://www.efa.org/

Heart/Stroke

American Heart Association: http://www.americanheart.org/

American Stroke Association: http://www.strokeassociation.org/

Hospice

Hospice Foundation of America: http://www.hospicefoundation.org/

National Hospice and Palliative Care Organization: http://www.nho.org/

Mental Illness
National Alliance for the Mentally Ill (NAMI): http://www.nami.org/
National Mental Health Association: http://www.nmha.org
Muscular Dystrophy
Muscular Dystrophy Association: http://www.mdausa.org
Multiple Sclerosis
Multiple Sclerosis: http://www.msfacts.org/
Osteoporosis
National Osteoporosis Society: http://www.nos.org.uk/
Parkinson's Disease
American Parkinson Disease Association: http://apdaparkinson.com/
Spinal Cord
National Spinal Cord Injury Association: http://www.spinalcord.org/
Vision
Glaucoma Research Foundation (GRF): http://www.glaucoma.org/
Macular Degeneration International: http://www.maculardegeneration.org/
(Some of these references also are found on http://www.patientadvocacy.org/links.html)

NEW SITES:

Congressional Quarterly: http://www.cq.com This subscription site provides very specific
and excellent information about what is happening on the Hill with bills.
C-span: http://c-span.org This is an excellent resource for more current bills.
New York Times: http://www.nytimes.com/ The *New York Times* provides information
about political issues.
Washington Post: http://www.washpost.com The *Washington Post* provides excellent information about recent policies.
Yahoo: http://www.Yahoo.com The news section provides information, particularly
about recent bills.

CHAPTER REVIEW QUESTIONS

1. Define the ethical responsibility of a therapist to be involved in advocacy.
2. Relate the basic skills of advocacy and how they affect each other:
   a. Self-reflection
   b. Knowledge
   c. Assertive communication
3. Provide an example of therapist advocacy on each of the following levels:
   a. client
   b. professional
   c. organizational
4. Review the features of an effective legislative lobbying campaign:
   a. legislative visit
   b. letter writing
   c. testimony provision

CHAPTER DISCUSSION QUESTIONS

1. Discuss how any recent changes in health care have made therapists consider the importance of advocacy skills in professional practice.
2. Reflection has been emphasized as an important component of effective advocacy. Why are passion about an issue and self-motivation important to advocacy over the long term?
3. Discuss an experience you have had in trying to effect reform or bring about institutional change. What did you learn from this experience?

REFERENCES

Alberi, R.E., and M.L. Emmons. 1978. *Your Perfect Right: A Guide to Assertive Behavior,* 3rd ed. San Luis Obispo, CA: Impact Publishers.

AOTAction Network. 2000. *Helping to Ensure the Future of OT Through Congressional Action.* Bethesda MD: American Occupational Therapy Association.

American Occupational Therapy Association, n.d. Public affairs division. Bethesda MD: AOTA.

American Occupational Therapy Association. n.d. AOTPAC Fact Sheet. http://www.aota. org/members/area1/links/LINK12.asp?PLACE=/members/area1/links/LINK12 .asp (accessed March 14, 2007).

———. 2000b. How a bill becomes a law. In *Public Policy 101,* ed. C. Metzler and C. Willmarth. Bethesda MD: American Occupational Therapy Association.

———. 2000c. Guidelines for a site visit for members of the U.S. Congress. In *OT Advocate Packet.* Bethesda MD: American Occupational Therapy Association.

———. 2000d. Tips for writing a letter to your member of Congress. In *OT Advocate Packet.* Bethesda MD: American Occupational Therapy Association.

———. 2000e. Tips for meeting with your members of Congress. In *OT Advocate Packet.* Bethesda MD: American Occupational Therapy Association.

———. 2000f. *http://www.aota/org* (accessed December 17, 2007).

———. 2000g. AOTA expands your influence. *http://www.aota/org/* (accessed December 17, 2007).

American Physical Therapy Association. 1999. Right to care: A physical therapist's guide to creating positive change in managed care. *PT Magazine* 7(1): 8-page insert.

———. n.d. Federal Regulatory Affairs. http://www.apta.org/AM/Template.cfm?Section= Federal_Regulatory_Affairs1&Template=/TaggedPage/TaggedPageDisplay.cfm& TPLID=180&ContentID=30165 (accessed March 7, 2007).

———. n.d. Grassroots. http://www.apta.org/AM/Template.cfm?Section=Grassroots1& Template=/TaggedPage/TaggedPageDisplay.cfm&TPLID=185&ContentID=18609 (accessed March 7, 2007).

———. 2002a. APTA Code of Ethics. *https://www.apta.org/PT_Practice/ethics_pt/code_ethics* (accessed December 17, 2007).

———. 2002b. Guide for professional conduct. *https://www.apta.org/PT_Practice/ethics_ pt/pro_conduct* (accessed December 17, 2007).

———. 2002c. PT advocacy. *http://www.apta.org/Advocacy* (accessed December 17, 2007).

————. 2002d. House of Delegates Policies. *http://www.apta.org/Home/Members/governance/governance* (accessed December 17, 2007).

American Public Health Association. 2000. Face to face meetings with policymakers. *http://www.apha.org/legislative* (accessed December 17, 2007).

Callahan, S. 2000. Educational innovations: Incorporating a political action framework into a BSN program. *J Nurs Ed* 39(1): 34–36.

Coile, R.C. 2000. Health care 2000: Top 10 trends for the new century. In *Russ Coile's Health Trends 2000,* Special Report, January: 1, 4–12.

Commission on Standards and Ethics (SEC), and S. Peloquin. 2005. Occupational therapy code of ethics. *Am J Occupa Ther* 59(6): 639–42.

Connolly, J. 1999. APTA battles the BBA. *PT Magazine* 7(7): 46–55.

Davis, C.M. 1998. *Patient Practitioner Interaction: An Experiential Manual for Developing the Art of Health Care,* 3rd ed. Thorofare, NJ: Slack.

Dodge, J. Effective Advocacy in Nebraska. Presented (2005, April, 26) at Persuading others to rally around the Cause. Nebraska Appleseed and Voices for Children.

Evert, M.M. 1995. Presidential address: Our journey together. *Am J Occupa Ther* 49(10): 1065–67.

Foose, D. 1999. Elder abuse: Stepping in and stopping it. *PT Magazine* 7(1): 56–62.

Griffith, D. 1999. Capital watch: Take action in your state. *PT Magazine* 7(3): 16–17.

Joint Commission on Accreditation of Healthcare Organizations. 2007. *Disclosing Medical Errors: A Guide to An Effective Explanation and Apology.* Oakbrook Terrace, IL: Joint Commission Resources, Inc.

Lamb, A. 2004, September, 20. Lobbying 101, *OT* Practice 9, 17, 16–19.

Lohman, H., L. Gabriel, and B. Furlong. 2004.The bridge from ethics to public policy: Implications for occupational therapy practitioners. *Am J Occupa Ther* 58(1): 109–12.

Lohman, H. 2003. Critical analysis of a public policy: An occupational therapist's experience with the patient bill of rights. *Am J of Occupa Ther* 57(4); 468–72.

Loukas, K.M. 1999. Representing you! *OT Pract* 4(11): 9–10.

Lozano, P., V.M. Biggs, B.J. Sibley, T.M. Smith, E.K. Marcuse, and A.B. Bergman. 1994. Advocacy training during pediatric residency. *Pediatrics* 94(4): 532–36.

Namerow, M.J. 1982. Implementing advocacy into the gerontological nursing major. *J Geront Nurs* 8(3): 149–51.

Sachs, D., and R. Linn. 1997. Client advocacy in action: Professional and environmental factors affecting Israeli occupational therapists' behavior. *Can J Occupa Ther* 64 (4): 207–15.

Scott-Lee, S.J. 1999. Lobbying for occupational therapy. *OT Pract* 4 (8): 5, 12.

Vermithrax, D. 2000. Lobbying/advocacy techniques. *http://www.trytel.com/~aberdeen/techniq.html* (accessed December 17, 2007).

Weingarten. 1996, October, 8. Writing a Member of Congress. Computing Research Association. http://www.cra.org/govaffairs/advocacy/writecong.html (accessed March 7, 2007).

Wynn-Gilliam, K. 2000. APTA mobilizes on manipulation: Association at work series. *PT Magazine* 8(2): 34–38.

Learn to write to your congressperson. *http://www.learn2.com/*

Tips on writing a letter to a legislator. *http://www.propeop*

Appendix

Table I.   History of the Individuals with Disabilities Education Act (IDEA)

1975: Public Law 94–142, 89 Stat. 773, Part B of the Education for All Handicapped Children Act of 1975	Authorized special education for children with disabilities. Considered rights of children, assisted states with special education, and evaluated the effectiveness of these educational efforts.
1980: Public Law 94–142	"Mandated programs and services for children 3 to 21 years that were consistent with state law" (U.S. Department of Education 2005, p. 4).
1986: Public Law 99–457, 100 Stat. 1145, Education of the Handicapped Act Amendments of 1986	Authorized education for children with disabilities aged three to five years (Part B), as well as early home-based intervention for families and toddlers, birth to three years (Part H). Included occupational and physical therapy as primary interventions.
1990: P.L. 101–476, 104 Stat. 1103, Education of the Handicapped Act Amendments of 1990	Changed the name of the act to Individuals with Disabilities Education Act (IDEA). Changed the terminology in the act from *handicap* to *disability*. Added autism and traumatic brain injury as conditions to be considered. Strengthened guidelines for early intervention programs. Included rehabilitation and social services under related services. Added a transition plan to the IEP.
1997: P.L. 105–17, 111 Stat. 37, Individuals with Disabilities Education Act Amendments of 1997	Maintained related services (occupational and physical therapy, etc.). Encouraged access to general curriculum for children with disabilities. Strengthened parental role. Changed evaluations to include discrepancies between child's performance and expectations of curriculum and general classroom. Ensured usage of qualified state personnel. Included verbiage asserting that utilization of paraprofessionals was consistent with state laws and regulations. Included related services in the division of special education. Included participation of related service personnel in child's IEP if personnel are involved in providing education services to child. Restructured IDEA into four parts: (a) general provisions, (b) assistance for education of all children with disabilities, (c) infants and toddlers with disabilities, and (d) national abilities to improve the education of children with disabilities.

(continued)

Table I.   History of the Individuals with Disabilities Education Act (IDEA) *(Continued)*

2004: PLl08–446	Alignment with No Child Left Behind Act of 2001 to encourage greater student accountability. Included several changes in the IEP process dealing with short-term objectives, reporting of progress, transitions with the IEP (age 16, part C to part B and between schools), and participation in the IEP conference. Two pilot programs related to the IEF were initiated. One involved a reduction in paperwork and the second involved a multiyear IEP conference. Several changes included in the bill, one of which stipulated that parents may be legally responsible if their course of action is found to be frivolous or improper, tightened up due process procedures. Several changes were related to disiplinary actions. The four parts of this bill remained with some internal changes: (a) General Provisions, (b) Assistance to States for Education of All Children with Disablities, (c) Infants and Toddlers with Disablities, and (d) National Activities to Improve Education of All Children with Disabilities.

From: APTA 2000; Mellard 2000; Nichcy 2000; Nichcy 2004, ttp://www.nichcy.org/reauth/2004IDEA SUMMARY-12.04.doc; Stephens and Tauber 1996; *www.caselink, U.S. Department of Education 2005.*

Table II.   History of Legislation Related to Developmental Disabilities

1963: P.L. 88–156, 77 Stat. 273, Maternal and Child Health and Mental Retardation Planning Amendments of 1963	Precursor to modern act. Established a federal program for maternity and infant care for high-risk mothers.
1963: P.L. 88–164, 77 Stat. 282 Mental Retardation Facilities and Community Mental Health Centers Construction Act of 1963	Precursor to the modern act. First major federal initiative for building of facilities for mentally ill and mentally retarded.
1970: P.L. 91–517, 84 Stat. 1316, Developmental Disabilities Services and Facilities Construction Amendments of 1970	Changed terminology "mental retardation" to "developmental disabilities." Expanded definition of individuals substantially handicapped to include those with mental retardation, cerebral palsy, epilepsy, and other neurological conditions. Changed focus from institutions to communities. Provided grant money to state-designated agencies and for university-affiliated programs (UAFs).

(continued)

Table II.   History of Legislation Related to Developmental Disabilities *(Continued)*

1975: Developmental Disabilities Assistance and Bill of Rights Act (P.L. 94–103, 89 Stat. 486)	Expanded upon earlier legislation by adding more diagnostic conditions, including autism, learning disabilities, and other conditions related to mental retardation that affect intellectual functioning. Required that disability occur before age of 18 and be chronic. Funded UAFs. Included with Title II a bill of rights for people with mental retardation and other developmental disabilities. Established protection and advocacy programs.
1978: P.L. 95–602, 92 Stat. 2455, Rehabilitation Comprehensive Services, and Developmental Disabilities Amendments of 1978	Expanded age requirement to 22. Changed definition of disability by making it general and based on functional limitations rather than specific handicaps. Established priority service areas for states.
1984: Developmental Disabilities Act of 1984 Amendments and reorganized (P.L. 98–527, 98 Stat. 2662)	Ensured that people with developmental disabilities (DDs) received appropriate services, and established systems to monitor services. Added statement of purpose specifying that programs help people with DDs achieve their maximal potential with integration into the community. Established employment as a priority.
1987: Developmental Disabilities Assistance and Bill of Rights Amendments of 1987 (P.L. 100–146, 101 Stat. 840)	Established focus on capacities, rather than limitations, for people with DDs. Clarified and enhanced roles of state planning councils and protection and advocacy systems.
1990: Developmental Disabilities Assistance and Bill of Rights Act of 1990 (P.L. 101–496, 104 Stat. 1191)	Clarified and enhanced roles of state planning councils.
1994: Developmental Disabilities Assistance and Bill of Rights Act Amendments of 1994 (P.L. 103–230, 108 Stat. 284)	Established language more consistent with other federal acts, such as the ADA, the IDEA, and the Technology Related Assistance Act. Established funding regulations for state grants. Strengthened and clarified state planning councils, protection and advocacy systems, and UAPs.
2000: Amendments (actually passed in 1999) Consolidated Appropriations Act, 2000 (P.L. 106–113, 113 Stat. 1501)	Established guidelines for allocation of grants with the developmental disabilities councils to bring about permanent improvements. Included new programs to assist states in strengthening family support and for development of curriculum with scholarship and availability for direct support workers.
2007	Up for reauthorization.

K. Boyd et al. 1996. Developmental Disabilities Act; J. Perinchief. 1996. Service management; P. J. Graney. 2000. RS20194; K. L. Reed. 1992. History of federal legislation for people with disabilities; Hightower-Vandamm. 1979. Nationally speaking.

Table III.   History of the Older American's Act

1992 Amendments	Developed rights and advocacy systems to protect older Americans.
	Changed the position of the commissioner of the Area Office on Aging (AoA) to assistant secretary for aging in the Office of the Secretary.
2000 Amendments	Added family caregiver support, which allows state agencies to provide counseling and respite services to caregivers.
	Added more state flexibility.
	Consolidated several categorical programs.
2006 Amendments	"Enhanced federal, state, and local coordination of long-term care services provided in home and community-based settings.
	Supported state and community planning to address the long-term care needs of the baby boom generation.
	Provided a greater focus on prevention and treatment of mental disorders.
	Outreach and service to a broader universe of family caregivers under the National Family Caregiver Support Program.
	Increased focus on civic engagement and volunteerism.
	Enhanced coordination of programs that protect elders from abuse, neglect and exploitation" (Carbonell 2006 p.1).

Table adapted from Administration on Aging. n.d. Older American Act. http://www.aoa .gov/about/legbudg/oaa/legbudg_oaa.asp (accessed October 11, 2007); The Center for Social Gerontology. http://www.tcsg.org/law/oaa/reauth.htm (accessed October 11, 2007); Statement of Josefina G. Carbonell: Older Americans Act Amendments of 2006. http://www .aoa.gov/OAA2006/Main_Site/resources/news/passage.aspx (accessed October 27, 2007); American Office on Aging. 2004. *Summary of key changes in the 2000 amendments.* http://www .aoa.gov/about/legbudg/oaa/legbudg_oaa_summary.asp (accessed October 27, 2007).

Table IV.   Key Public Policy Related to Work since the 1970s.

1973: PL 93-112, 87 Stat. 355 Reha-bilitation Act of 1973	Modern rehabilitation act. Has sections including affirmative action in employment (section 503) and nondiscrimination in facilities (section 504).
1984: PL 98–524, 98 Stat. 2435 Carl D. Perkins Vocational Education Act	Provided state funding for vocational programming. Act continues to be amended.
1990: PL 101-336, 104 Stat. 324 Americans with Disabilities Act of 1990 (ADA)	Civil rights act, which, among other things, provides protection in employment.
1999: H.R. 3433 Ticket to Work and Work Incentives Improvement Act	Allows people with disabilities to keep their federal health insurance benefits (Medicare and Medicaid) if they become employed. Helps people with disabilities be employable to reduce dependence on benefits and assistance and to maximize people's financial self-sufficiency.

Dunn. 2000. Personal communication; Reed. 1992. *The beginning of occupational therapy*; Johansson. 2000. *Disability advocates say more could be done*; Rothstein. 1992. *Disability and the Law*.

Table V.   History of the Rehabilitation Act (RA)

1920: Smith–Fess Act (Vocational Rehabilitation Act) Ch. 219, 41 Stat. 735	Precursor to modern act. Provided counseling and guidance, vocational training, and job placement. Limited support services were available for prosthetics and transportation. Is the root of the Vocational Rehabilitation Act. The Smith–Fess act was amended several times until the modern act became law in 1973.
1943: Barden–LaFollette Act (Vocational Rehabilitation Act) Ch. 190, 57 Stat. 374	Precursor to modern act. Amendment to PL 66236. Added more diagnoses, including psychiatric diagnoses. Began covering rehabilitation services. Established an Office of Vocational Rehabilitation.
1954: Ch. 655, PL 83–565, 68 Stat. 652 Hill–Burton Act (Vocational Rehabilitation Act Amendments of 1954)	Precursor to modern act. Intent was to expand building of hospitals. These amendments addressed many areas, including expanding rehabilitation facilities, making facilities more assessable, and financing therapy education. Funded research and program development. Provided funding for occupational therapy, physical therapy, and other services.
1965: PL 89–333, 79 Stat. 1282 Vocational Rehabilitation Act Amendments of 1965	Precursor to modern act. Replaced the Office of Vocational Rehabilitation with the Vocational Rehabilitation Administration. Provided construction money to rehabilitation facilities and increased the scope of covered diagnoses to the more severely disabled as covered by the Vocational Rehabilitation Act. Considered for the first time the impact of

(continued)

Table V.   History of the Rehabilitation Act (RA) *(Continued)*

	social disability. Established the National Commission on Architectural Barriers, which studied architectural design.
1973: PL 93–112, 87 Stat. 355: Rehabilitation Act of 1973	Is the current act. Included mandated services for more severe disabilities and added concepts of "consumer empowerment and choice, integration, independence and self sufficiency" (National Disability Rights Network 2006, p.1)
1974	Attempted to change focus from considering only employability.
1978: PL 95–602, 92 Stat. 2955 Amendments to the Rehabilitation Act of 1973, Rehabilitation Comprehensive Services, and Developmental Disabilities Amendments of 1978	Included 504 and 505 regulations. Added independent living with Title VII. Created the National Institute of Handicapped Research. Added a Protection and Advocacy for Individual Rights program.
1984: PL 98–524, 98 Stat. 2435 Carl D. Perkins Vocational Act	Authorized more funding for state vocational education and programs.
1986: PL 99–357, 100 Stat. 761 Carl D. Perkins Vocational Education Act Amendment	Dealt with state allocation of funds. Addressed technology. Specifically included people with severe disabilities, such as those with persistent mental illness.
1992: Amendments (PL 102–569, 106 Stat. 4334)	Mandated that state vocational rehabilitation agencies provide for individual choices of services and service providers, focused on careers rather than jobs, and made the assumption that people with disabilities are employable. Addressed rehabilitation services to underserved minority populations.
1998: Amendments (PL 105–220, 112 Stat. 936)	"Reauthorized as title IV of the Workforce Investment Act" (National Disability Rights Network 2006, p.1) Made vocational rehabilitation programs part of state workforce investment systems. Reorganized the way employment services were provided by adding more coordination between state and federal programs. Partnered state rehabilitation agencies with agencies from the Department of Labor to create "one-stop centers." Enhanced section 508: Strengthened federal government's existing obligation to ensure that technology be available to people with disabilities. Added complaint procedure and reporting requirements. Added more consumer involvement in individual plans and implemented an Individualized Plan of Employment (IPE), which established employment as the final outcome.

(continued)

Table V.   History of the Rehabilitation Act (RA) *(Continued)*

	Also implemented a Comprehensive System of Personal Development (CSPD), which created higher standards for practitioners working with people in the system. Required national certification for being a rehabilitation counselor. Allowed people receiving Social Security Disability (SSI) or Supplemental Security Income (SSI) to be eligible for vocational rehabilitation services (National Disability Rights Network 2006, p.1).
2005+	Workforce Investment Act (WIA), of which the Rehabilitation Act is a part, has been up for reauthorization several times, but never was passed into a new law. Some issues of concern associated with the attempted reauthorizations are to better meet the needs of the visually impaired; to strengthen accessibility and quality of work training; to realize the potential of merging funding for vocational rehabilitation into a general employment block service grant; to achieve better coordination between various acts that affect the employment of people with disabilities, such as with the Work Incentives Act and the IDEA; to strengthen programming for youths making the transition to work; to add complaint procedures for clients; and to increase funding. The 1998 amendments, however, remain unchanged until the act is reauthorized.

Bristo. 1996. *Achieving Independence;* Conyers and Ahrens 2003; Dunn. 2000. Personal communication; Reed. 1992. History of federal legislation for peoples with disabilities; Rothstein. 1992. *Disability and the Law;* Jacobs. 1996; Larkin, Alson, Middleton, and Wilson. 2003. *http://www.access-board.gov/ sec508/Section; National Disability Rights Network. 2006.* The Workforce Investment Act & the Rehabilitation Act. *http://www.napas.org/* (accessed February 4, 2007); The WorkForce Alliance. 2005. TWA letter regarding H.R. 27. http://www.workforcealliance.org/site/preview.asp?cid={93353952-1DF1-473A- B105-7713F4529EBB}&key=6eICJQNrHiE&staging=0&go=http://www.workforcealliance.org/site/lookup.asp?c=ciJNK1PJJtH-*-b=1145013 (accessed February 20, 2007); National Council on Disability. 2005. National Council on Disability Recommendations Workforce Investment Act Reauthorization. http://www.ncd.gov/newsroom/publications/2005/workforce_investment.htm (accessed February 20, 2007); American Council of the Blind (ACB). 2005. Rehabilitation Reauthorization. http://www.acb.org/washington/vr-factsheet-2005.html (accessed February 20, 2007). The Commission on Rehabilitation Counselor Certification (CRCC). http://www.crccertification.com/ (accessed February 20, 2007).

Table VI. **History of the Assistance Technology Act**

Section G of the Education of the Handicapped Act	Precursor to modern act. Addressed access to existing technology, but did not address development of technology.
Section 508 of the Rehabilitation Act Amendments of 1986 (P.L. 99–506, 100 Stat. 1807).	Precursor to modern act. Addressed access to existing technology, but did not address development of technology.
The Technology-Related Assistance for Individuals with Disabilities Act of 1988 (The Tech Act) (P.L. 100–407, 102 Stat. 1044)	Focus on advocating for and modeling of changes in systems that would increase access to and funding of assistive technology. Addressed lack of information about technology, lack of training, and lack of accessibility to technology. Established grant money for state technological assistance programs. Focused on providing funds for technological development.
Technology-Related Assistance for Individuals with Disabilities Amendments of 1994 (P.L. 103–218, 108 Stat. 50).	Increased focus on advocacy as a strategy for systems change. Expanded program authorizations. Continued authorization of grant money for state technological assistance programs, some of which remained unfunded.
Assistive Technology Act of 1998 (P.L. 105–394, 112 Stat. 3627).	Shifted focus to system capacity building to address assistive technology needs of individuals with disabilities. Mandated state activities include public awareness, interagency coordination, technical assistance and training, and outreach. Title III created opportunities for microloan programs for individuals to purchase assistive technology devices or services. Repealed 1988 Act.
Improving Access to Assistive Technology for Individuals with Disabilities Act of 2004 (PL 108-364)	Eliminated sunset provisions on funding. Made services provided by the states more consistent. Required states to provide at least two of the following: alternative financing programs for the purchasing, leasing, technical support and repairs of equipment, as well as assessment and training with equipment usage; equipment demonstration centers; equipment loan programs; or equipment reutilization programs. Includes state protection and advocacy systems to provide legal assistance to consumers on issues related to assistive technology. Included in the bill was funding for research. (No funds are currently appropriated.)

Schultz. 2000. Personal communication; Reed. 1992. *The beginnings of occupational therapy;* Reyes-Akinbileje. 1999. CRS Report for Congress; Shultz 2007.

Glossary

Access   The ability to obtain a health care service when you need it.

Accreditation   A voluntary quality-assurance and improvement process whereby an organization is rated against accepted standards of performance.

Actuarial analysis   The insurance process that predicts the risk of covered events in the risk pool and calculates a premium, called actuarial adjustment, for pool members.

Advocacy   The process of identifying issues and participating in policymaking and policy change.

Alternative medicine   A form of health care that has emerged in contrast to the bioscientific, allopathic model of care that dominates in the United States.

Assignment of benefits   The process whereby a patient transfers insurance benefits directly to the provider from the insurer.

Assistive technology   Equipment, software, and devices that enable persons with disabling conditions to become more independent in their environments.

Barriers   Physical, social, and attitudinal obstructions to full participation in society for persons with disabling conditions.

Benchmarking   The measurement and comparison of performance over time or against a known standard.

Beneficiary   The recipient of the benefits from an insurance contract.

Benefit period   The length of time from day of admission to the hospital to 60 days post-hospital or SNF discharge. Used in determining deductible and co-insurance payments for the Medicare program.

Biomedical model   A perspective on disablement that locates the problem in the person with the disabling condition and the solution in medical care services.

Bundling   The collation of fees for individual, but related, services into one new fee category.

Capitation   A payment mechanism for health care whereby a provider is paid a flat fee per month for each covered member in a health plan.

Case management   The process of eligibility determination and coordination of services for a person receiving multiple health care services.

Case mix adjustment   A system of classifying patients for payment purposes by clinical characteristics and anticipated resource utilization.

Case rate   A negotiated payment based on a visit, a day, or an episode of care.

Categorical eligibility   One of the methods by which one qualifies for Medicaid; mandated in all states. Includes low-income women and children, wards of the state, and persons with disabilities (receiving SSI payments).

Certification   Approval by a physician of a therapy plan of care for a Medicare beneficiary; a form of professional regulation that protects the title of the provider.

Chiropractic   A form of manipulative and body-based alternative medicine centered on the nervous system's role in health maintenance.

Clinical practice guideline   A statement of the process of care based on the best available evidence of the effectiveness and efficiency of care.

Clubhouse model   The social model as used in community-based settings as a form of mental health treatment.

Coalition   A group of individuals or organizations that come together to participate in advocacy; a prerequisite for effective advocacy.

Community rating   A process of actuarial adjustment that assigns a premium rate based on people living in a geographic region.

Complementary medicine   Alternative medicine procedures that are used as an adjunct or in addition to allopathic medical care.

Consolidated billing   The requirement for an SNF to bill for all Medicare Part A services; prevents contractual providers (e.g., therapists) from independently billing for their care.

Consumer-directed health care   A health insurance product that consists of a high-deductible form of health insurance and a health savings account.

Conventional medicine   Another term for the bioscientific, allopathic medical care model that is dominant in the United States.

Cost-based reimbursement   A retrospective method of health care financing whereby a provider reports the costs of providing care and is paid by an insurer.

Cost limits   Payment mechanisms utilized in insurance contracts to share or limit the costs of health care. Includes plan limit, first-dollar coverage, co-insurance, co-payment, and deductible.

Cost shifting   Associated with underpayment of the true costs of caring for Medicare beneficiaries, which are then paid by private insurers who pay artificially high prices for care.

Credentialing   A process used by insurers and some health care organizations to ensure that providers achieve minimum standards of education and experience.

Custodial care   The kind of care given in a facility that provides long-term residential and skilled health care services.

Defined benefit plan   Health insurance plan in which the sponsor predetermines the benefits. Typical of most forms of health insurance today.

Defined contribution plan   Health insurance plan in which the sponsor (e.g., business or government) predetermines the level of funding offered to eligible beneficiaries. Benefits are provided on the basis of this funding and excess beneficiary contributions.

Deinstitutionalization   The predominant philosophy guiding mental health treatment since the early 1960s.

Direct access   The ability of a patient to obtain physical therapy and occupational therapy services without requiring a referral from another provider.

Disablement   A process whereby a person who experiences an illness or injury develops a set of impairments, functional limitations, and disabilities. Associated with the medical rehabilitation model.

Dual eligibility   Exemplified by persons who qualify for both Medicare and Medicaid coverage—typically, low-income elderly persons or persons with disabilities.

Dualism   System consisting of two sources of health policymaking: government and private enterprise. A unique feature of the U.S. health care system.

Empowerment   A social attitude and philosophy which provides an environment and skills that enable people with disabling conditions to make and act upon individual choices.

Enabling factors   System characteristics that predispose a person to be able to access health care services (e.g., availability of insurance, provider location).

Entitlement   A statutory guarantee to a set of benefits for eligible persons.

Epidemiology   The science of public health; the systematic monitoring and investigation of disease and injury.

Evidence-based practice   A process of delivering health care based upon the best available evidence of effectiveness and efficiency.

Fee for service   Payment mechanism for health care whereby a provider is paid an amount of money for each procedure performed.

Fee schedule   A list of services performed, together with an associated payment amount for each service.

Financing   The methods of paying for health care. Broadly speaking, includes private insurance, out-of-pocket payments, and government insurance programs.

Formal care   Health care that is part of the personal health care system consisting of a mix of acute, subacute, and long-term care facilities and related health care personnel.

Gatekeeper   A primary care provider in a health maintenance organization, usually a physician, who provides primary care and coordinates or controls access to the rest of the health care system.

Global budgeting   Payment mechanism for health care whereby a provider is given a lump sum of money to care for a population for a period of time, usually a year.

Gross domestic product   Total output of goods and services in the United States in a year.

Health disparities   Differences in health status or health care based upon geographic or demographic characteristics of a population.

Health savings account   A tax-protected pool of money set aside by a person to pay for out-of-pocket health care costs; usually associated with a high-deductible form of health insurance.

Health services   Related policy and systems that organize, finance, and deliver health care.

Hospitals   The institutional core of the acute medical care system; site of most tertiary and quaternary care in the United States.

Humane philosophy   A movement that began at the beginning of the 20th century and described the need to provide care and services for persons with mental illness.

Inclusion   A social philosophy that minimizes barriers and empowers persons with disabling conditions to achieve full participation in society.

Independent living   A social movement that (1) promotes access to adequate housing, education, and employment for persons with disabling conditions and (2) acts to prevent discrimination against such persons.

Informal care   Personal health care provided by nonprofessional workers, primarily family and friends.

Integrated health care system   A combination of primary care, secondary care, tertiary care, and quaternary care made possible through a process of vertical or horizontal integration.

Intermediary   Medicare claims processor and reviewer.

Intermediate care   Care given by a facility that provides residential services; a minimum level of professional care focusing on periodic monitoring and basic personal care.

Interpersonal excellence   A component of health care quality that includes the caring and affective elements of patient care.

Level of care   A stage of the informal or formal care system; often considered to be part of a "continuum of services."

Leverage   A position of dominance in an economic market that forces other players to negotiate on terms favorable to the person in the dominant position.

Lobbying   The process of redressing grievances to elected representatives; a First Amendment right in the United States.

Marginalization   A social process that isolates and stigmatizes persons with disabling conditions from the general population.

Market   The set of interactions between buyers and sellers involved in the exchange of economic resources (i.e., money, goods, and services).

Matrix system   An organizational structure in a hospital that matches a product-line team to a discipline-specific management structure.

Means-tested requirement   Requirement whereby Medicaid and SCHIP eligible beneficiaries must meet certain income and asset levels.

Medical negligence   An act (or failure to act) by a health care professional that causes an injury or other adverse event to a patient.

Medically necessary   Sometimes termed medical "necessity." The determination by a provider with physician status that a health care intervention is required. A prerequisite for all forms of health care insurance reimbursement. Associated with the certification and recertification process in Medicare.

Medically needy eligibility   A state-option qualification for Medicaid based on demonstrated medical need and, in some cases, income or asset level.

Medicare assignment   An agreement between a provider and Medicare to accept (participate in) the fee schedule as payment in full for services (minus the appropriate deductible and co-insurance).

Medigap   A term for private supplemental insurance plans that provide benefits for services not covered by traditional Medicare.

Moral hazard   Financially irresponsible behavior regarding insurance and experienced as favorable selection and adverse selection.

Need factors   Elements entering into the presence of a medical condition that predisposes a person to access health care services.

Office on Aging   Locale of a government program that provides various community supports for older people with health and social needs.

Outcome   The results of a health care intervention.

Panel   A group of providers selected by a managed care organization to provide services to plan members. May be open or closed.

Patient-focused care   Developed initially in hospitals, a redesign of health care services from the perspective of the patient.

Patient privacy   Condition whereby the patient's identity and records are kept confidential from the general public; a requirement of law.

Patient safety   A basic expectation of health care quality whereby the patient is protected from unnecessary harm or from harm that can be anticipated.

Pay for performance   Collection of incentive payment systems that reward high-quality health care or penalize poor-quality health care.

Peer review   Process whereby a therapist's activity is examined and compared with accepted standards of practice.

Peer review organizations   Medicare-sponsored organizations that perform quality-control, investigatory, and patient-education functions.

Penetration   The percentage of the insurance market that is controlled by managed care.

Personal care services   Home-based attendant care services that assist persons with disabilities with community integration (e.g., bathing, dressing).

Physician-hospital organization   An integration of physician practices and the hospital to create leverage and compete with managed care organizations.

Premium   An amount of money paid by a beneficiary each period into a risk pool in order to qualify and pay for insurance benefits.

Presumptive eligibility   Used in the Medicaid program to provide temporary benefits until permanent eligibility can be determined.

Primary care   The most common form of health care in the United States. Care for common, episodic illnesses. Occurs primarily in outpatient settings.

Process   The delivery of health care services, including physical therapy and occupational therapy. It has two components: technical excellence and interpersonal excellence.

Product-line teams   Reorganization of patient care services away from traditional discipline-specific services to patient-focused teams (e.g., a joint-replacement team).

Professional regulation   A voluntary or mandatory process of ensuring the competence of health care providers. It has three levels: registration, certification, and licensure.

Prospective payment   A form of health care payment whereby providers are paid a set fee or rate prior to the delivery of services. Case-based payment, capitation, and Medicare Part A payment mechanisms are examples of prospective payment schemes.

Public health model   Model of health care for populations that focuses on the identification of disease and injury, and intervention for the agent, host, and environment.

Quality improvement   A process that identifies quality issues, sets goals to improve performance, and measures progress towards those goals.

Quaternary care   High-technology health care for uncommon, acute, and chronic disorders (e.g., organ transplantation). Associated with academic medical centers.

Reflection   A process of self-examination that is critical to understanding the personal motivations that affect the advocacy process.

Related services   Services for students defined in the Individuals with Disabilities Education Act and that are mandated to assist those students in accessing a public education; include occupational therapy and physical therapy.

Risk   An insurance term that identifies the likelihood of a person or group incurring a loss (i.e., a need for benefits).

Secondary care   Care for common, chronic-type disorders (e.g., diabetes mellitus, hypertension).

Safety-net provider   A health care provider that provides care to a large or predominantly uninsured or underinsured population.

Social disability   A perspective on disablement that locates the problem in the policies, systems, and attitudes of those who are not experiencing disablement.

Social insurance   A form of government-sponsored health insurance whereby people paying premiums (taxes) are not eligible for benefits. Benefits are paid to those who have a defined social need. Examples are Medicare and Medicaid.

Special education   Primary and secondary education for children from birth to age 21 who have disabilities.

Spend-down   A process whereby a person with potential Medicaid eligibility "spends down" his or her assets to a certain level in order to gain eligibility for the program.

Spousal impoverishment   Associated with the spend-down program in Medicaid, this provision allows the spouses of Medicaid beneficiaries to remain in the community.

Standard   An accepted or, in some cases, optimal level of practice or performance.

State option   Eligibility criterion for Medicaid that can be included or excluded by the states (e.g., medically needy eligibility).

Structures   The stable elements of the health care system (e.g., physical structures, human resources).

Swing-bed unit   A ward in which subacute care is given, typically in a hospital, to patients recovering from an acute illness or injury.

Technical excellence   A component of health care quality that considers the knowledge and expertise of the provider in the health care encounter.

Tertiary care   A technologically sophisticated level of care associated with inpatient hospital stays.

Testimony   Information provided to public policymakers in verbal and written form, as well as in response to questions.

Underinsured   People with health insurance, but who have impaired access to health care due to fewer plan benefits.

Underwriting   The insurance process that examines individual characteristics to determine eligibility and cost of insurance.

Uninsured   People who have impaired access to health care due to lack of health insurance.

Universalism   A philosophy of disablement that emphasizes the common experience of disability and advocates policies that reduce barriers and reinforce inclusion.

Vested   Property whereby, after payment of taxes into the Medicare trust fund for 40 quarters, a person is eligible for Part A benefits upon reaching retirement age, experiencing permanent disability, or develping end-stage renal disease.

Vocational rehabilitation   A process of assessment, education, training, and support for persons with disabling conditions in order to prepare them for the workforce.

Voluntary agency   Not-for-profit organization that provides advocacy, education, and limited personal health care for persons with illness or disease. For example, the National Multiple Sclerosis Society.

Waiver program   The program that allows states to apply to the federal government in order to establish new and innovative Medicaid programs.

Index